Society and Medication: Conflicting Signals for Prescribers and Patients

Society and Medication: Conflicting Signals for Prescribers and Patients

Edited by
John P. Morgan
City University of New York
and Mount Sinai School of
Medicine

Doreen V. Kagan
City University of New York

LexingtonBooks
D.C. Heath and Company
Lexington, Massachusetts
Toronto

Library of Congress Cataloging in Publication Data

Main entry under title:

Society and medication: conflicting signals for prescribers and patients.

Based on papers presented at a conference titled Proper Prescribing: Conflicting Signals, May of 1981 in New York City.
Includes index.
1. Drugs—Prescribing—Congresses. 2. Drug utilization—Congresses. 3. Drugs—Side effects—Congresses. I. Morgan, John P. II. Kagan, Doreen V. [DNLM: 1. Prescriptions, Drug—Congresses. QV 748 P 965 1981]
RM138.P76 1983 615.5'8 81-48145
ISBN 0-669-05290-6

Published simultaneously in Canada

Printed in the United States of America

International Standard Book Number: 0-669-05290-6

Library of Congress Catalog Card Number: 81-48145

This book is dedicated to
Louis Lasagna, M.D.,
mentor, friend, and all-around guiding light.

Contents

Tables and Figures

Tables

Figures

Preface and Acknowledgments

John P. Morgan

The era of scientific therapeutics has begun only recently. At least, I believe it has begun. The pharmacohistorian, writing in 2005, may not be able to contain his derision when describing the medication characteristics of our time. Reading therapeutic texts, promotional literature, or most journals would give the impression that the decisions to prescribe and the choices of drug are made usually by practitioners on clinical grounds. The practitioner evaluates the symptoms and signs and chooses a chemical that, taken faithfully, will combine properly with biological tissue and be therapeutic. The fact that I can recite this sequence indicates that it may occur. However, I fear that it does not occur often, and then, even when the choices are rational in our current context, many a psychological or mythological slip intervenes between the medicinal cup and the lip.

In the nineteenth century, physicians in the United States were prone to utilize morphine for a large number of complaints—particularly common diarrheal disorders. Physicians also widely utilized opioids for sedative-hypnotic and analgesic purposes. Our perspective indicates that, even though the drugs were often effective symptomatically, prescribers were not very aware of the danger of dependence. (Even this remark indicates a certain commitment to contemporary fashion. I lack data that prove Americans so treated had a high incidence of dependence.) Nowadays, the uses of opioids vary enormously from those cited here and are equally uninformed.

I am asked occasionally to see patients who are being treated for serious pain. The urban university hospital in which I work is staffed by medical scientists, skilled clinicians, and house officers who apparently cannot learn the proper dose of meperidine. I see the patients who are invariably in pain because of an inadequate 50–75 mg. oral dose of meperidine, and I increase the dose or switch to a proper dose of methadone.

Now, for the first time, often the patient not only experiences pain relief but also, for the first time, vomits secondarily in reaction to the presence, in adequate dosage, of opioid at the chemoreceptor trigger zone. My application of rational dosing may help if I can get the patient to hold on while the nausea lessens, but I occasionally find later that the patient again is treated with inadequate medication as if he and the physician prefer symbolic drug administration to the real thing. I should also note that it is generally I who am angered by the undertreatment; patients not always are.

There may be patients who, for a variety of reasons, do not want the full analgesia that skillful manipulation of opioids may produce.

Both physicians of the nineteenth century and of 1981 used opioids on a basis predicted by irrational, almost magical, beliefs that easily override both scientific knowledge and rational therapeutics. The wrongheadedness of the nineteenth century was based on the perhaps excusable belief that symptomatic relief was not accompanied by serious side effects (a magical and foolish belief in drug benevolence). Current undertreatment is based on a wrongheaded belief that underdosage is best because proper dosage will make patients into addicts (a magical and foolish belief in drug seductiveness).

We should not be surprised that forces of the prescientific era would carry over into the scientific one. A cultural traffic in chemicals has always both served and been influenced by magical, mythological, and psychological forces. One should not forget this because the chemicals are now prescribed and dispensed by people in clean white coats in white-tiled rooms and because the orally transmitted customs and rules for drug use are now codified and administered by state and federal legislative and administrative entities.

The only unusual issue about the complex forces influencing the complex social event of prescribing is our unwillingness as physicians to deal cogently with these issues. We sense that the use of central-nervous-system depressant benzodiazepines may not have much to do with the rules of clinical medicine, but we seem to have little language to discuss the problem other than the words *anxiety, neurosis, drug dependence,* and the like. We need much more to discuss and understand facts such as that female physicians prescribe benzodiazepine differently than male physicians, that men receive benzodiazepines twenty-five times as often as women for the diagnosis of alcohol abuse, and that more benzodiazepines are given in the summer than in the fall. These factors, reflecting social forces, are of course amenable to scientific study. They are as important, if not more important, than gamma-butyric acid (GABA) receptors and the presence or absence of microsomal enzyme induction.

Students of medicine (and practitioners seeking postgraduate education) are taught about drugs almost solely from a biological-reductionistic viewpoint. My bias is that ten hours of instruction in some of the nonclinical issues I have discussed may be as valuable as more hours spent in the latest details of the serum levels and dose-response curves.

In May 1981, a group of scientists interested in both clinical and nonclinical issues met in New York City for a conference titled Proper Prescribing: Conflicting Signals. The conference was cosponsored by The Sophie Davis School of Biomedical Education at the City College of New York, Mount Sinai School of Medicine, The Arnold and Marie Schwartz College of Pharmacy and Health Sciences, Long Island University. The chapters in this book grew out of the papers presented at that conference and are directed toward a broader perspective of drug use and prescribing than the usual clinical perspective.

As the era of scientific therapeutics progresses, it will carry along with it the social, political, economic, and psychological dimensions that have always accompanied the complex ritual of chemical and drug use. This book highlights the fact that increased understanding of prescribing occurs only as the forces of biological and clinical sciences grow and improve.

Prescribing is everyone's interest and no one's specialty. I hope this book might be a first step toward the development of prescribing as a discipline of interest and study.

The editors express appreciation and acknowledge the valuable contribution of the conference steering committee: Patricia J. Bush, Ph.D.; Donald W. Light, Ph.D.; Mike Mulvihill, Dr.Ph.; David L. Rabin, M.D., M.Ph.; T. Donald Rucker, Ph.D.; Leroy L. Schwartz, M.D.; Mickey C. Smith, Ph.D., R.Ph.; Michael Weintraub, M.D.; Albert I. Wertheimer, Ph.D.; and Charles Winick, Ph.D.

Additionally, the following organizations supported the conference financially: Burroughs Wellcome Co.; The Center for the Study of Drug Development, Department of Pharmacology, University of Rochester Medical Center; The Dow Chemical Company; *Drug Therapy Journal;* McNeil Pharmaceutical; *Medical Marketing and Media;* Merrell National Laboratories; Merck Sharp & Dohme; Norwich-Eaton Pharmaceuticals; Ortho Pharmaceutical Corporation; Pennwalt Corporation; Pfizer Pharmaceuticals; The Princeton Institute for Health Policy; The Proprietary Association; Roche Laboratories; A.H. Robins; Sandoz Pharmaceuticals; Schering-Plough Corporation; Smith Kline & French Laboratories; E.R. Squibb & Sons, Inc.; Syntex Laboratories, Inc.; The Upjohn Company; and Warner-Lambert Company.

Part I
National Perspectives

1 An Empirical Overview of the Prescription-Drug Market

Albert I. Wertheimer

Everything about the prescription-drug market can be described in one word—*huge*. That would include sales, research activities, marketing prowess, political clout, international nature, and so forth. The Pharmaceutical Data Service (PDS) estimates 1980 outpatient prescriptions to total 756,323,000 for new prescriptions, coupled with another 651,424,000 refill prescriptions, for a total outpatient count of 1,407,747,000 prescriptions. That is nearly 5 prescriptions for each man, woman, and child in the United States. These 1.4 billion prescriptions had a price tag of $7.058 billion at acquisition cost.[1]

If we double that figure, we might estimate retail outpatient sales of prescription drugs to approach $14.5 billion. This figure, coupled with the estimated sale and usage of prescription drugs in hospitals and other health-care institutions, generates 9 percent of the health-care expenditures in the United States. Recall also that this excludes the over-the-counter (OTC) market of nonprescribed drugs, which adds another 50 percent to the prescription-sales figures.

In 1977, the U.S. Census of Manufacturers reported 757 establishments primarily engaged in the manufacture of ethical (restricted to sale only on a doctor's prescription) and proprietary drugs. Only 292 of these employed 20 or more workers.[2] For 1977, industry sales (shipments) were approximately $11.3 billion and gross fixed assets were $3.8 billion. These figures are for firms in industry 2834, Pharmaceutical Preparations, of the Standard Industrial Classification (SIC) system. Pharmaceutical Manufacturer's Association (PMA) member firms traditionally have accounted for over 90 percent of the industry's sales of human-dosage-form drugs. The overall trend is one of fewer, larger firms generating greater revenues and utilizing more-productive assets.[3]

About 1,000 basic pharmaceutical chemical entities are on the market, represented by a great range of dosage forms. Many of these drugs are produced by more than one manufacturer. Drug-manufacturing facilities are concentrated largely in New York, New Jersey, Pennsylvania, Indiana, Illinois, Michigan, Missouri, Ohio, California, and Puerto Rico. Through networks of distribution centers and wholesale distributors, pharmaceutical products produced in these and other states are available to patients in more than 7,000 hospitals and 60,000 pharmacies.[4]

For the period 1965–1978, total worldwide annual sales of the U.S. pharmaceutical industry grew over 300 percent, from $3.9 billion to $16 billion. The major source of this growth came from greater foreign sales. Domestic annual sales increased 220 percent, but foreign sales grew 560 percent for the period. In 1978, foreign sales represented 41 percent of total sales compared with only 25 percent in 1965.[5]

While total industry sales have continued to grow, the percentage of total sales accounted for by specific classes of product has undergone relative changes. Table 1–1 shows that sales of drugs acting upon the central nervous system led all other categories in both 1972 and 1978 with 26 percent and 23.6 percent respectively. During the six-year period, however, sales of central-nervous-system drugs as a proportion of total sales declined by 9.2 percent, while sales for other product classes such as vitamins, respiratory-system drugs, anti-infectives, and cardiovascular drugs experienced relative increases.

Foreign sales of U.S. companies, by product class, show rankings different from domestic sales. Anti-infectives predominate, with drugs for the central nervous system in second place, followed by respiratory-system, neoplasm, and endocrine drugs.

Although the core products of the pharmaceutical industry are ethical human-use drugs, members of the industry manufacture other important products as well. These are classified by the federal government under SIC codes 2831, Biologicals (excluding veterinary products), and 2833, Medicinals and Botanicals. Sales of these products have increased over 267 percent during the five years from 1972 to 1977, with 1977 sales reaching $3 billion.[6]

In the distribution of human-use-dosage-form ethical pharmaceutical sales in the United States, drug wholesalers represent the largest customer group for the industry, purchasing directly 51.4 percent of total industry sales in 1978. Retail pharmacies constitute the next largest customer group, purchasing 22.8 percent directly. Retailers also buy drugs from the wholesalers and are the largest customer class dispensing pharmaceuticals directly to the patient. In 1978, hospitals of all types of ownership (private and federal, state, and local government) purchased 22.6 percent of the manufacturers' output directly. Hospitals also purchase drugs from wholesalers and dispense to patients.[7]

The patterns of drug distribution are changing, as shown by the trends for the 1968–1978 period. From 1968 through 1972, retailers accounted for nearly 30 percent of direct manufacturer sales, while wholesalers averaged about 47 percent and private hospitals only 13 percent. Since 1972, wholesalers have increased their share significantly to over 50 percent of direct sales, private hospitals grew to 16 percent, and retailers fell off to 23 percent.[8]

Table 1-1
Manufacturers' Percent Share of Domestic Sales of Ethical Drugs for Human Use, by Product Class, 1972 and 1978

	Relative Share of Sales		*1972–1978 Percent Gain or Loss of Market Share*
	1972	*1978*	
Central nervous system	26	23.6	− 9.2
Anti-infectives	12.8	15	+ 17.2
Gastrointestinal and genitourinary	10.7	11.8	+ 10.3
Neoplasms and endocrine	12	9.7	− 19.2
Vitamins and nutrients	7.6	9.6	+ 26.3
Cardiovasculars	8.4	9.4	+ 11.9
Respiratory system	6.6	7.8	+ 18.2
Dermatologicals	3.3	2.9	− 12.1
Other	12.6	10.2	− 19
Totals	100	100	

Source: Pharmaceutical Manufacturer's Association, *Prescription Drug Industry Factbook* (Washington, D.C., 1980).

Retail sales measure the value of drug products dispensed to the customer primarily through independent and chain retail pharmacies. The value of retail prescription sales includes the cost of the product to the pharmacy as well as the retail markup or charge for professional dispensing services.

Closely tied to retail sales is the volume of prescriptions dispensed. Table 1–2 shows trends in the number of prescriptions from 1975 through 1978. As may be seen, the total number of prescriptions has been declining during this period. In 1978, 1.4 billion prescriptions were dispensed, down almost 7 percent from the 1.5 billion dispensed in 1975. The decline in new prescriptions during the 1975–1977 period appears to have been reversed, however, in 1978. Also, the increasingly larger sizes of prescriptions—that is, more product per prescriptions—partly explain the downward trend in total prescriptions.

Merck Sharp & Dohme (MSD) was the number-one company in the pharmaceutical industry last year as measured by sales volume (at acquisition cost) of prescriptions dispensed in community pharmacies, according to a report by PDS.[9] In second place was Smith Kline & French (SK&F), followed by Roche, Parke-Davis, and Ayerst. Altogether, the top twenty companies accounted for 66 percent of the retail pharmacy prescription

Table 1-2
Number of U.S. Prescriptions, 1975-1978

Year	*New Prescriptions*	*Refills*	*Total*
1975	749,715,000	753,548,000	1,503,263,000
1976	748,933,000 (percent change, less than 1)	724,952,000	1,473,885,000
1977	733,925,000 (percent change, −2)	690,622,000	1,424,547,000
1978	751,045,000 (percent change, +2)	658,131,000	1,409,176,000

Source: Pharmaceutical Manufacturer's Association, *Prescription Drug Industry Factbook* (Washington, D.C., 1980).

market, in terms of acquisition cost, PDS reports.[10] The twenty companies in order were:

1. MSD,
2. SK&F,
3. Roche,
4. Parke-Davis,
5. Ayerst,
6. Upjohn,
7. Wyeth,
8. Searle,
9. Pfizer,
10. Lilly,
11. Squibb,
12. Abbott,
13. Burroughs Wellcome,
14. Dista,
15. Ciba,
16. McNeil,
17. Schering,
18. Syntex,
19. Lederle,
20. Ortho.

On an individual basis, SK&F's Tagamet was the number-one product last year in retail pharmacy sales, as measured by acquisition cost. Altogether, the top twenty products accounted for 27 percent of the retail pharmacy prescription market, at acquisition cost. The top 20 were:

1. Tagamet (SK&F),
2. Inderal (Ayerst),
3. Valium (Roche),
4. Motrin (Upjohn),
5. Dyazide (SK&F),
6. Clinoril (MSD),
7. Keflex (Dista),
8. Aldomet (MSD),
9. Lasix (Hoechst),
10. Naprosyn (Syntex),
11. Ortho-Novum (Ortho),
12. Indocin (MSD),
13. Persantine (Boehringer-Ingelheim),
14. Tylenol with codeine (McNeil),
15. Diabinese (Pfizer),
16. Slow-K (Ciba),
17. Davocet-N (Lilly),
18. Aldoril (MSD),
19. Mellaril (Sandoz),
20. Hygroton (USV).[11]

Table 1–3
Leading Drugs, by Dollar Volume versus Prescription Volume

Dollar Volume	Number of Prescriptions
1. Tagamet	1. Valium
2. Inderal	2. Inderal
3. Valium	3. Dyazide
4. Motrin	4. Lanoxin
5. Dyazide	5. Tylenol with codeine
6. Clinoril	6. Lasix
7. Keflex	7. Dimetapp
8. Aldomet	8. Motrin
9. Lasix	9. Tagamet
10. Naprosyn	10. Darvocet-N
11. Ortho-Novum	11. Dalmane
12. Indocin	12. Aldomet
13. Persantine	13. Ortho-Novum
14. Tylenol with codeine	14. Actifed
15. Diabinese	15. Keflex
16. Slow-K	16. Slow-K
17. Darvocet-N	17. Empirin with codeine
18. Aldoril	18. Premarin
19. Mellaril	19. Benadryl
20. Hygroton	20. Dilantin

Source: U.S. Department of Health and Human Services, *Health United States, 1980* (Hyattsville, Md., 1981), p. 540.

When product rankings based on dollar volume are compared with those based on number of prescriptions dispensed, differences show up—attributable, of course, to differences in cost. Table 1–3 shows how the top twenty in this list compare with the top twenty in acquisition cost.

Shipments should continue to rise at the 10 percent annual rate of the past six years. Growth will be fueled by new drugs for previously untreatable ailments, by the relatively low price of drug care, and by increased usage by an aging population. However, a continued high level of government interference will exert pressure on margins and restrict the development of new and profitable compounds. Programs designed to foster the use of generic substitutes for ethical drugs will place further pressure on margins.

Regulations in the United States have encouraged overseas marketing of many important drugs prior to their introduction in the United States. On average, the major U.S. pharmaceutical companies derive about 45 percent of their revenues from foreign markets. Future results overseas may be limited by government efforts to control drug prices and by currency fluctuations. Also, foreign pharmaceutical companies are developing strong marketing and research organizations, thereby presenting tough competition for U.S. firms.

According to estimates from the Department of Health and Human Services' (DHHS) Health Care Financing Administration (HCFA)[12], drug costs continue to decline as a percentage of total health-care costs. In 1979, only 8 percent of the health-care dollar was spent for drugs and medical sundries, compared with 8.15 percent in 1978 and 8.23 percent in 1977. The HCFA further estimates that prescription drugs represent 56 percent of this category; thus, only 4.48 percent of the U.S. health-care dollar was spent on prescriptions in 1979. This declining trend is continuing, despite the fact that entirely new medicines, which tend to supplant hospitalization and surgery, are being introduced for conditions not previously treatable by drugs.

However, consumers are particularly aware of the cost of drugs and are very sensitive to price increases because only a small share of drug costs is covered by third-party payment. The out-of-pocket spending by consumers for drugs is more than twice the outlays for hospitals and almost as much as doctor bills. The pharmaceutical share of the health-care dollar has been declining since 1960 but is expected to rise during the 1980s, partly because of greater utilization by an increasingly older population. Use of drugs will be stimulated by greater demand for drugs that are used in the treatment of chronic conditions and increased efficiency and cost-effectiveness of drug treatment.[13]

Research

The pharmaceutical industry has invested over $13 billion in pharmaceutical research and development (R&D) since the early 1940s. These efforts have led to the discovery of more than 1,000 new chemical entities.

Company-financed R&D for human-use ethical pharmaceuticals was budgeted at $1.5 billion for 1979, a 14 percent increase over the $1.3 billion spent in 1978. Research by U.S. firms abroad accounted for $222 million, or 17 percent of the 1978 total.[14]

Companies finance almost all their own R&D, although to a very limited degree they also conduct research under contract for the federal government. These government-funded, company-conducted projects involved annual expenditures ranging from $7 million to $14 million over the last fifteen years. In 1978, federally financed R&D amounted to $7 million, or less than 1 percent of the industry total.[15]

The annual ratio of company-funded domestic R&D to domestic sales has varied between 10.5 percent and 12.1 percent since 1965 and has remained stable at 11.5 percent for the years 1976, 1977, and 1978.

In spite of the deceleration in new drug discoveries, the United States has maintained a strong leadership in drug innovation and still accounts for 64 percent of the new chemical entities introduced in this country since 1940. Switzerland is the second largest originator with 7 percent, followed by the United Kingdom and West Germany. In the United States over 90 percent of the new drug discoveries have originated in private-industry laboratories.[16]

Anti-infectives, with a listing of 189 products, is the largest therapeutic class for new chemical entities. Hormones follow with 86 products, then cardiovascular preparations, gastrointestinal preparations, and ataraxics respectively.[17]

Patent activity is another measure of the intensity of successful pharmaceutical research. A new drug may be the subject of several different patents. Patents may be obtained for new chemical entities, for novel manufacturing processes, and for new uses of existing compounds. Noteworthy, is the decrease in the relative share of patents originating in the United States that were issued for drugs and medicines, from 67 percent in 1963 to 54 percent in 1977.

Structure

Four-firm concentration rates measure the percentage of the market the four leading firms of its kind comprise. Analyzing 4-digit SIC industrial classification codes for 1972, only 145 of the 453 measured had lower concentration rates. However, low concentration does not necessarily predict high competitiveness. And yet, the relatively low index of concentration in sales is noteworthy since there has been a marked trend toward concentration in drug-industry R&D as well as in the introduction of new products. For the years 1959 through 1962, an average of 109 firms per year introduced new pharmaceutical products. For the years 1971 through 1977, the average had dropped to 47.[18]

By any number of measures of research and invention, including the size of R&D budgets and the innovational output of the largest firms, there has been a trend toward fewer companies successfully engaging in new product development; but a trend toward concentration in sales does not seem to have occurred.

As with any industrial sector, the concentration rate for share of the market is higher when the industry is subdivided into subcategories. Thus, there is greater concentration on the part of the machine-tool industry that produces drill presses than there is for makers of machine tools in general. When the pharmaceutical industry is analyzed according to major product classes (for example, anti-infectives, anti-inflammatory agents, analgesics), no clear evidence exists of a trend toward greater concentration. Indeed, an examination of the share held by the top four firms of these relevant markets shows a slight decline for the five-year period 1967–1971 compared to that of the previous five years. It is evident that firms have been entering new therapeutic submarkets, and this appears to have offset the trend toward concentration in the innovation of truly new products.[19]

Earnings

For many years the earnings of the U.S. pharmaceutical industry consistently have been among the top three or four for major manufacturing industries. However, the spread between the pretax return on equity for pharmaceuticals and the comparable return for all manufacturing has been declining.

Pricing

Manufacturers' prices for pharmaceuticals have tended to resist inflationary pressures. The ethical pharmaceutical component of the Producers Price Index (PPI) includes about fifty items and fifteen therapeutic classes. In 1979 the annual average of these fifteen categories was 141.2 percent, an increase of 1,216 percent above the 1977 average and a cumulative rise of only 41.2 percent since 1967, the base year. By comparison, the comprehensive All Commodities PPI for 1979 had risen 21.2 percent from 194.2 percent and was 135.4 percent above the 1967 level.[20]

Surveys of the average prescription price have varied according to the methodology employed and stores sampled. For 1978, for instance, the estimates vary from \$6.57 in the *Lilly Digest,*[21] which surveys independent community pharmacies, to \$5.54 in the *American Druggist,*[22] which surveys both chains and independents. The National Prescription Audit estimate was \$6.44, up from \$5.98 in 1977 and \$5.60 in 1976.

Moderate changes in the price of the average prescription can be explained in part by nonprice factors; the most important of these is the continuing increase in the size (number of doses) of the average prescription. Firestone has calculated the effect of this change in size on the price of the prescription.[23] He finds that the typical 1978 prescription, when adjusted for size, costs only 20 percent more than the 1960 prescription. This compares with a doubling in price, for the same eighteen-year period, for a prescription not adjusted for size.

Current Issues

Paper New-Drug Applications

Ethical-drug companies, already hurt by the slow Food and Drug Administration (FDA) approval of new drugs and by regulatory uncertainties, ironically may be adversely affected by moves to accelerate part of the FDA's operations. In December 1980, the FDA said it will allow drug manufacturers to cite existing studies to show that their generic versions of brand-name drugs are safe and effective. The change could reduce generic-drug approval-processing time to less than three months, from the present six to 18 months on average. The new paper new-drug-application (NDA) policy would allow manufacturers of generic copies of existing drugs to obtain FDA approval to market identical, or so-called me-too, drugs without conducting their own clinical tests. This policy appears to clash with the FDA's standing practice of continuing examination of new drugs that it has approved for marketing. Recent legal decisions have favored the new policy, however. Federal courts have ruled that the FDA, and not the marketer, has a burden of proof to show why unapproved drugs should not continue to be sold in the marketplace. The FDA must present evidence that a generic drug is not safe and effective before it can be removed from the marketplace. Marketing of unapproved drugs is thus allowable if there are no probable dangers. This permits the marketing of me-too drugs without costly and time-consuming FDA approval and case-by-case institution of condemnation actions. The PMA, the drug industry's trade organization, has challenged this policy.

A second change in FDA policy would end the requirement to submit scientific reports for third and subsequent copies of a drug. The proposed changes would hurt innovative drug companies relative to generic producers because a reduction in regulatory paperwork and research requirements for generics would decrease the cost of producing generic compounds and thus would increase the advantageous pricing flexibility available for generic producers. Also, a decline in approval time for generic drugs would shorten the exclusive marketing period that innovators have under their patents and would decrease the profit margins achieved from developing a new drug.

Generic Drugs

The major pharmaceutical firms have not been ignoring the generic threat. Some companies have cut prices on multisource products, while others have offered extended dating on products. Most generic houses cannot afford to offer 180-day dating because their profit margins are low relative to the major drug manufacturers, and they could not finance a large retail inventory. Some major drug firms such as Squibb, SK&F, and Pfizer have responded to generic competition by adding generic products to the branded items they offer. Price wars have developed, with some generic houses terminating the sale of certain products. Despite the tough brand competition, generic prescription sales in 1979 soared 59 percent from those of the prior year. Also, generic prescriptions continue to grab a greater share of the total market. In 1978, generics accounted for about 10 percent of the total dollars spent on prescriptions; that market share currently stands at 15 percent, or more than $1.5 billion in manufacturers' sales. By 1990, generics are expected to account for 25 percent of the $28 billion U.S. market forecast for ethical drugs.

Branded products still clearly dominate the market in terms of the number of prescriptions filled, but these prescriptions declined close to 3 percent during 1979. However, as can be seen from table 1–4, generics advanced almost 2 percent during this time. This trend can be traced directly to mandated drug-product selection laws now on the books in most states. The laws exist because of pricing variations. In terms of average prescription prices, generics are less expensive than branded drugs. During 1979, patients paid an average of $7.03 per prescription, 9.2 percent above the prior year's level. The average price of a generic prescription rose only 4.6 percent to $5.03, while branded drugs increased 9.9 percent to $7.35.

Both federal and state governments have encouraged the use of generic pharmaceuticals in the hope of generating cost savings for both themselves (through lower Medicaid reimbursements) and consumers. At the state level, this has taken the form of substitution laws that either allow or compel pharmacists to fill prescriptions generically. The prescriber now has the authority to provide substitution in the forty-eight states with substitution laws. The pharmacist is required to substitute in nine states unless the prescriber prohibits it. The pharmacist is required to dispense a lower-priced

Table 1–4
Prescription-Drug Volume

Product	*Prescription Volume (millions)*	*Percent Change (1978–1979)*	*Percent Share*
Branded	1,200.9	– 2.8	87.9
Generic	165	+ 1.9	12.1
Total	1,365.9	– 2.2	100

Source: Standard and Poor, *Standard and Poor's Industry Surveys: Health Care, Drugs, and Cosmetics* (New York, 1981), p. 18.

or the lowest-priced product in thirty-seven states. He must obtain the patient's consent in sixteen states, and he must dispense only products listed in a state-managed formula in twenty-seven states.

Substitution has helped to reduce U.S. leadership in the R&D of human pharmaceutical products. Fewer U.S. firms are engaged in the R&D of drugs since the return on investment has decreased with the rise in generic usage.

The rapid rise in generic sales is also partly attributable to increased market participation by multinational companies, to increased public confidence in the quality of generics, and to the government's emphasis on increased competition in the drug area.[24]

Patents

The compounds for which patents are expiring include the following:

Company	*Product and Generic Name*	*Patent Expiration Date*	*Indication*
American Home	Atromid-S (clofibrate)	1983	Lipid-lowering agent
	Inderal (propranolol HCI)	1983	Antiarrythmic
	Serax (oxazepam)	1984	Tranquilizer
Bristol-Myers	Salutensin (hydroflumenthiazide with reserpine)	1983	Antihypertensive
Eli Lilly	Keflin (cephalothin sodium)	1982	Antibiotic
MSD	Indocin (indomethacin)	1981	Anti-inflammatory
	Aldorin (methyldopa with hydrochlorothiazide)	1984	Anti-hypertensive
Pfizer	Geopen (carbenicillin disodium)	1981	Antibiotic
	Diabinase (chlorpropamide)	1982	Antidiabetic
	Vibramycin (doxycycline)	1982	Antibiotic
Schering-Plough	Valisone (betamethasone valerate)	1984	Corticosteroid

Source: National Wholesale Druggist's Association, *Annual Report* — 1980, White Plains, N.Y.

Unresolved Issues

Modified patent-life legislation is pending in Congress. Volume-purchase plans are being considered by a few states. Drug coverage for Medicare has been postponed for the moment. Patent licensing is being considered from the Canadian experience. Finally, national health insurance is awaiting better times.

Conclusions

While the market has some depressing features, most vital signs are encouraging. Drug-utilization review (see chapter 3) is correcting some previous problems, and better prescribing is taking place. Drugs remain the first line of therapy.

Notes

1. *American Druggist,* April 1981, p. 3.
2. U.S. Bureau of the Census, *Drug Manufacturing Establishments, 1977, Census of Manufacturers' Preliminary Reports,* for SIC 2831, 2833, 2834 (Washington, D.C., June, December 1979), pp. 1–4.
3. Pharmaceutical Manufacturer's Association, *Prescription Drug Industry Factbook* (Washington, D.C., 1980), p. 160.
4. Ibid. p. 24.
5. Ibid., p. 19.
6. U.S. Bureau of the Census, *Statistical Abstracts of the United States* (Washington, D.C., Government Printing Office, 1981), p. 793.
7. Pharmaceutical Manufacturers' Association, *PMA Annual Survey, 1978–79* (Washington, D.C., 1979), p. 7.
8. National Wholesale Druggists Association, *Annual Report, 1980* (White Plains, N.Y., 1981), p. 12.
9. *American Druggist,* p. 3.
10. Ibid., p. 12.
11. Ibid.
12. U.S. Department of Health and Human Services, *Health United States, 1980,* (Hyattsville, Md., 1981), p. 339.
13. Pharmaceutical Manufacturer's Association, *Prescription Drug Industry Factbook,* p. 341.
14. Ibid., p. 545.
15. J. Feder, J. Holahan, and T. Marmor, eds., *Conflicting Goals and Policy Choices* (Washington, D.C.: Urban Institute, 1980), p. 88.
16. Pharmaceutical Manufacturer's Association, *Prescription Drug Industry Factbook,* p. 35.
17. Ibid., p. 531.
18. Standard and Poor's, *Standard and Poor's Industry Surveys: Health Care, Drugs, and Cosmetics* (New York, N.Y., 1981), p. 18.
19. Ibid., p. 221.

20. U.S. Bureau of the Census, *Statistical Abstracts,* p. 462.

21. Eli Lilly & Company, *The Lilly Digest* (Indianapolis, 1980).

22. Hearst Magazines, *American Druggist* (New York, 1980).

23. John Firestone: Mimeograph. Study prepared for Pharmaceutical Manufacturer's Association (Washington, D.C., 1980).

24. M.W. Raffel, *The. U.S. Health System: Origins and Functions* (New York: Wiley & Sons, 1980), p. 104.

2 Variations in Physician Prescribing Patterns

David L. Rabin

One reflection of the post–World War II growth in biomedical knowledge has been the rapid rate of growth of prescriptions in the past thirty years. So great has been the growth that it has given rise to the concern that we are an overmedicated society. The development of effective anti-infective, anti-inflammatory, hormonal, and psychoactive drugs enormously increased the therapeutic power of the physician. The exercise of this power is reflected in the continued increase in prescriptions. Prescriptions dispensed by community pharmacies increased from 363 million in 1950 to 1.47 billion in 1976, a fourfold increase in a quarter-century.[1] During a similar time period, there has been but a slight increase in physician visits, from 815 million in 1968[2] to 1 billion in 1978.[3] The increase in prescriptions is then in part due to an increase in the intensity of prescribing for patients seen. This increase in intensity of prescribing can be seen in the increase in prescriptions per person per year, from 2.4 in 1950 to 6.9 in 1976.[4]

This rapid and continuing increase initially was viewed with detachment since it appeared to be associated with decreased infectious-disease deaths. The replacement of death from infectious disease by death from chronic disease, however, moderated the sense of societal benefit from increased therapy. The increased cost of medical care and public awareness of side effects of therapy further raised public concern. Public concern for the volume of sedatives, hypnotics, tranquilizers, estrogens, and oral contraceptives prescribed was paralleled by professional concern for the prescribing patterns for these drugs as well as for antibiotics.

Changes in the established patterns of care sometimes occur before there is wide recognition of change. There has been a change in the pattern of prescribing drugs. From table 2–1 we see that from 1965–1970, there was an increase of 32.4 percent in prescription dispensed and from 1970–1975 of 17.5 percent [4]—that is, the annual rates of growth were diminishing gradually.

For five of the past six years, there has been a decrease in the number of prescriptions dispensed. In total, between 1975 and 1980, the total number of prescriptions decreased 7.2 percent.[5] At the same time, there was a leveling off in the number of physician visits per person, now 4.8 visits per person per year, indicating a slight decrease in prescriptions dispensed per

Table 2-1
Total Number of Prescriptions and Five-Year Percent Change, 1965–1980

Year	*Total Prescriptions*	*Five-Year Percent Change*
1965	966,914,000	
1970	1,279,872,000	32.4
1975	1,503,265,000	17.5
1980	1,394,308,000	−7.2

Source: IMS America, *National Prescription Audit* (Ambler, Pa., 1965, 1970, 1975, 1980).

person per year.[6] A portion of this decrease can be attributed to an increase of 68 percent in the prescription size between 1960 and 1979, but the change in the annual pattern of increase is unmistakable.[7] This shift from ever-increasing prescriptions per year to diminishing increases and now annual decreases in prescriptions has occurred despite the presence of medical and demographic factors that could have been expected to lead to increased prescriptions.

Factors Tending to Increase Prescribing

The U.S. population is expanding in size and increasing in age. In the decade 1970–1979, there was an 11 percent increase in total population and a 28 percent increase in those over age 65, those with most illness and medical need.[8] Since the proportion of patients seeing a physician continued to increase from 70.7 percent in 1970 to 75.4 percent in 1978, the increase in population size should be reflected in an increase in numbers of prescriptions.[9] With a disproportionately aging population, there should be, as well, increasing short- and long-term disability in the population. With increasing disability there should be increased medical need for therapy. National statistics on disability confirm an increase in disability rates for those over 65, as well as for the total population.[10] It is surprising that rates increased for nearly all age and sex groups. For the total population, indicators of short-term disability are bed days and restricted-activity days. Bed days per 100 persons increased from 6.3 to 7.1 days per year between 1966 and 1976. During the same period, other restricted-activity days increased from 9.3 to 11.1. An indicator of long-term-care disability is the number of persons who find it impossible to perform their chief activity because of long-standing disability. This rate, too, increased from 213 to 355 persons per 10,000 persons from 1966 to 1976.

In the recent past, effective medical therapy for several common diseases also has increased. Examples are therapy for hypertension, peptic ulcer, cancer, and musculoskeletal disease. There is also evidence for both cancer and hypertension that a larger proportion of affected people is being treated with medical therapy than previously.[11]

Factors Tending to Better Prescribing

The increase in prescriptions led to studies on physician prescribing practices. These studies identified physician characteristics associated with better prescribing—for example, Stolley et al.;[12] Schaffner and Ray;[13] Shosteck;[14] and Rabin, Bush, and Fuller.[15] The studies showed that better physician prescribing is associated with younger age,[16, 17, 18] specialization, [19, 20] particularly in internal medicine more pharmacology teaching;[21] health-maintenance-organization (HMO) and group practice;[22, 23] and urban location.[24]

Over the past decade, major changes occurred in the characteristics of practicing physicians in the directions associated with better prescribing patterns. These changes should be reflected in national prescribing practices. From 1970 to 1978, the percentage of actively practicing physicians who were specialists increased from 53 per 100,000 population to 78.6. The increase was even greater for those who were internists or who received postgraduate training in internal medicine. The percentage of actively practicing physicians who are internists increased from 13.5 percent in 1970 to 19.3 percent in 1978. Additionally, there has been a rapid growth in the specialty of family practice that began in 1968.[25] Physicians entering this specialty spend three years of postgraduate training, part of which is in internal medicine.

Over the past fifteen years, there has been a substantial increase in both the number and size of medical-school classes. About 15,000 physicians now graduate each year; therefore, every two years we produce an equivalent of 10 percent of all currently practicing physicians. As a result of the increase in the number of physicians, the ratio of physicians to population increased from 14.2 per 10,000 persons in 1960 to 19.7 per 10,000 in 1980.[26] The number of practicing physicians increased nearly one-third in the past decade. The large increase in physicians entering practice has led to a decrease in the average age of physicians as indicated by an increase in the proportion of practicing physicians who are less than 35 from 13.8 percent in 1970 to 27.4 percent in 1979.[27]

There has also been a change in pharmacology teaching. Surveys by the Association of Medical Schools for Pharmacology indicate that in the 1970s there was a return to traditional teaching of pharmacology to departmental rather than integrated basic-science courses.[28] The change is felt to provide for better, more-rigorous teaching in pharmacology. Further, about 30 percent of departments now do some pharmacology teaching in the clinical years. This is felt to be an important change, tying the basic science of pharmacology to its application in complex clinical situations, demonstrating dramatically the significance of pharmacology to clinical practice.

There has also been a change in patterns of practice with a larger number of physicians in HMO and group practice. The proportion of physicians in group practice increased from 16.4 percent in 1969 to 25.8 percent in 1980.[29] The proportion of physicians practicing in HMOs increased substantially in the past decade from 1 percent to nearly 15 percent of practicing physicians by 1979.[30] Most of these are physicians in independent-practice associations.

Data are thus available to suggest that there has been a considerable change in the educational patterns of practicing physicians, the age and specialization of practicing physicians, and their practice organizations in the past decade. These changes are consistent with previous associations found between physician practice and better prescribing. Therefore, there is reason to believe that as these characteristics change, there would be an improvement in the prescribing practices of physicians. This improvement might be a partial explanation of the slowing of the rate of increase in prescribing and, more recently, the actual decrease in the number of prescriptions.

Indication of Improved Prescribing

A decrease in the number of prescriptions of itself, while reassuring to those concerned with quality of prescribing, is only the grossest index of better prescribing. Is there other evidence to indicate that prescribing has changed for the better? There has been much professional debate and societal pressure to increase generic prescribing. To this end, a number of states repealed antisubstitution laws. The problems of cost of prescribing and the risks and benefits of generic prescribing have appeared in the medical literature. Physicians have been encouraged to prescribe generically since cost is less, allegedly at no or little increase in risk to patients. In association with the decrease in the number of prescriptions, there has also been a substantial increase in the proportion of prescriptions written generically. From 1974 to 1980, for example, the proportion of generic prescriptions has increased 24.9 percent.[31] More important, however, is the fact that there have been particularly great reductions in the prescribing of drugs in those drug categories that have been the focus of professional and societal concern (see figure 2–1). These changes have been in the high-volume prescription categories of drugs: hypnotics, tranquilizers, estrogens, and antibiotics. A decrease in the prescribing of these drugs could account for much of the decrease in prescriptions.

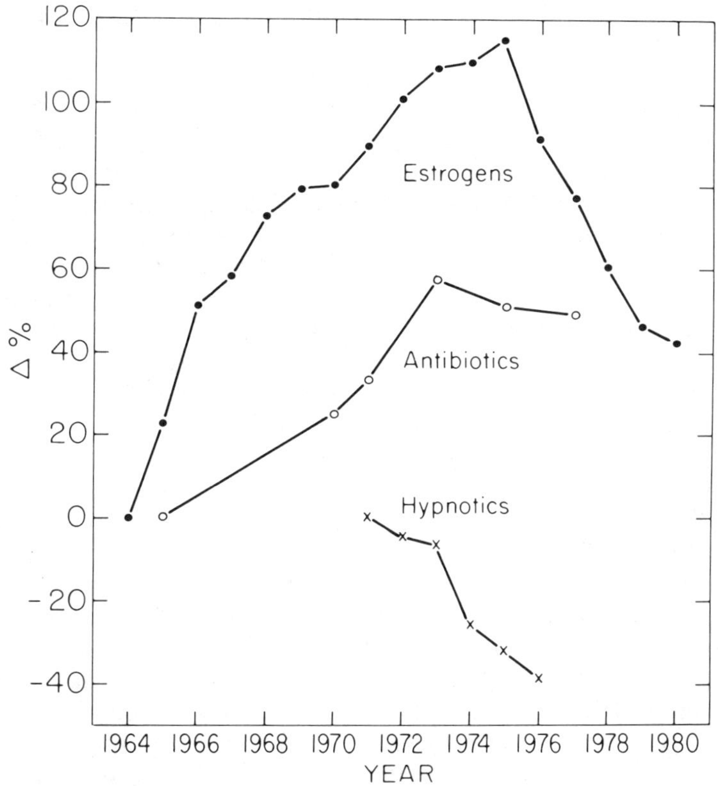

L.B. Burke, D.L. Crosby, and C.S. Lao, "Estrogen Prescribing and Menopause," (Unpublished manuscript presented at the 105th APHA meeting, Washington, D.C., November 2, 1977; Updated June 23, 1978); NIDA, *Sedative Hypnotic Drugs: Risks and Benefits* (Bethesda, Md.: August 1977); and M.J. Finkel, "Magnitude of Antibiotic Use," *Annals of Internal Medicine* 89 (1978):791–792.

Figure 2–1. Percentage Change in Retail Prescriptions for Estrogen, Hypnotic, and Antibiotic Prescriptions, by Years, 1964–1980

Changes in the prescribing of hypnotics are well documented. After many years of increase, there was a decrease in the volume of hypnotics prescribed of 41 percent between 1971 and 1976.[32] There also has been moderation of the rate of increase and now a decrease in the prescribing of tranquilizers as well. Valium , which remains the most commonly prescribed drug, has experienced a decrease in prescriptions from 61.9 million in 1975 to 33.9 million in 1980.[33] Furthermore, the decrease in prescriptions has been associated with evidence of increasing discrimination in prescribing. Thus, there has been not only a decrease in prescribing of hypnotics but also a proportional increase in the prescribing of relatively safer benzodiazepines as contrasted to the barbiturates and other hypnotic preparations. During the period 1971–1976, the total decrease in barbiturate hypnotics was over 75 percent.[34] The proportion of benzodiazepine hypnotics dispensed of all hypnotics increased fourfold from 1971–1976.

There also has been a substantial decrease in the number of prescriptions for estrogens, following the controversy regarding the efficacy and safety of estrogens since some researchers believe they increase the risk of cancer when used in postmenopausal women. From the year 1964 to 1975, there was a continual increase in the number of estrogen prescriptions. In 1976 there began an abrupt and substantial annual decrease in prescriptions of 72.7 percent to 1980 from a 1975 total of 27.3 million prescriptions.[35]

Similarly, there has been a decrease in prescribing of systemic antibiotics. After many years of increase, there was, by 1973, a total of 207.2 million prescriptions for certain oral antibiotics. By 1975, the total decreased to 192.5 million and, by 1977, to 186.7 million—in all, a 9.9 percent decrease.[36]

Summary

The gradual lessening in the rate of increase of prescriptions and now a decrease in dispensing rates medically reflects more-discriminating prescribing. The supposition is substantiated further by an increase in generic prescribing and a decrease in prescribing of commonly prescribed products known to be potentially deleterious. At the same time, there has been an increase in prescribing for once neglected common diseases like hypertension.

The decrease in prescribing, and an increase in the appropriateness of prescribing, has occurred while the characteristics of practicing physicians have changed to those more associated with better prescribing. This change has occurred despite the fact that the population served in the United States has increased in size and medical need.

It is impossible to determine the absolutely appropriate level of prescribing. There is little doubt that there continues to be problems in prescribing. These problems relate both to overprescribing of drugs like antibiotics for conditions like the common cold, as well as underprescribing of preventive medications like vaccines for unimmunized children and adults. As knowledge of the risks associated with the taking of certain medications increases and the efficacy of taking other medication is increasingly apparent, there should continue to be changes in prescribing patterns. Inevitably, these changes will occur with some delay from the time that there is medical consensus that a particular pattern of prescribing is more appropriate. This review of changes in prescribing in the past decade suggests, however, that currently practicing physicians may be more discreet in their use of medical therapy. As the physician characteristics associated with these apparent improvements in prescribing are becoming more evident in the practicing population, there is reason to believe that therapy of patients also will continue to improve.

Notes

1. P.R. Lee, "America Is an Overmedicated Society," in *Controversies in Therapeutics,* ed. L. Lasagna (Philadelphia: W.B. Saunders, 1980), pp. 4–15.

2. National Center for Health Statistics, Current Estimates from the Health Interview Survey—United States 1968, Rainbow Series 10 (60):23, Hyattsville, Md.

3. National Center for Health Statistics, Current Estimates from the Health Interview Survey—United States 1978, Rainbow Series 10 (130):30, Hyattsville, Md.

4. P.R. Lee, "America Is an Overmedicated Society," pp. 4–15.

5. Dalton, C. Pharmaceutical Research Services, IMS America. Personal communication, April 1981.

6. NCHS, "Current Estimates—1978," p. 4.

7. T. Firestone, "From 1960 through 1979 the Doses per Average Rx Jumped by 68.2%," *Pharmacy Times,* September 1980, pp. 106–109.

8. U.S. Bureau of the Census, *Current Population Reports,* Series P25, no. 870.

9. National Center for Health Statistics, Current Estimates from the Health Interview Survey—United States 1978, Rainbow Series 10 (130):4; and Series 10 (85):4, Hyattsville, Md.

10. A. Colvez and M. Blanchet, "Disability Trends in the United States Population 1966–76: Analysis of Reported Causes," *American Journal of Public Health* 71 (1981):464–471, 1981.

11. J. Stamler et al., "Hypertension Screening of One Million Americans—Community Hypertension Evaluation Clinic (CHEC) Program: 1973–1975," *Journal of the American Medical Association* 235 (1976): 2299–2306.

12. P.D. Stolley et al., Relationship between Physician Characteristics and Prescribing Appropriateness," *Medical Care* 10 (1972):17–28.

13. W. Schaffner, W. Ray, and F. Federspiel, " Surveillance of Antibiotic Prescribing in Office Practice," *Annals of Internal Medicine* 89 (1978):796–799.

14. H. Shosteck, *The Antibiotic Prescription Patterns of Primary Care Physicians, Final Report,* DHEW Contract #223-75-3007 (Washington, D.C., March 1979).

15. D.L. Rabin, P.J. Bush, and N.D. Fuller, "Drug Prescription Rates before and after Enrollment of a Medicaid Population in an HMO," *Public Health Report* 93 (1978):16–29.

16. Stolley et al., "Relationship between Physician Characteristics and Prescribing Appropriateness," pp. 17–28.

17. Schaffner, Ray, and Federspiel, "Surveillance of Antiobiotic Prescribing," pp. 796–799.

18. Shosteck, *Antibiotic Prescription Patterns.*

19. Stolley et al. "Relationship between Physician Characteristics and Prescribing Appropriateness," pp. 17–28.

20. Schaffner, Ray, and Federspiel, "Surveillance of Antibiotic Prescribing," pp. 796–799.

21. Stolley et al., "Relationship between Physician Characteristics and Prescribing Appropriateness," pp. 17–28.

22. D.L. Rabin, P.J. Bush, and N.D. Fuller, "Drug Prescription Rates before and after Enrollment of a Medicaid Population in an HMO," *Public Health Report* 93 (1978):16–29.

23. J.P. Lo Gerfo, E. Larson, and W.C. Richardson, "Assessing the Quality of Care for Urinary Tract Infection in Office Practice. A Comparative Organizational Study," *Medical Care* 16 (1978):488–495.

24. Schaffner, Ray, and Federspiel, "Surveillance of Antibiotic Prescribing," pp. 796–799.

25. F.D. Moore, and S.M. Lang, "Board Certified Physicians in the United States: Specialty Distribution and Policy Implications of Trends during the Past Decade," *New England Journal of Medicine* 304 (1981):1079–1080.

26. Department of Health and Human Services, *Health United States—1980,* DHHS Pub. no. (PHS) 81-1232 (Washington, D.C., December 1980), p. 188.

27. American Medical Association, *Physician Distribution and Medical Licensure in the US, 1979* (Chicago: AMA Center for Health Research, 1979).

28. Minutes of the Winter Meeting, January 6–8, 1978, Association for Medical School Pharmacology, Key Biscayne, Florida. 1 March 1978.

29. AMA, *Physician Distribution.*

30. Department of Health and Human Services, *National HMO Census of Prepaid Plans, 1979* (Washington, D.C., 1979).

31. Dalton, personal communication.

32. National Institute on Drug Abuse, *Sedative-Hypnotic Drugs: Risks and Benefits* (Bethesda, Md., August 1977).

33. V. Cohn, "US May Require Labeling of Food Giving Salt Content, *Washington Post,* 19 June 1981, p. A16.

34. AMA, *Physician Distribution.*

35. L.B. Burke, D.L. Crosby, and C.D. Las, "Estrogen Prescribing and Menopause," unpublished manuscript (Washington, D.C. Department of Health and Human Services, 1980).

36. M.J. Finkel, "Magnitude of Antibiotic Use," *Annals of Internal Medicine* 89 (1978):791–792.

3 Drug-Utilization Review: Moving Toward an Effective and Safe Model

T. Donald Rucker

An increasing interest in the nature and quality of medical care received by patients has resulted in the recent development of more than a dozen techniques for assessing this area.[1] One methodology in this evaluation armamentarium is drug-utilization review (DUR). For the purpose of this discussion, DUR is defined tentatively as a formal program for assessing data on drug use against explicit, prospective standards and, as necessary, introducing remedial strategies to achieve some desired end.

Since it is estimated that nearly 3 billion drug orders are initiated annually in the United States, the potential role of DUR in improving patterns of prescription use becomes an important topic for analysis.[2] Our task is made difficult, however, by the absence of a fully developed and tested theoretical model for implementing quality assurance within a fragmented, heterogeneous delivery system. Further, study is encumbered by the complexity of our subject (readers are encouraged to consult the sources listed in the notes at the end of the chapter), the variability in scope and objectives of contemporary programs, the paucity of operating units in contrast to pilot or developing projects, the lack of knowledge about current DUR efforts (does the literature describe 15 or 88 percent of our experience base?), coupled with the proliferation of terminology, often without significant distinction.[3] Our task is also confounded by the prevalence of utilization studies "which provide for only minimal feedback to the involved practitioners" and exclude "any follow-up phase . . . to ascertain if any changes in drug use have occurred."[4]

Nevertheless, sufficient work has been undertaken in both the general and specific models to warrant a critique of DUR at this time.[5] Although a few studies documenting limitations in prescribing practices appeared in the early 1950s, investigators did not start to focus more extensively on this question until the middle 1960s.[6] Subsequently, several review programs, with varying levels of sophistication, were established, and by late 1971, one informal survey was able to identify five programs that were in operation.[7]

While physicians have provided leadership in examining selected services furnished in hospitals,[8] and while pharmacists have contributed to the literature on DUR,[9] most of the impetus for adopting quality-assurance procedures has been generated by insurance carriers[10] and government-sponsored health-insurance programs.[11] Since 1980, the Joint Commission on the Accreditation of Hospitals has assumed a stimulus role,[12] but implementation as a requirement has been deferred.[13]

Needs Assessment

The gap between some parameters of rational drug therapy and actual prescribing practices constitutes one of the major weaknesses of our health-care-delivery system. After intensive study of this phenomenon, Silverman and Lee concluded that "the problem of irrational prescribing can no longer be ignored, covered up, or dismissed as trivial, for it represents not merely an unwise expenditure of funds but a serious hazard to health and even life.[14]

These limitations are prevalent throughout the system.[15] In the ambulatory sector, one investigation reported that between 25 and 35 percent of the 200 drugs dispensed most frequently through community pharmacies were deficient in terms of relative safety and/or efficacy.[16] Indeed, the therapeutic credentials of 38 of these chemical agents were so questionable that eight superior hospital formularies by-passed them altogether in 1980.[17] (These particular formularies ranked highest in a 1976 study that collected data from fifty-two hospitals with 500 beds or more.[18])

Moreover, as the figures in table 3–1 indicate, even a preeminent HMO is not immune from suboptimal prescribing practices.

Significant shortcomings also have been documented in nursing homes and hospitals.[19] Despite the adoption of a Medicaid regulation that requires that pharmacists review patient medication orders every thirty days in skilled-nursing facilities,[20] the findings presented in table 3–2 imply that more-systematic procedures like a DUR program are needed. Most investigations, though, have concentrated on drug use in hospitals, with little attention being devoted to those of outside of medical centers. One study of nine facilities concluded that 4 to 7 percent "of all discharges reflected morbidity caused or exacerbated by inappropriate drug therapy."[21] Another study documented the significance of indirect costs—"the inappropriately prescribed groups had more than 150 percent days of inefficient care than the appropriately prescribed groups."[22]

Philosophical and Conceptual Factors

On the one hand, some medical spokespersons have great difficulty in embracing virtually any type of review activity. This position stems from

Table 3–1
Drugs Most Frequently Encountered by Pharmacists as Potential Drug-Therapy Problems, September 1977 to March 1978

	Rate of Problems per 100 Prescriptions for Each Drug or Group of Drugs Dispensed	
Drug or Group of Drugs	*Mean*	*Standard Deviation (months)*
Anticonvulsants	14.9	11.3
Antihistamines	5.3	2.3
Antihistamine combinations	1.7	1
Antihypertensive vasodilators	14.1	1.9
Anti-inflammatory (nonsteroid)	6.8	3.1
Anti-inflammatory (steroid)	4.5	1.7
Barbiturates	9	2.3
Benzodiazepines	7.4	3.3
Beta-adrenergic blockers	12.6	1.7
Digitalis glycosides	11.8	2.4
Diuretic (combinations)	10.6	2.4
Diuretic (K depleting)	10.3	1.1
Diuretic (K sparing)	5.3	3.8
Diuretic (loop)	10.3	4.9
Estrogens	3.9	1
Iron	5	1.6
Meprobamate	7	3.3
Methyldopa	18.8	3.7
Persantine	9.3	3
Salicylates	4.1	1.6
Salicylate combinations	9.4	3.4
Thyroid and related drugs	10.9	1.3
Tricyclic antidepressants	11	2.8
Uric-acid inhibitors	12.1	4.7

Source: Pharmacy Department, Group Health Cooperative of Puget Sound, Washington. D.B. Christensen et al., "Documenting Outpatient Problem Intervention Activities of Pharmacists in an HMO," *Medical Care* 19 (1981):109. Reprinted with permission from *Medical Care,* January 1981.

the contention that "the practice of medicine, although based upon scientific discovery, techniques and technologies, is still very much an art."[23] If programs for monitoring prescribing practices are to be carried out, they should concentrate on establishing the frequency of unexpected, severe reactions caused by drugs and avoid limitations on treatment options or the application of theoretical nationwide standards.[24]

On the other hand, some experts have been able to cross this philosophical chasm.[25] Azarnoff notes that the latitude to prescribe "has been

Table 3-2
Rank Order of Colorado Drug-Utilization Criteria Showing Most Deficiencies across Ten Nursing-Home Facilities

	Deficiency Rate	
Criterion	*Percent*	*Number*
Flurazepam ordered for three months continuously	98.5	(64/65)[a]
Hematinics prescribed and no stool for occult blood taken	95.5	(21/22)
Hematinics prescribed and no urinalysis done	95	(19/20)
Diuretics prescribed and weekly weight not done	94.4	(152/161)
Urinary antiseptic prescribed without initial urinalysis	91.7	(11/12)
Duration of phenothiazines, six months or more	89.6	(69/77)
Urinary antiseptic prescribed and no urine pH in last month	87	(20/23)
One or more antiarthritics combined with acetyl-salicylic acid	78.6	(33/42)
Diuretics prescribed and no weekly blood pressure	67.7	(111/164)
Antihypertensive prescribed and no weekly blood pressure	66.3	(139/203)
Hematinics prescribed without initial hemoglobin and hematocrit or complete blood count	65	(13/20)
Diuretics prescribed and no electrolytes ordered in last ninety days	64.6	(104/161)

Source: Constructed from data contained in the Colorado PSRO Demonstration Final Report, as reported in *The PSRO and the Nursing Home: An Assessment of PSRO Long-Term Care Review* (Santa Monica, Calif.: The Rand Corporation, August 1979), table 6.4.
Note: Criteria with less than 10 cases excluded.
[a]Numbers cover only those facilities with one or more deficiencies (number of deficiencies/ number of cases appropriate for review).

granted to all physicians without regard to qualifications and ability." In the absence of "monitors and controls, significant problems in drug utilization, which are detrimental to the patient, have arisen."[26] Indeed, Donabedian contends that "constant monitoring will have to be maintained, for without it medicine cannot see itself, nor know where it is going."[27]

Once the monitoring concept has been accepted, and DUR identified as the preferred administrative vehicle,[28] an implementing mechanism must be created. Although sponsorship, construction of review procedures, and access to a data base stand as critical elements in this process, it is necessary first to treat several prerequisites.

Level of Review

Most investigations and projects have stressed limitations in prescribing practices while giving little or no attention to the subsequent functions of dispensing and consumption. Since deficiencies have been recorded in these latter areas as well,[29] including hospitals,[30] DUR programs that overlook these related levels seem destined to produce suboptimal results to say nothing of wasting funds, directly and indirectly, by conducting a single-focus program.

Program Objectives

Another major question concerns the determination of program objectives. The three primary options pertaining to policy and resource allocation are (1) improvement in the quality of care,[31] (2) conserving program funds or personal expenditures, and (3) maintaining program integrity—that is, controlling problems of fraud and benefit abuse. In setting priorities, government plans and insurance schemes have favored (2) and (3).[32] However, professionally developed DUR efforts usually have stressed (1), often to the exclusion of other goals.

The extent to which these three objectives might be accommodated simultaneously within a single program can be treated only briefly in this chapter. However, either deductive reasoning or experience gained under professional standards review organizations (PSROs) suggest extreme difficulty in eliciting sustained cooperation from peer-review committee members, and probably most practitioners as well, when pressures exist to make quality-of-care considerations subservient to budgetary matters.[33]

If quality of care is to be emphasized as a major goal, DUR will need discriminating techniques to ensure that the potential benefits of drug therapy are maximized while its risks are held to reasonable limits. Additional issues, however, will require resolution. One issue involves ranking prescribing problems based upon factors such as frequency, severity, and ultimate impact, if unresolved, on both patient health and system cost. Since no program is likely to have access to unlimited resources, priorities will be required.

Another matter pertains to the proportion of staff time and resources that will be devoted to minimizing excess and bad prescribing relative to underprescribing (that is, ordering subtherapeutic amounts of a drug per day or a duration of therapy insufficient to attain the desired result).[34] If the committee is effective in addressing this problem, DUR may, in many but not all such cases, become a means of increasing outlays for prescribed medications. However, the research necessary to promulgate comprehensive standards has not been carried out and the net economic implication of this potential event has not been established.

In turning to the matter of cost containment, a patient-oriented DUR program seems likely to manifest a significant potential for reducing health-insurance outlays and total personal health-care expenditures. First, if examples of over- and bad prescribing exceed those of underprescribing, successful implementation will produce a decrease in utilization levels. Second, by emphasizing prescribing within the drugs-of-choice model, individuals will receive a higher proportion of pharmaceutical preparations whose relative safety and efficacy properties are probably superior to alternatives available in the market. Ingestion of such agents will maximize the probability of recovery within the shortest time while minimizing the likelihood of adverse effects. Although out-of-pocket drug cost may rise in some instances (like when an optimal product is under patent protection), total social cost incurred during the treatment period should be minimal.

Important savings also can be realized after the therapeutic parameters of rational drug therapy have been satisfied. Practitioners can consider ordering and dispensing a product that is available from a low-cost supplier when a multiple-source preparation is indicated as well as a more-economical agent (for example, a nonnarcotic analgesic or a noncephalosporin) within a particular therapeutic category. Consequently, if the DUR program has been effective in confining prescribing practices to the quality-assurance model, then a foundation will have been established for subsequently eliciting clinician support in the cost-containment area. A plan that seeks to transform a prescriber into a drug economist, however, runs the risk that neither sound prescribing nor fiscal conservation will be achieved.[35]

In addition to the emphasis placed on the quality of care and containment of costs, DUR activities covering insured ambulatory patients certainly will be confronted with the issue of program integrity. The latter pertains to the process of claims auditing to determine the accuracy of records submitted by providers seeking reimbursement, individuals who are not entitled to protection or who are obtaining services excluded from coverage, and benefit patterns of persons who seem to be abusing their contractual relationship.[36] In order to implement this last goal, the DHHS has promulgated screening standards for the Medicaid program that identify patients who receive, for example, more than ten narcotic analgesics or twenty psychostimulant prescriptions per year. Similar controls applied to particular products also alert the administrator when a given patient has, for example, more than fifteen orders for Dalmane or twenty for Triavil filled during the same time period.[37]

Implementation of program-integrity controls raises several important questions related to the operation of DUR: How should the responsibility for preparing study criteria and screening standards be shared between peer-review committees and full-time staff engaged by the insurance scheme? Can distinctions between questionable drug use and abuse be made with validity and reliability?[38] What types of referral procedures will be required to follow patients who seem to be moving from one category to the other?

What type of administrative structure is likely to maximize the effectiveness of both the audit and quality-of-care functions?[39]

While some investigators have addressed these concerns, further research is needed.[40] For our purposes, let it be noted that centralized review activities may be advocated since the same data base—providers and beneficiaries—is the focus of both quality assurance and claims auditing. Unless these functions are coordinated closely, however, the duplication of effort may lead to prohibitive administrative expenses. Conversely, separation of certain responsibilities may be indicated since providers conditioned by the fear of gestapo tactics (real or imaginary) generated by the surveillance staff would seem to be unsympathetic candidates for educational efforts instituted by the review committee.

Administrative Procedures

Although the parameters of a DUR program will be shaped ultimately by the factors discussed in the last section and in this one, we must introduce a more-rigorous outline of our subject. The DUR concept implies a continuous administrative function consisting of the following minimum components:

Authority exercised within an organized structure that provides resources for conducting review responsibilities;

Comprehensive criteria (elements) that serve as the framework for studying drug-use patterns;

Explicit, prospectively determined standards (norms) that delineate the acceptable limits of use within each criterion;

Accurate documentation of drug and medical experience (performance) data;

Objective assessment of such data by committee members, including provisions that permit any practitioner in question the opportunity to offer contrary evidence;

Adoption of appropriate intervention strategies to minimize deviance between drug-use practices and standards (desired values) recognized by the committee;

Periodic evaluation of both the norms employed as well as program effectiveness.

Additionally, a model program should be expected to feed back experience to professional schools so that physician and pharmacist training can be modified, as necessary, to help minimize prescribing/dispensing problems in the future.[41] In summary, DUR purports to be a self-corrective system, one that "knows its goals, can measure how far its performance is from its goals, and has incentives to apply this information to improving its performance."[42]

Authority

The ability of a DUR program to carry out its assigned responsibilities depends upon an adequate support system—power to organize a committee, to generate data, and to develop remedial techniques—provided by sponsoring entities such as hospitals, HMOs, and insurance carriers. Given the political uncertainty surrounding PSROs, the potential role of this legislative creation in influencing DUR is difficult to predict.

Contemporary programs have placed administrative responsibility in a review committee. While there seems to be agreement that the membership should be dominated by health-care professionals, the question has been raised as to whether or not private practitioners (in the peer-review role) or professional auditors, who are employed by the sponsor, should direct program activities.[43]

In considering the types of qualifications needed for committee deliberations, it seems apparent that physicians and pharmacists possess the scientific and technical background necessary to make professional judgments about problems of drug use. While several programs have operated with a ratio of six pharmacists to one physician, optimal committee size and composition at this time seem related more to personal and pragmatic factors than sound theory.[44] Reliance on the former might be reduced, however, if fundamental research was initiated to help determine professional and personal qualifications, nomination and selection procedures, tenure, and incentive structure that might lead to effective committee performance.

Study Criteria

The following list presents selected criteria that may be employed in initiating DUR efforts within the area or prescribing practices. Similar points of reference should be developed to cover dispensing services, regardless of site, and patient compliance.[45]

Therapy of choice is/is not drug therapy.

Patient condition:

With controls on single and multiple conditions, and then on drugs, list conditions within the categories labeled, unlabeled, and contra-indicated.

Having identified particular patient susceptibility, specify drugs likely to produce allergic reaction.

List instances for which delayed drug therapy may be indicated.

Polypharmacy:

Classify drugs according to probability and severity of interaction.

Identify oral combination products that can be recognized as acceptable therapy.

Define role of adjunctive therapy.

Eliminate duplicative prescribing.[46]

Figure proportion of oral combination agents prescribed to total orders written for oral products, per doctor.

Given a formulary based upon the drugs-of-choice concept, enumerate drugs prescribed that are external to this guideline (total and per doctor). Calculate proportion of prescriber's orders that are drugs of first/second choice and marginal drugs.

Determine breadth of drug-selection index—too few agents ordered/too many?

Determine drug quantity; is it insufficient or excessive:

per dose?

per day?

per order?

per treatment period?

For drug quantity, when appropriate, were titration principles followed?

Were instructions for ingestion:

Complete/incomplete?

Appropriate/inappropriate?

Was the dosage form the optimal form ordered?

Were laboratory test results obtained, as appropriate, that corroborate:

Initiation of drug therapy?

Continuance of drug therapy?

Withdrawal of drug therapy?

Delineate guidelines for appropriate use of compounded medications.

Describe prescribing based upon limitations in patient examinations:

Telephone prescribing,

Anticipatory prescribing.

Make an analysis of drugs ordered but not dispensed.

Define situation-specific parameters:

Agents that should be prescribed rarely in ambulatory settings;

Agents that should be prescribed rarely by non-board-certified practitioners;

Guidelines (both positive and negative) according to type of prescriber (for example, dentist, podiatrist, physician's assistant, nurse practitioner, pharmacist);

Proportion of controlled substances ordered;

Unique guidelines derived from official labeling, such as patient age and the role of drug holidays.

Having formulated criteria within the context of the rational drug-therapy model, develop criteria to determine prescribing effectiveness in minimizing total drug cost and total patient cost per treatment period.

Although no current program is known to have reached the scope suggested here, patient care seems unlikely to be optimized unless this broad screen is adopted, preferably within twenty-four to thirty months after operations have commenced. When experience data are run against acceptable standards, some criteria may prove to be redundant. If this desired end is attained, then screens on these items can be ordered more infrequently.

Standards

Development and professional endorsement of acceptable/desirable norms covering drug use for each criterion represent a key responsibility of the DUR committee.[47] It also highlights an area of some controversy since even experts may have difficulty in agreeing on how to measure good or bad prescribing.[48] Our ultimate objective, of course, is to codify the parameters of scientific knowledge so that the therapeutic benefits of prescription therapy can be maximized and their negative consequences minimized. A prudent committee, therefore, would be expected to deter codification when the evidence is more shallow than firm.

Development of standards by "local practitioners might perpetuate individual biases or suboptimal prescribing behavior."[49] In addition, replication of function is likely to make the cost of DUR excessive as well. Should DUR programs proliferate more through haphazard incrementalism than coordinated design, then these risks may be substantial. Consequentially, some methodology—perhaps a consortium of professional organizations—is needed to identify bona fide experts in drug therapy and to enlist their efforts in generating the needed protocols.

This task of preparing standards is feasible. Every marketed drug product contains guidelines specified by the official label. In addition, numerous parameters of rational drug therapy have been set forth for a diverse group of pharmaceuticals by Maronde,[50] Brandon et al.,[51] West,[52] Henricks,[53], and Kabat et al.[54] Similar standards have been prepared for antibiotics and psychotropics.[55]

Because it would be impractical to develop guidelines for monitoring all products on the market (perhaps more than 15,000 legend items),[56] a formulary constitutes one of the basic screening tools in the DUR process. The task of identifying agents as the drugs of choice (preparing a formulary) represents a good example where locally developed standards might be superseded by the collective insight of expert panels. Although one study found significant weaknesses among formularies prepared by fifty-two large medical centers,[57] these data do not necessarily lead to the conclusion that a single national formulary is the preferred alternative. Formularies developed on a regional basis in Italy have been evaluated favorably,[58] and a somewhat similar approach would merit intensive scrutiny in the United States.[59]

Experience Data

When DUR is conceived of as a local issue, the scope and timeliness of the records available for review will be determined by the policies and client base of the sponsoring organization. Since diagnostic information and clinical laboratory results provide an essential point of reference for interpreting certain drug-use practices (such as those for phenylbutazone), the committee's perception will be facilitated, or impaired, by the confluence that can be arranged between the primary sources of data.[60] Moreover, because the overwhelming quantity of unorganized information "doomed individual chart review as a practical method for medical audit,"[61] expert staff assistance is required to control and format computerized performance data for committee use.

Regardless of the breadth of the information base, the accuracy with which data are compiled stands as one of the key ingredients governing DUR success. If one assumes that at least 95 percent of the desired modifications in practitioner behavior will be realized through voluntary compliance, then it appears that nothing is likely to erode cooperation faster than the inability of review committees to control standards of care derived from subjective evidence and unreliability in performance data. This perspective is amplified by Azarnoff's admonition warning against any regulation where the decision "would perpetuate irrational therapy" while restrictions "imposed improperly would stifle therapeutic innovation."[62]

Most contemporary programs analyze prescription orders or drug claims on a retrospective basis. Frequently, a delay of at least several months can be anticipated between data of order and application of remedial measures. An expansion of the role of prospective concurrent review can be advocated in order to provide improved care on a more timely basis and to reduce the workload of the committee.[63] This innovation, of course, does not abolish the review function but merely shifts forward certain components with the result that they now become an integral part of the decision-making algorithm employed by the practitioner. While implementation of this concept is neither universal nor imminent, pharmacists, among others, have documented that benefits can be obtained through computer-assisted drug audits and drug-therapy monitoring.[64]

Finally, experience indicates that sampling has limited utility in supporting the documentation function.[65] This limitation stems from the fact that a patient-oriented rather than population-oriented process is concerned not so much with estimation as with the accumulation of sufficient data to verify deviant behavior and to adopt specific remedial procedures.

Interpretation of Practice Patterns

During this critical phase of evaluation, committee members will be concerned with validating the facts associated with particular cases, assessing review methods,[66] and rendering professional judgment concerning the importance of observed deviations. One of the ways in which committee credibility can be established is to concentrate initially on practice patterns that are patently irrational.[67]

While many instances of nonconformance automatically will be placed on the agenda for remedial attention, others should be examined more closely "to ascertain whether or not a problem does indeed exist."[68] Thus, more-intensive or prolonged study may be indicated for cases such as those where:

The illness episode, rather than the drug order, represents the more-appropriate frame of reference.

Patients have multiple conditions, or have been given a tentative diagnosis.

The drug of interest was recently marketed.

Prescribers work on the frontier by creating new medical knowledge.[69] When documentation has been completed, the norms used for committee reference may have to be revised.[70] The committee might also approve protocols for investigating drug use covering unlabeled conditions.

Practitioners use methods that purport to be innovations when they really lack scientific justification.

Nonclinical factors influence prescribing decisions.[71]

If committee activities prove successful in minimizing questionable and completely unacceptable drug usage, practitioners will retain flexibility in making many professional judgments. These areas of discretion include, among others, relative risk-benefit ratios when multiple products are involved in the therapy of choice,[72] as well as factors related to patient condition. Since an underlying assumption of the DUR concept holds that some 90–95 percent of the protocols employed in an evaluation of drug-therapy decisions have been derived from objective evidence, positive results may be anticipated if due caution is exercised in dealing with the residual.

Restraint also seems essential in interpreting empirically derived utilization statistics from examination of profiles. It should be apparent that data indicating, for example, drug-prescribing rank, comparative per capita drug-use figures (by sex or age), or tabulations of heavy prescribers possess little or no power for proving the case of irrational prescribing. While certain experience profiles may serve to alert monitors, the full review process, which incorporates normative measures, must be carried out. Thus, DUR committees would be expected to adopt a policy of neutrality concerning utilization levels and trends so long as prescribing and use patterns conform to the duly authorized standards of appropriate care.

Intervention Techniques

In order for the DUR function to effect changes in practitioner behavior, the committee will need to prepare a statement for external use that specifies its philosophy, objectives, and operating procedures and internal administrative guidelines including protocols for decision making with particular reference to intervention strategies.

Perhaps the most essential component involves a simple statement, to be forwarded with every communication directed to practitioners, that outlines the composition of the committee, including professional qualifications of each member; its objectives, which at a minimum, should be to facilitate attainment of rational drug therapy; the desire to focus on solving problems rather than personalities[73]; and the willingness to receive contrary evidence should its judgment be questioned.

If the committee is to pursue the option that seems most appropriate to the problem under consideration, a range of strategies will be required,[74] and an illustrative set is furnished in the following hierarchical listing that implies that informal, educational methods be followed for a reasonable period of time before more-stringent sanctions are adopted.[75]

Informal emphasis

Offer verbally to have DUR committee member, or independent expert, visit prescriber to discuss prescribing problem either in general or in particular.

Distribute drug bulletin that delineates general prescribing problems and preferred alternatives.

Send letter to the practitioner that defines the particular prescribing problem and that recommends preferred alternative(s) or furnishes general educational material covering a given therapeutic category.

Send letter to the practitioner that documents that a problem has been observed and that warns that scrutiny by the committee will continue.

Forward detailed letter that defines the problem and that invites the prescriber to an informal discussion sponsored by the full committee.

Formal emphasis

Send letter that defines the prescribing problem and that requires that the prescriber appear before the DUR committee, which will conduct a formal hearing.

Document problem and refer to:

Chief of service (if problem arose in a hospital),
Local medical society,
Insurance-plan administrator.

Threaten to invoke sanctions.

Prepare full report and request that disbarment proceedings be initiated by:

Local/state medical society,
State licensure board,
Hospital executive committee and/or insurance program.

Further, these measures should be supplemented by a bilateral incentive system that stresses rewards for better performance (covering both financial and nonfinancial recompense) as well as penalties for persistent deviance. Few, if any, DUR programs have been implemented within the context of such a comprehensive framework. Moreover, one investigator concerned with quality-assurance methods has noted that there is considerable evidence "that positive reinforcement with feedback and education result in more permanent change of behavior than does punishment."[76]

If the review committee can reduce the incidence of irrational prescribing, this impact could act as a significant buffer to the imposition of across-the-board regulations promulgated by a third party. Practitioners already have been subjected to restrictions such as a maximum thirty-day supply per prescription, a limit of five prescriptions per month for a single patient, and even a ceiling on the number of drug orders that can be initiated during a particular time period. If DUR cannot be shown to be a workable concept for structuring therapeutic choices, however, clinicians should be prepared to confront a bureaucratic onslaught that may also limit reimbursement to one or two of the cheapest products found in each therapeutic category.

Additional Functions

Periodic updating of committee standards is necessary if these guidelines are to be consonant with the latest scientific developments. Some regional mechanism with particular expertise in comparative drug therapy, like a fully staffed drug information center, might be created to furnish this technical assistance.[77] Such a center might also acquire resources to conduct an external evaluation of DUR programs—say, every two to three years—if this service is not provided by an alternative organization. Finally, practitioner training might benefit significantly if the experience, both positive and negative, of DUR programs could be summarized and fed back to the educational institutions. While these responsibilities may seem more peripheral than central to decision making on an aberrant profile, the scope and effectiveness of these independent-staff services may represent a key element in moving toward optimal drug use.

Cost-Effectiveness

As a general principle, expenditures should be incurred to improve patient health status as long as the cost is less than the benefits. The task of establishing the true economic cost of operating a particular DUR program, though, is fraught with complexity. While certain direct expenses may be estimated with some accuracy, these outlays constitute only a portion of the total.[78] Others expenses, which are more elusive, include joint costs (few resources are assigned exclusively to DUR activities), indirect expenses, amortization rate for start-up expenses and capital outlays, and implicit charges for any donated services.

Even if reliable expenditure data can be compiled, the differences between communities in terms of economic and medical resources, patient conditions, and professional views on how medicine should be practiced, to say nothing of unique DUR program features, may vitiate the utility of comparative statistics. In addition, the dynamics of both health-care-delivery techniques and the pricing of inputs may combine to render cost-effectiveness analysis more specious than rigorous.

Rather than to pursue such imponderables and unknowns, let us observe here that many DUR programs have reported an improvement in prescribing practices,[79] while they also have effected a reduction in drug expenditures.[80] Further, analysis should not overlook the possibility that a relatively small expenditure for DUR may be able to generate significant savings, especially in nondrug areas. One reason for this possibility is that the majority of prescribing problems often is associated with a minority of physicians.[81] Since the law of diminishing returns will be confronted ultimately, the cost of moving from a success rate of 95 percent to 99 percent, however, could command resources that no society can afford.[82].

If national policy seeks to maximize the benefits of contemporary therapeutic modalities including drugs, while minimizing the cost of achieving this end, greater progress may be attained if sufficient resources are allocated to the development of a holistic model for optimizing health-care delivery. This model, of course, would attempt to specify the most efficient and effective quality-assurance techniques.

One foundation for reaching this goal is thought to lie in the development of a comprehensive, computerized medical-information data base that is controlled by the health professions. Proposals for addressing this issue with respect to prescribed medications were outlined in 1971 and 1974,[83] while more-general and -advanced systems were described in 1977 and 1978.[84] One of the most important characteristics of this national network is that it would incorporate prospective and concurrent methods for evaluating patient care. In addition, this unique computer system would be integrated with, but not controlled by, health-insurance carriers or intermediaries. If such a coordinated information system became fully operative, then retrospective DUR programs might sustain a workload reduction of some 90–95 percent within five to seven years.

Given the structural modifications for the delivery and measurement of health-care services implied here, investigations can be initiated to document the comparative advantages of competing quality-assurance methods such as continuing-education programs for practitioners,[85] consumer education,[86] ad hoc drug-therapy audits,[87] intensive drug-therapy monitoring,[88] medical-care audits,[89] as well as DUR and others. Of course, assessment of patient outcomes under these techniques would become an important part of the research design.

Limitations of the DUR Model

The previous discussion has presented some suggestions concerning ways in which an organized DUR activity could mitigate instances of irrational prescribing while simultaneously helping to reduce the direct and indirect costs of illness. Traditional models, however, may be subject to one or more systemic or operational weaknesses. This section focuses on selected constraints without reference to their relative importance or empirical dimensions. Such an agenda, I hope, will stimulate investigators, practitioners, and potential sponsors to document these problems more completely and to suggest methods that may be used to control their significance.

Paper Tiger?

Some critics have charged that a system of peer evaluation leads to private deliberations among the review-panel members with the end result that this process does more to protect professional colleagues than to help patients to derive maximum benefit from available medical knowledge. These commentators advocate, on the one hand, that membership on review committees be expanded to include public representation, that the whole process be removed from practitioner control,[90] or that summary information be "disseminated to the public in a manner reasonably calculated to be constructive and understandable."[91] On the other hand, Silverman and associates contend that professionals should be given some interval (perhaps several years) to develop reasonably smooth working relations before public representatives are allowed to participate in the DUR function.[92]

The claim also has been made that review committees too often are administrative eunuchs who lean heavily on informal, educational methods to stimulate voluntary cooperations on the part of deviant practitioners. Without a more-powerful array of sanctions, coupled with a propensity to invoke them when necessary, many irrational practices, it is believed, are likely to be perpetuated.

External Constraints

One of the most significant structural weaknesses inherent in the DUR concept lies in its inability to confront prescribing or dispensing problems that arise from sources external to the treatment model. Let us assume that most irrational practices related to drug use can be dichotomized, as illustrated in the following list:

Major Control	*Little or No Control*
Practitioner did not know the drug(s) of choice for a given medical condition;	Complexities in drug nomenclature such as look-alike, sound-alike names;
Prescription written for sub-optimum dosage form or strength;	Conflicting signals—for example, experts disagree on the therapeutic properties of a particular agent;
Pharmacist dispenses 25 mg. rather than 50 mg. tablet.	Product contains ingredient(s) in subtherapeutic amount.

Research is required to ascertain the actual composition and significance of this list; a superior source for launching such a study has just been published.[93]

It can be observed that educational efforts sponsored by a DUR program have the greatest chance of minimizing irrational practices emanating from the major-control category. Similarly, it seems improbable that a conventional DUR effort will be able to exert a positive influence on basic constraints found within the little-or-no-control classification. In my view, these systems problems could account for as much as 33 percent, or more, of the cases that would be of concern to a DUR committee.

We are thus confronted with the likelihood that DUR programs will be incapable of precipitating modifications at the systems level because they are not recognized as such; because if discerned, such problems have been dumped into that residual barrel of inaction—the hope/pray/finesse/curse model—and because if discovered and confluence is established with a key organization at a nonregional level—drug producer, third-party insurance plan, central nomenclature body, regulatory agency, professional association, or school—a random admonishment seems unlikely to produce meaningful change.

Can the DUR format be altered to overcome this limitation? One possibility may be found in an expansion of objectives to include problem identification as well as problem resolution. This enlarged functional perspective would permit such programs to provide data to help to establish the percentage of committee problems falling in the two categories noted in the preceding list and to identify for both investigators and concerned organizations the difficulties that are not readily solved at the local level. While DUR programs are not designed to effect changes at the systems level, the investigation process could gather data easily on underlying factors that impede optimal drug use.

Suboptimal Reform

Two of the major limitations of the traditional DUR program—retrospective review and a data base limited to prescription records—were noted in the central portion of this chapter. Both concerns suggest that a more-comprehensive analytical model is needed to ensure that optimal benefits are received from drug therapy.

In a similar fashion, the DUR concept might be strengthened or altered if we knew more about the process of professional decision making relative to different practice settings and perceptions formed due to association with administrative bodies. For example, negative practitioner attitudes toward DUR could be anticipated if practitioners are disenchanted with duplicate review activities (some hospitals may have several programs underway simultaneously), excessive paper work commonly required to complete insurance claims or patient charts, reimbursement levels set below actual or perceived costs of production, and/or delayed payment sustained from participation in a third-party program. With respect to the last three items, it should be noted that prescriber attitudes toward DUR might be conditioned by factors external to the review mechanism and even the drug-insurance scheme. Regardless of the causal pathways, a suboptimal theoretical/operational model may impair DUR effectiveness.

A broader analytical model can be justified also when it is recognized that DUR represents an adjunctive option or alternative to one or more of the following: caveat emptor; practitioner education, both professional and postgraduate; patient/consumer education; mandatory periodic relicensure; a host of ad hoc restrictions on prescribing as mentioned briefly previously; and competing quality-assurance methods. Moreover, recent interest has been expressed in "a unified approach to quality assurance and risk management" within a hospital.[94]

Despite the length of this discussion, numerous additional areas merit attention. Some of these include the posture that a committee might adopt in evaluating the use of placebo therapy,[95] the need for uniform data elements,[96] the reliability of diagnostic information, methods to ensure the confidentiality of patient records,[97] practitioner regression after initial stimulus from DUR, shared professional jurisdiction covering both practice and DUR implementation, a financing mechanism to ensure continuity of the DUR function, potential catalysts that might be enlisted to support the DUR concept (or its superior surrogate), and the status of patients not covered by a DUR program.

Prognosis

Can DUR be regarded as a workable option for improving the use of prescribed medications? On the one hand, if the index for prognosis is measured by the number of mature operating units, the number of investigators who have accumulated significant knowledge about our subject, the political climate, or professional enthusiasm for the concept, then a pessimistic conclusion seems inescapable.

On the other hand, if the index is based upon documented shortcomings in drug-use practices, the feasibility of developing and applying standards of good care, the possibility of focusing remedial efforts on a minority of clinicians, or the underlying pressures militating toward social progress, then a more-optimistic argument may be tenable.

Regardless of how these conflicting forces evolve, practitioners should contemplate that prescribed drugs represent the single therapy ordered most frequently in medical practice today and that some form of validation of its appropriateness is inevitable as technical and nontechnical knowledge about prescribing increase.

Notes

1. Institute of Medicine, *Advancing the Quality of Health Care* (Washington, D.C.: National Academy of Sciences, August 1974), p. 13.

2. This figure embraces drug dispensing and administration for all inpatient and ambulatory-care settings pertaining to both the private and government sectors. It also recognizes that 5–10 percent of the prescription orders may not be filled.

3. This problem obtains with respect to both concept (the literature refers to DUR, drug-use review, and drug-usage review) and technique (performance data may be called norms).

4. M.H. Stolar, "Drug Use Review: Operational Definitions," *American Journal of Hospital Pharmacy* 35 (January 1978):77.

5. For the general models, see P.Y. Ertel and M.G. Aldrige, *Medical Peer Review: Theory and Practice* (St. Louis: Mosby, 1977); A. Donabedian, *The Definition of Quality and Approaches to Its Assessment* (Ann Arbor, Mich.: Health Administration Press, 1980; and for the specific models, see J.M. Gregory and D.E. Knapp, "State of the Art of Drug Usage Review," *American Journal of Hospital Pharmacy* 33 (1976):925-928; and W.N. Kelly, J.A. White, and D.E. Miller, "Drug Usage Review in a Community Hospital," *American Journal of Hospital Pharmacy* 32 (1975):1014–1017.

6. HEW Task Force on Prescription Drugs, *Approaches to Drug*

Insurance Design (Washington, D.C.: Government Printing Office, 1969), pp. 73–74; and M. Silverman, P.R. Lee, and M. Lydecker, *Pills and the Public Purse* (Berkeley, University of California Press, 1981), p. 109.

7. T.D. Rucker, "The Role of Computers in Drug Utilization Review," *American Journal of Hospital Pharmacy* 29 (February 1972):128.

8. S. Shindell, "Hospital Utilization-Review Mechanisms," *Journal of the American Medical Association* 196 (1966):130–136; H. Jick et al., "Comprehensive Drug Surveillance," *Journal of the American Medical Association* 213 (August 1970):1455–1460; and R.F. Maronde et al., "A Study of Prescribing Patterns," *Medical Care* 9 (September–October 1971): 383–395.

9. D.C. Brodie, *Drug Utilization and Drug Utilization Review and Control,* DHEW Pub. No. (HSM) 72-3002 (Rockville, Md., 1971); W.H. Campbell, R.E. Johnson, and D.B. Christensen, "A Procedural and Conceptual Analysis of Drug Use Review," *Drugs in Health Care* 2 (Fall 1975):211–230; and D.A. Zilz, "Drug Insurance and the Quality of Care," *Proceedings of the National Conference on Drug Coverage under National Health Insurance,* DHEW Pub. No. (PHS) 78-3208 (Washington, D.C.: National Center for Health Services Research, 1977), pp. 19–23.

10. "Paid's New Cost-Cutting Alternative," *Drug Topics* 120 (1 March 1976):16–18; and F.Y. Yarborough and M.F. Laventurier, "Peer Review Works via a Committee of 7: 6 Pharmacists Plus One Physician," *Pharmacy Times* 40 (March 1974):58–63.

11. HEW Task Force, *Approaches to Drug Insurance Design,* p. 64.

12. Joint Commission on Accreditation of Hospitals, *Accreditation Manual for Hospitals* (Chicago, 1980), pp. 151–154.

13. Ibid., pp. 208–209.

14. M. Silverman, and P.R. Lee, *Pills, Profits and Politics* (Berkeley: University of California Press, 1974), p. 300.

15. P.R. Lee, "America Is an Overmedicated Society," in *Controversies in Therapeutics,* ed. L. Lasagna (Philadelphia: W.B. Saunders Co., 1980), pp. 7–11.

16. T.D. Rucker, "The Top-Selling Drug Products: How Good Are They?" *American Journal of Hospital Pharmacy* 37 (June 1980):836.

17. See T.D. Rucker, "Superior Hospital Formularies: A Critical Analysis," *Hospital Formulary* 17 (September 1982): 465–524. Aldoril, Ambenyl, Apresazide, Benylin, Butisol sodium, Ceclor, Choledyl, Dexchlorpheniramine, Diethylpropion, Dimetane exp - DC, Equagesic, Fastin, Fiorinal with Codeine, Hydergine, Hydropres, Librax, Libitrol, Lorazepam, Methyclothiazide, Metolazone, Naldecon, Neosporin ophth, Norgesic Forte, Norinyl-1/50-21, Ornade, Parafon Forte, Phenergan exp, Phenergan VC exp, Phenergan VC exp with Codeine, Phentermine, Pyridium, Regroton, Salutensin, Ser-Ap-Es, Stuartnatal 1 + 1, Synalgos-DC, Tussionex,

and Tuss-Ornade. Products included in a single formulary include: Actifed-C expectorant, Amitriptylline/Perphenazine, Anusol-HC, Brompheniramine exp, Cyclobenzaprine, Donnatal, Fenoprofen, Fiorinal, Nitroglycerinoral capsules, Propoxyphene Napsylate, and Propoxyphene HCl compound.

18. T.D. Rucker and J.A. Visconti, *How Effective Are Drug Formularies?* A Descriptive and Normative Study. (Washington, D.C.: ASHP Research and Education Foundation, 1979).

19. For nursing homes, see Silverman, Lee, and Lydecker, *Pills and the Public Purse,* pp. 114–118. For hospitals, see Campbell, Johnson, and Christensen, "Procedural and Conceptual Analysis," p. 212; and M. Castle et al., "Antibiotic Use at Duke University Medical Center," *Journal of the American Medical Association* 237 (27 June 1977):2819–2822.

20. J.E. Knoben, "Drug Use Review," in *The Practice of Pharmacy,* eds. D.C. McLeod and W.A. Miller (Cincinnati, Harvey Whitney Books, 1981), p. 91.

21. A.A. LeRoy and M.L. Morse, "Impact of Inappropriate Drug Therapy on Hospital Admission Study," *Journal for Medicaid Management* 1 (Fall 1977):82.

22. D.A. Knapp et al, "Drug Prescribing and Its Relation to Length of Hospital Stay," *Inquiry* 17 (Fall 1980):258.

23. J.H. Sammons, "New Controls on Physician Prescribing Are Not Needed," in *Controversies in Therapeutics,* ed. L. Lasagna (Philadelphia: W.B. Saunders Co., 1980), p. 543.

24. Ibid.

25. For example, R.H. Brook, "Studies of Process-Outcome Correlations in Medical Care Evaluations," *Medical Care* 17 (August 1979):868–873; and A. Donabedian, "The Quality of Medical Care," *Science* 200 (26 May 1978):856–864.

26. D.L. Azarnoff, "Monitoring and Control of Physician Prescribing Are Needed," in *Controversies in Therapeutics,* ed. L. Lasagna (Philadelphia: W.B. Saunders Co., 1980), p. 534.

27. Donabedian, "Quality of Medical Care," p. 863.

28. M. Laventurier, "Guidelines of Drug Utilization Review of the San Joaquin Pharmaceutical Society," *California Pharmacist* 18 (February 1971):8–15.

29. R. Jang et al., "An Evaluation of the Quality of Drug-Related Services in Neighborhood Pharmacies," *Drugs in Health Care* 2 (Winter 1975): 21–38.

30. D.C. Brodie et al., "Model for Drug Usage Review in a Hospital," *American Journal of Hospital Pharmacy* 34 (March 1977):251–254.

31. The related issue of which type of measure(s)—structure, process, or patient outcome—should be used to assess program results is a signif-

icant topic that requires separate analysis. Where prescription drugs are involved, process rather than outcome variables will probably dominate because few medical problems will permit the practitioner to control all the factors that influence patient health status. For one general discussion of this subject, see A. Donabedian, *Needed Research in the Assessment and Monitoring of the Quality of Medical Care,* National Center for Health Services Research, DHEW Pub. no. (PHS) 78-3219, July 1978.

32. D.C. Brodie, "Drug Utilization Review/Planning," *Hospitals* 46 (1 June 1972):112.

33. W.A. Knaus, "PSRO Update: Where We Stand Now," *American Medical News,* (20 June 1977):8.

34. R.M. Marks and E.J. Sachar, "Undertreatment of Medical Inpatients with Narcotic Analgesics," *Annals of Internal Medicine* 78 (February 1973):173–181; and Lee, "America Is an Overmedicated Society," p. 12.

35. T.D. Rucker, "Comparative Approaches to Cost Constraints in Pharmaceutical Benefit Programs: Commentary," in *Impact of Public Policy on Drug Innovation and Pricing,* eds. S.A. Mitchell and E.A. Link (Washington, D.C.: American University, 1976), p. 188. See also chapter 21.

36. "How Federal Probers Will Seek to Uncover Medicaid Drug Fraud," *American Druggist* 174 (July 1976):16, 18–19.

37. "What Project Integrity Is," *Nebraska Mortar and Pestle* 40 (June 1977):31.

38. R.F. Maronde et al., "Prescription Data Processing—Its Role in the Control of Drug Abuse," *California Medicine* 117 (September 1972): 22–28.

39. J.P. Morgan, "Watching the Monitors: 'Paid' Prescriptions, Fiscal Intermediaries and Drug-Utilization Review," *New England Journal of Medicine* 296 (3 February 1977):256.

40. S.H. Rosenberg et al., "An Eclectic Approach to Quality Control in Fee-for-Service Health Care: The NYC Medicaid Experience," *American Journal of Public Health* 66 (January 1976):21–30; and L.E. Bellin, "Realpolitik in the Health Care Arena: Standard Setting of Professional Services," *American Journal of Public Health* 59 (May 1969):820–825.

41. Rucker, "The Role of Computers," p. 132.

42. C.M. Jacobs, and T.H. Christoffel, *Measuring the Quality of Patient Care: The Rationale for Outcome Audit* (Cambridge, Mass.: Ballinger Pub. Co., 1976), p. 3.

43. L.E. Bellin, "PSRO—Quality Control? Or Gimmickry? *Medical Care* 12 (December 1974):1017–1018.

44. Yarborough and Laventurier, "Peer Review Works."

45. For examples that might be applied to the dispensing model, see

Jang, Knapp, and Knapp, "Evaluation of the Quality of Drug-Related Services," p. 24. For examples pertaining to patient compliance, see D.L. Sackett and R.B. Haynes, "Compliance with Therapeutic Regimens," in *Perspectives on Medicines in Society,* eds. A.I. Wertheimer and P.J. Bush (Hamilton, Ill.: Drug Intelligence Publications, 1977), p. 335–357.

46. Analysis of insurance claims revealed that one beneficiary "had visited 15 different physicians and obtained 15 prescriptions for an amphetamine. Each physician was unaware that other physicians were similarly prescribing until so informed by Blue Shield" (Blue Shield of Michigan, "Prescription Drug Program Utilization, 1969–1971," Research Report, vol. 2, p. 21). This example illustrates that an effective DUR program must be concerned with both patient compliance and patient deception.

47. W.A. Miller, "Quality Assurance of Pharmacy Services," in *The Practice of Pharmacy,* eds. D.C. McLeod and W.A. Miller (Cincinnati: Harvey Whitney Books, 1981), p. 377.

48. Morgan, "Watching the Monitors," p. 254.

49. Knoben, "Drug Use Review," p. 87.

50. R.F. Maronde, *Drug Utilization Review with On-Line Computer Capability,* ORS/SSA, DHEW Pub. no. (SSA) 73-11853 (Washington, D.C., May 1972), pp. 51–81.

51. B. Brandon et al., "Drug Use Screening Criteria," *American Journal of Hospital Pharmacy* 34 (February 1977):146–151.

52. S.K. West et al., "Drug Utilization Review in an HMO," *Medical Care* 15 (June 1977):508.

53. J.N. Henricks, *Audit Criteria for Drug Utilization Review* (Bethesda, Md.: American Society of Hospital Pharmacists, 1981).

54. H.F. Kabat et al., *Drug Utilization Review in Skilled Nursing Facilities* U.S. Department of Health, Education & Welfare (Washington, D.C., November 1975).

55. C.M. Kunin and H.Y. Efron, "Audits of Antimicrobial Usage, Guidelines for Peer Review," *Journal of the American Medical Association* 237 (7 March 1977):1001–1008; B.E. Blom and N.C. Moore, *Psychotropic Drug Therapies,* Mental Health Audit Criteria Series (Chicago, InterQual, 1978); O.B. Towery and A.B. Brands, *Psychotropic Drugs: Approaches to Pharmacologic Drug Use* (Washington, D.C.: DHEW Pub. no. (ADM) 79-758, 1979), pp. 47–69; and Committee on Therapeutics, New York State Office of Mental Health, "Psychotherapeutic Drug Manual" (Albany, March 1981).

56. G. Karr, "Monitoring Drug Utilization—Modification of Prescribing Habits," *Canadian Journal of Hospital Pharmacy* 30 (January–February 1977):13.

57. Rucker and Visconti, *How Effective Are Drug Formularies?,* pp. 109–110.

58. G. Tognoni et al., "Drug Utilization Studies and Change of Thera-

peutic Practice,'' in *Epidemiological Evaluation of Drugs,* eds. F. Colombo et al. (Littleton, Mass.: PSG Pub. Co., Inc., 1977), pp. 22–23.

59. T.D. Rucker, ''Effective Formulary Development—Which Direction?,'' *Topics in Hospital Pharmacy Management* 1 (May 1981):42–43.

60. C.F. Muller, ''The Study of Prescribing as a Technic of Examining a Medical Care System,'' *American Journal of Public Health* 57 (December 1967):2121.

61. S. Kelman, *Improving Doctor Performance* (New York: Human Science Press, 1980), p. 69.

62. Azarnoff, ''Monitoring and Control,'' p. 539.

63. Rucker, ''Role of Computers,'' p. 132.

64. G. Gilroy et al., ''Integration of Pharmacy into the Computerized Problem-Oriented Medical Information System (PROMIS)—A Demonstration Project,'' *American Journal of Hospital Pharmacy* 34 (February 1977):155–162; and R.B. Stewart, ''Drug Therapy Monitoring,'' in *The Practice of Pharmacy,* eds. D.C. McLeod and W.A. Miller (Cincinnati: Harvey Whitney Books, 1981), pp. 73–80.

65. Rosenberg et al., ''An Eclectic Approach,'' p. 22.

66. Jacobs, and Christoffel, ''Measuring Quality of Patient Care,'' p. 30.

67. Rosenberg et al., ''An Eclectic Approach,'' pp. 28–29; and HEW Task Force, *Approaches to Drug Insurance Design,* pp. 64, 70.

68. F.B. Palumbo et al., ''Detecting Prescribing Problems through Drug Usage Review: A Case Study,'' *American Journal of Hospital Pharmacy* 34 (February 1977):153.

69. Azarnoff, ''Monitoring and Control,'' p. 539.

70. Morgan, ''Watching the Monitors,'' p. 251.

71. Campbell, Johnson, and Christensen, ''Procedural and Conceptual Analysis,'' p. 212.

72. D.E. Knapp and P.D. Oeltjen, ''Benefit-to-Risk Ratio in Physician Drug Selection,'' *American Journal of Public Health* 62 (October 1972): 1346–1347.

73. T.D. Rucker, ''The Need for Drug Utilization Review,'' *American Journal of Hospital Pharmacy* 27 (August 1970):657.

74. Jacobs and Christoffel, *Measuring Quality of Patient Care,* p. 98.

75. Campbell, Johnson, and Christensen, ''Procedural and Conceptual Analysis,'' p. 223.

76. R.J. Haggerty, ''Quality Assurance: The Road to PSRO and Beyond,'' *Pediatrics* 54 (July 1974):93.

77. Rucker, ''Effective Formulary Development,'' pp. 42–43.

78. D.A. Knapp and F.B. Palumbo, ''Dollar Costs of Conducting Drug Use Review,'' *Journal of the American Pharmaceutical Association* NS17 (April 1977):231–233.

79. Knoben, ''Drug Use Review,'' p. 92.

80. M. Laventurier, "A Prototype Pharmacy Foundation Peer Review Program," *California Pharmacist* 19 (1972):36–38; and R.F. Maronde, "Drug Utilization Review," *Hospital Formulary Management* 9 (June 1974):46–47.

81. R.F. Maronde, "Drug Utilization Review," in *Perspectives on Medicine in Society,"* eds. A.I. Wertheimer and P.J. Bush (Hamilton, Ill.: Drug Intelligence Publications, Inc., 1977), p. 171.

82. A. Donabedian, *Needed Research in the Assessment and Monitoring of the Quality of Medical Care,* DHEW Pub. no. (PHS) 78-3219 (Washington, D.C.: National Center for Health Services Research, July 1978), p. 9.

83. T.D. Rucker, "Schematic of Drug Information System," *Proceedings: Computer-Based Information Systems in the Practice of Pharmacy,* 19–21 July 1971, pp. ii, 24–26; and T.D. Rucker, "Drug Use: Data, Sources, and Limitations," *Journal of the American Medical Association* 230 (11 November 1974):889–890.

84. Gilroy et al., "Integration of Pharmacy," pp. 155–162; and E.R. Gabrieli, "Medical Information System, Health Records, and Knowledge Banks," *Medical Instrumentation* 12 (1978):245–247.

85. T.D. Rucker, "Drug Information for Prescribers and Dispensers: Toward a Model System," *Medical Care* 14 (1976):156–165.

86. R. Greene, *Assuring Quality in Medical Care* (Cambridge, Mass.: Ballinger, 1976), p. 279.

87. C.W. Greenlaw, "Antimicrobial Drug Use Monitoring by a Hospital Pharmacy," *American Journal of Hospital Pharmacy* 34 (1977): 835–838.

88. Stewart, "Drug Therapy Monitoring," pp. 73–80.

89. R.C. King and A.M.K. Cheung, "Drug Therapy Review as Part of a Medical Audit Process," *American Journal of Hospital Pharmacy* 35 (1978):578–580.

90. "National Health Care Quality Control: The Alternatives," *Health Perspectives* 2 (July–August 1975):3.

91. Institute of Medicine, *Advancing the Quality of Health Care,* p. 33.

92. Silverman, Lee, and Lydecker, *Pills and the Public Purse,* p. 111.

93. N.M. Davis and M.R. Cohen, *Medication Errors: Causes and Prevention* (Philadelphia: George F. Stickley Co., 1981).

94. P.W. Keys, "Drug-Use Review and Risk Management," *American Journal of Hospital Pharmacy* 38 (1981):1534; and J. Tremblay, "Another View," 39 (1982):578–579.

95. T.D. Rucker, "Public Policy Considerations in the Use of Psychotherapeutic Drugs," *Drugs in Health Care* 1 (1974):12.

96. M.B. Forbes, L.B. Burke, and J.K. Jones, "Need for Uniform Data Elements in Hospital Drug Use Review," *American Journal of Hospital Pharmacy* 38 (1981):711–715.

97. L. Lasagna, *Controversies in Therapeutics* (Philadelphia: W.B. Saunders & Co., 1980), p. 533; P.M. Rabinowitz, *Talking Medicine* (New York: W.W. Norton, 1981), p. 274; and Rucker, "Role of Computers," pp. 132–133.

Part II
Regulatory Perspectives

4 U.S. Drug Development: Regulatory Issues and Trends

J. Richard Crout

Some social movements and institutions apparently are destined to be small but influential—small because they are somewhat iconoclastic and unpopular and influential because they speak the truth, or at least come close enough to the central truth that they must be listened to even if they are occasionally controversial. I would characterize those health-care professionals who are concerned about rational prescribing as one of these movements. They are destined to be unpopular, but they are also likely to be influential because of the quality and cogency of the questions they ask and the importance of the topic.

This book is in that tradition in that it attempts to explore the diverse views on what constitutes rational prescribing practices in order to arrive at some kind of central truths.

Nature of Regulatory Agencies

My first reflection about regulation is that it is difficult. There are several reasons for this. First, during the past decade, regulatory agencies have become the focus for the discussion of important public-policy issues. Second, most regulatory agencies have no natural political constituency—they do not offer favors to anyone. To some extent, the FDA does not fit into this mold. The agency does occasionally approve an NDA for which physicians and the drug industry are grateful. However, certain other regulatory agencies, by their nature, have nothing positive to offer the industry they regulate. The best example of this is the Environmental Protection Agency (EPA), which is hard pressed to do anything but deliver bad news as far as industry is concerned. By their nature, regulatory agencies also limit freedom. There is no way that regulation cannot come into conflict with perhaps the greatest of U.S. values—that is, the commitment to freedom. Finally, regulatory agencies occasionally use tools that are blunt and gross, which open us to the attack of: Why are you doing such a dumb thing?

Legal and Moral Imperatives

My second reflection—one that scientists do not like to hear—is that the regulatory process is set in law. The actions of regulators are guided by a set of legal principles that is intended to serve the public at large. The first moral imperative of the regulator is to do the greatest good for the greatest number of people—that is, to think in terms of public policy. The second moral imperative is to be correct—that is, to make no mistakes. While the public trusts regulators to be right, regulators have no moral imperative to be fast. That does not mean that regulators have to be paralyzed or inefficient in their ability to make decisions. It means that any decision made requires an extraordinary amount of consultation, of thinking over all the possible ramifications, so that they are certain it is the correct one. The regulators must make the right decision for the right reasons and must also be able to explain their reasoning to various groups. These are difficult criteria to meet, and I submit that they are very different from the standards that most scientists are asked to meet, for example, when they publish papers.

This means, then, that those who wish to communicate with a regulatory agency, or to participate in the regulatory process, have to find out what laws, regulations, and policies govern the agency in question because these are the ground rules that must be followed. It is also very important for scientists who must deal with the government to be able to distinguish what is a law from what is a regulation or policy because these distinctions determine who is empowered to make a decision or to change things as well as how difficult it will be to change them. Changing a policy can be fairly easy; altering a regulation is a little harder. However, only Congress can change a law.

The same evidence that influences scientists in general is also persuasive to regulators. Regulators tend to be convinced by arguments that are civil, to the point, and incisive. They tend not to be persuaded by pressures like hundreds of letters from practitioners that seem obviously to have been generated by a particular drug firm or by congressional inquiries on behalf of constituents with a problem before the agency. It has been my experience, fortunately, that regulators want to respond to the rational insofar as they perceive it and to avoid the political. However, since regulators cannot always avoid becoming embroiled in political issues, they have to have what I call a keel—a commitment to make decisions on the basis of evidence. If these regulators can maintain that commitment to the evidence, they can cope with a variety of arguments and comments attempting to persuade them to make decisions on different bases.

The Power of Regulation

Regulation does change behavior. I was brought up to believe in the power of rationality and of education to persuade. I was raised to believe that if you could convince someone of something, this would automatically lead to a change in behavior, most likely for the better. However, this is not the only way that change comes about in the real world. Much evidence suggests that, in fact, dramatic or really meaningful social change arises because some external force compels people to change their behavior. Then, afterward, people change their attitudes to reconcile them with their behavior. Taking the example of racial discrimination, there is no doubt that if the U.S. government had followed the general premise that discrimination could be eliminated only by changing people's attitudes, many centuries would have passed before any changes in discriminatory practices would have occurred. In reality, changes occurred in the United States because the Supreme Court forced people to change their behavior—that is, to make alterations in access to public facilities and schools. These changes in behavior, then, facilitated changes in our attitudes. The important lesson for us to learn is that regulation is a powerful tool for changing behavior, even of those whose attitudes are opposed to change. Thus, it is important to use regulation wisely when it is necessary and when the goal is consonant with U.S. life, laws, and values. It is interesting that supportive attitudes will commonly ensue later, even from former opponents.

Misuse or Abuse by the Few

The most difficult problem in drug regulation in general, is how to handle misuse or abuse by the few because regulatory action may lead to the many paying for the sins of the few. Misuse, for example, of the principle of informed consent and some of the ethics of medical investigation have resulted in our current extensive system for monitoring clinical research. Abuse of drugs by the few has given rise to the Federal Controlled Substances Act and all the problems surrounding the manufacture, distribution, and dispensing of controlled substances. Intransigent or deviant physicians are the cause of the most serious problems of overprescribing and misprescribing and are of concern to all members of the health-care field. A difficulty arises, however, from the fact that no societal consensus exists on how to handle these problems. Every one of the solutions is an emotional issue. Drug regulatory laws, for example, are aimed at products, at controlling human behavior. Those who would use such laws to limit human behavior are venturing into a highly controversial area. One need only look at the issue of gun control, for example, to get a feeling for the political thicket that entangles the proposed use of product regulation to limit product use. Consider the reaction of the drug industry, pharmacists, or physicians to any suggestion that the distribution of a particular drug should be limited.

Thus, in my opinion, the greatest unsolved problem in regulatory medicine is how to regulate the use of drugs and the procedures employed by medical professionals—particularly, how to handle the deviant or the intransigent physician and still preserve the freedom of those professionals to provide the best care for their patients. Over the last ten years, this problem has been debated in congressional committees and discussed in numerous forums like this book. To my knowledge, there is still no consensus whatever on a political solution, or a technical solution, for this problem. Even if we could devise a method for regulating certain aspects of professional behavior, a group of people, asking whether this would be a change for the better, undoubtedly would arise.

Effects of U.S. Regulatory Decisions Abroad

Another observation I would make about regulatory activities, which is a trend that has developed over the past decade, is that everything that we do has repercussions throughout the world. This is particularly true for the FDA, but I am sure it applies to other U.S. regulatory agencies as well. The United States is still the world's largest single market. Thus, the approval of a drug in the United States is equivalent from a marketing standpoint to approval in all of the countries of the European Economic Community. Approval of a drug in the United States is also very important to developing countries and, in fact, provides entree to essentially every country in the world.

In much the same way, regulatory decisions in the United States that are adverse to a drug have important ramifications worldwide. A drug can be withdrawn quietly from the market in a Scandinavian country or Australia, for example, but not in the United States; we are too visible. As a result, every important adverse decision by the FDA must be contested; industry may lose a world market if it loses a regulatory battle in the United States. This is one reason for the contentiousness of our drug regulatory system, although certainly not the only reason.

Effects of Foreign Decisions on the FDA

Conversely, the decisions of regulatory bodies in other countries influence U.S. regulation. U.S. regulators are sensitive to the fact that a drug has been approved or withdrawn from the market in other countries. If we know that Canada and the United Kingdom have approved a particular agent, we may tend to give it a higher priority. I do not think that regulators change their standards or their opinion of the evidence because of approval in other countries, but it is often a reason for paying closer attention to a drug.

I would also add that there is a growing convergence around the world in regulatory decision making, not because of any great international plan but largely because during the past decade, U.S. regulatory officials and their counterparts in various countries have learned to share their ideas and, in so doing, have reached more of a common philosophy. Foreign regulatory agencies have adopted certain U.S. policies, a move that has resulted in drug approval times getting a little longer in other countries, while at the same time, the approaches of our foreign colleagues have tempered U.S. approaches.

Future Changes

My view of the future is that the basic regulatory system we have now will remain. We are living in a deregulatory environment, but the political forces that are being brought to bear on the FDA at the present time are not asking for radical or fundamental changes. They are asking mainly for improvement in the approval process—to do what the FDA does but to do it better, faster, and more efficiently.

Shorter Approval Times

I think the basic task ahead is to streamline the bureaucracy—that is, to improve administration of the review process. The FDA is trying to do that, and it may well succeed. If it is successful, I think the most important benefit would be the shortening of drug-approval times by a year or, at best, by a little more than that. At present, there is an average of two years between the submission of an NDA and its approval by the agency. If the pharmaceutical industry submitted perfect NDAs, and if FDA reviewers were totally efficient, the two years could be reduced to six months. However, given that these two phenomena are unlikely to occur, potential for vastly shortening drug-approval times by streamlining administrative procedures is not great. I do not mean to imply that we should not attempt to shorten approval times but that it is not possible to effect revolutionary changes by tinkering with the administrative process.

Similar Drug-Development Times

Although I believe that the amount of time between submission and approval of an NDA will be reduced in the future, I think that there will continue to be a relatively long time for drug development and clinical testing. I do not believe that the FDA can shorten the drug-development-and-testing process and get drugs on the market much faster than it takes now without undercutting major current regulatory requirements. In chapter 6, Dr. William Wardell suggests that one possibility for decreasing the time required for testing a drug would be to substitute a postmarketing-surveillance program for the later phases of premarketing clinical trials. Other proposals have been to minimize toxicology requirements early in the drug-review process and to delegate the authority for monitoring the conduct of early research to a new set of institutional-review bodies so that studies would not come under the purview of the FDA until a later stage. I am neither advocating nor opposing these proposed changes. However, I am suggesting that these are the sorts of major changes that must be considered, with all of their political ramifications, if we wish to shorten the drug-development process by more than a year.

Exemptions from Drug Regulations

I think there will continue to be a conflict over substances that, for one reason or another, are desired by the public but that do not meet established efficacy or safety standards. Laetrile is a prime example of this. Cigarettes and saccharin are other examples. I would hope that Congress will not tear down our basic regulatory standards to accommodate such substances because those standards serve us well for the vast majority of drugs. My view is that the efficacy requirement will survive the debate over how to handle this problem. However, if some means of handling drugs like laetrile becomes a political necessity, I think the right solution is simply to exempt these products from the drug laws—as was done with vitamins in the 1970s—rather than to alter the fundamental structure of our regulatory system.

Reimbursement Mechanism

Finally, I think that at some point in the future the United States will discover the reimbursement mechanism as a regulatory tool. One of the ironies of our times is that Medicare and Medicaid are searching for ways to control costs, and yet they are reimbursing for laetrile. These two practices are not rationally reconcilable. When the irrationality of this situation is perceived, I think we will begin to use reimbursement, which is actually a much more-subtle, less-contentious, and more-powerful tool than marketing approval, to implement certain kinds of regulatory decisions.

Many countries currently use the reimbursement mechanism under their national health system as a tool to regulate health policy. Some day the political support for this now-controversial regulatory mechanism is likely to develop in the United States.

5 The FDA's Role in Appropriate Drug Use

Stuart L. Nightingale

The FDA's statutory authority to regulate the interstate marketing of drugs passed its seventy-fifth anniversary on 30 June 1981. On that date in 1906, President Theodore Roosevelt signed into law the first federal Food and Drugs Act that, among other things, made it illegal to manufacture or traffic in adulterated or misbranded drugs.

The pharmacologic climate in which the 1906 Food and Drugs Act came into being was one we can scarcely imagine today. In contrast to the handful of demonstrably useful drugs available to physicians at the turn of the century, literally thousands of nostrums, potions, elixirs, and tonics were being offered to the U.S. public. Neither gullible consumers nor the concerned physician had any basis on which to judge the value of most remedies, and all too often, we may be sure, their use did far more harm than good. How could it have been otherwise when alcohol, heroin, opium, and cocaine were widely employed, though rarely declared, in a pharmaceutical array that included products such as Warner's Safe Cure for Diabetes and Kick-a-poo Indian Sagwa?

While the FDA's drug-regulatory goal has not changed over the years—namely, to protect the public from adulterated or misbranded drugs—the scope of its responsibilities has become much broader, in conformance with the numerous additional authorities given the FDA under new legislation over the years. The FDA's responsibilities extend from monitoring and regulating research with products under FDA's jurisdiction to ensuring the reliability and validity of safety and effectiveness data. These responsibilities include protecting human research subjects and granting market approval with assurances that drug labeling and advertising are accurate and not misleading, so that practitioners can make the most appropriate use of the drug products available to them and their patients. The FDA has, therefore, an important role as a monitor, overseer, and source of information that is of great significance to prescribers in their efforts to make appropriate use of drugs in patient care.

Drug Labeling

Once the FDA approves a new drug for marketing, it has little control over the conditions under which the drug is used. What it can and does control is the information given prescribers by drug sponsors about approved drugs. Under the law, a drug may be labeled, promoted, and advertised only for those indications in which safety and effectiveness have been established and that the FDA has approved—so-called approved uses. These approved uses are determined on the basis of premarket studies including adequate and well-controlled clinical trials carried out under investigational new drug exemptions. While drugs in this stage of development cannot be marketed or promoted by the sponsor, in the very late stages of the investigation, it is possible for practitioners to obtain certain investigational drugs under what is known as a compassionate, or treatment, category. The FDA, on occasion, does authorize a drug sponsor to supply an investigational drug to a physician for use in treating a patient whose serious disease cannot be managed adequately by the use of available alternate therapy. Reports of adverse effects must be reported to the FDA in each instance.

Valid new uses for drugs already on the market often are discovered first through the serendipitous observations and therapeutic innovations of physicians. Before such advances can be added to the official labeling, however, data substantiating the new indication based on the legal standard of substantial evidence derived from adequate and well-controlled clinical trials must be submitted to the FDA for evaluation. This may take some time to occur, and without initiative on the part of the drug firm whose product is involved, it may not occur at all for certain uses. However, because the medical literature regularly presents reports of new, unlabeled uses for approved drugs, it is common for physicians to use drugs for unapproved indications before the FDA has the opportunity to approve their inclusion in labeling.

While drugs are approved for specific indications at the time they are marketed initially, using them for nonlabled indications or in dosage regimens other than those specified in official labeling is certainly not illegal. In fact, such unapproved, or more precisely, unlabeled, uses may be quite appropriate in certain circumstances as determined by sound medical practice. Regardless, the FDA does not have or seek the authority to regulate the practice of medicine. The latter is the province of the states and is controlled by state medical-practice acts.

The term *unapproved uses* is, of course, misleading. It subsumes a variety of situations, ranging from unstudied to carefully investigated drug uses—some salutory, others hazardous, some occurring very infrequently, others so common and so widespread as to constitute normal or usual medical practice. The FDA does have a significant responsibility and a clear legal obligation, however, to make sure that the claims made for approved drugs are supported by the findings of rigorous clinical investigations.

A different problem arises when a drug has been found to be either ineffective or unsafe for a particular indication—for example, the use of digitalis for weight control. In such cases, the official labeling may include a prominently displayed warning, a so-called box warning, that advises physicians that such use of the drug is hazardous and, in effect, disapproved. The inclusion of comments relative to such use in official drug labeling is relatively rare, and properly, should be an important deterrent to inappropriate prescribing. Legally, of course, there is no such category as a disapproved drug or indication.

The official labeling of an approved drug is a summary of information submitted to the FDA by the drug sponsor, usually the manufacturer, in support of an application for approval to market the drug. The drug-product package insert is the official labeling that is required by law. This labeling is referred to by the FDA as professional labeling. The *Physicians' Desk Reference* (PDR) is a commercial compendium of labeling for drugs that are listed in it. Thus, when a physician turns to the *PDR*, he or she is examining the summarized findings on which approval of the drug is based.

The critical role of drug labeling in providing prescribing information has highlighted the fact that improvements in the organization and content of drug labeling were needed. Two major and related steps are now being taken to make the labeling more helpful to the practitioner.

In June 1979, the FDA published in the *Federal Register*[1] a final regulation entitled, "Labeling for Prescription Drugs Used in Man," which spells out how labeling information contained in the package insert is to be organized by NDA sponsors into a well-defined format to present clearly and accurately sufficient information to facilitate proper use of the individual drug. Although the provisions detailing the specifics of the format and content are too extensive to be discussed fully, it should be noted that the section on clinical pharmacology has been expanded to include specific data on pharmacokinetics and other information pertinent to a drug's clinical use. The precautions section includes, where appropriate, information under the following subsections: general; information for the patient, which suggests what the physician may want to tell his or her patient about a drug in order to encourage compliance and to allay undue anxiety; laboratory tests; drug interactions; carcinogenesis; mutagenesis; impairment of fertility; labor and delivery; pediatric use; nursing mothers; and use in pregnancy.

The new section on adverse reaction defines an adverse reaction as an undesirable effect reasonably associated with the drug. Adverse reactions are listed in ways that are most useful to the practitioner—by organ system, toxicological mechanism, severity, or frequency. When information on frequencies of adverse reactions is available, it must be expressed in rough estimates of orders of magnitude that will provide physicians with clear and concise statements of the frequency of the reactions. For the first time, a separate section on drug abuse and dependence appears in the labeling, and a section on overdose is included.

Standards listed and explained in the *Federal Register* document have been developed for the kind of information to be included in each section of the revised drug labeling. They will eliminate the inclusion of extraneous and promotional information and require that information be given in explicit rather than general terms. The adoption of this new labeling format and content is proceeding according to schedule. Every newly approved drug is required to be labeled in accordance with the regulation, and the labeling for all previously approved drugs will be cast in the new format within the next few years.

A related step to improve the clarity and usefulness of drug labeling is the class-labeling program—the development of uniform labeling for drug products that fall within the same pharmacologic and therapeutic category. Thus, identical or closely related drugs that are marketed under different trade or generic names and for which, as of now, the information contained in the official labeling may be quite dissimilar, will be compared and contrasted to each other in regard to the new labeling format. The objective of class labeling is to permit the practitioner to select readily from among a class the optimal drug for a particular indication in a particular patient, without having to seek other sources of information. A class label is intended to incorporate all approved drug information in one document so that statements common to all members of a class do not have to be repeated and, even more important, so that true differences between drugs can be highlighted in the labeling for the class to which they belong. The first example of class labeling—for single-entity barbiturates—was published in the *Federal Register*[2] in November 1980. Some thirty-one other classes of drugs are scheduled to have class labeling within the next two years or so. This major change will help to eliminate the undesirable and confusing situation caused by the fact that drugs in the same class approved sometime later than the original members of the class may have quite different labeling, simply because later findings have been developed through research and incorporated in labeling.

Drug Advertising

Advertising is another major source of prescription-drug information. The FDA monitors such advertising to make certain that it contains balanced, accurate summaries of salient information that is consistent with approved labeling. Although drug advertisements that do no more than remind physicians of the name of a particular product are not required to include summaries of official labeling, any advertisement that describes or alludes to a drug's use in patient care must include, in addition to the generic name of the product and the name and address of the manufacturer, a brief but thorough summary of prescribing information including contraindications, warnings, and other pertinent material.

A prescription-drug advertisement that implies incorrectly that a drug is the treatment of choice or that suggests that a drug is useful for the treatment of a condition not included in the official labeling would be unacceptable.

The FDA does not preclear advertising and other promotional materials for prescription drugs, but manufacturers often voluntarily submit newly developed advertisements and promotional materials to the FDA to make sure that they meet the agency's regulatory requirements. As part of its program to monitor the information contained in prescription-drug advertising and promotion, the FDA reviews an extensive selection of professional journals and other publications, scientific exhibits, and advertising campaigns that may include films, recordings, brochures, and publications developed for continuing-education activities sponsored by the drug industry.

The Food, Drug, and Cosmetic Act provides a number of legal remedies to deal with advertising and promotional activities that amount to misbranding. These remedies are used infrequently, however, because manufacturers usually agree to distribute corrective promotional materials and, if necessary, to send "Dear Doctor" letters advising physicians of errors of fact or implication if the FDA asks them to do so.

Postmarketing Surveillance

Thus far, I have touched on drug-labeling and prescribing information that is developed by the drug industry and, thus, subject to FDA regulation. Other sources of information derive from activities of the FDA. Of particular importance is the information developed in the course of the FDA's activities in the postmarketing surveillance of drugs used in medical practice. Many kinds of information pertinent to safe and effective use of regulated products can be developed only through continuous monitoring of products in actual use. Although clinical testing of drugs prior to approval can disclose side effects and adverse reactions that have a comparatively high statistical probability, rare events—those that may occur only once in 10,000 chances or even less often—may be discovered only after a drug has been approved and has reached wide general use. Postmarketing surveillance also can disclose abuse of drugs whose clinical testing may have identified no such risk or identified only a minor potential for abuse. Of course, postmarketing surveillance offers the only certain means of assessing long-term effects that seldom can be gauged during preapproval clinical trials that normally last only a matter of months.

Postmarketing surveillance gives the FDA the means to ensure that drugs approved for marketing as safe and effective continue to meet this standard. Since safety is determined through a weighing of the potential risks and benefits of a drug for any given use, if experience shows a higher risk, the balance of risks and benefits may change. In that case, the FDA is able to alert physicians and, if necessary, to alter the labeling of the drug or take steps to remove it from the market.

Information on the extent and patterns of drug use are obtained from a variety of sources—manufacturers, drug-marketing and -distribution channels, and hospital-based drug-utilization audits. Data on adverse reactions come from reports to the FDA by individual physicians, hospitals, and occasionally, consumers. The *FDA Drug Bulletin* periodically includes report forms to facilitate adverse-reaction reporting by physicians, pharmacists, and other health professionals. Drug manufacturers are required to report adverse reactions to their products on a timely and regular basis. In all, the FDA receives about 12,000 adverse-drug-reaction reports each year, and the agency's data bank now includes some 110,000 entries. Drawing on this information, as well as on reports that appear in the published literature, the FDA plans to produce an annual summary of adverse reactions to drugs reported since 1969. This summary will be available through the National Technical Information Service.

The FDA supports a number of specific organ or system registries that not only collect and evaluate adverse-drug-reaction data but also consolidate new and earlier findings. A distinct advantage of these registries is that they are operated by health-care professionals who are specialists in the specific field involved. Registries currently funded or in the planning stage include a hepatic registry, operated by the Veterans Administration in the Washington, D.C., area; the tissue-reactions registry, operated by the Armed Forces Institute of Pathology, that gathers data on deaths and tissue specimens believed to be associated with adverse drug reactions; an ophthalmology registry, maintained by the University of Oregon, that assembles reports of ocular adverse reactions throughout the country; the radiocontrast media registry, now being reconstituted to assemble hospital data; the dermatology registry that is just getting under way and that will collect data on dermatologic reactions and reactions to dermatologic agents through reports to the American Academy of Dermatology; and a hematology registry that is now in the planning stage.

Other contract-supported postmarketing-surveillance data systems include a project to collect and analyze Medicaid data, multiple-case control approaches to assess potentially drug-related chronic disorders that would not usually be detected in spontaneous reporting systems, a system to monitor pediatric adverse reactions in hospitalized children, and a large project with several components including a data base of 40,000 hospitalized patients on whom all drug-event data have been collected.

Another significant source of information available to the FDA are surveys, registries, and findings of other government agencies including the National Center for Health Statistics, which compiles extensive data on potentially pertinent information such as hospitalization and outpatient health care; the Drug Abuse Warning Network (DAWN) system of the Drug Enforcement Agency and the National Institute on Drug Abuse; and the Center for Disease Control, which maintains a registry of birth defects.

That brings me to what is, I submit, a most important question: What does the FDA do with the postmarketing data it acquires through a multiplicity of sources and projects, and how is it of value to prescribers? Part of the answer is obvious from my earlier comments. The information developed through postmarketing surveillance of drug utilization and experience is a major source of necessary changes in official drug labeling.

When experience, for example, with the use of tetracycline in children demonstrated that the drug could cause permanent staining of teeth, the official labeling for tetracycline products used in pediatric practice was changed to include a specific warning of this adverse reaction. Unfortunately, the use of tetracycline in the most susceptible age group—children up to the age of eight years—continued, and in 1978, the FDA took steps to remove pediatric tetracycline drops from the market. Preparations of the drug in liquid form were allowed to remain on the market because they were needed in geriatric care. However, figures from the July 1978–June 1979 *National Disease and Therapeutic Index*[3] showed that 60 percent of the prescriptions for tetracycline liquid were being written for children age newborn to nine, while patients over age 65 accounted for only 6 percent of the prescriptions.

Because this adverse reaction is both significant and unequivocal, it was summarized, the labeling changes were highlighted, and the removal of pediatric formulations of tetracycline were recounted in two issues of the *FDA Drug Bulletin.*[4] This publication, whose major purpose is to provide precisely this kind of information to physicians, pharmacists, and other health professionals, is mailed several times a year to nearly one million practitioners. It exists primarily as a means whereby the FDA can discharge its responsibility to help inform prescribers and others concerned with the use of drugs of significant developments affecting the safe and effective use of approved products.

The most recent issue of the *FDA Drug Bulletin,*[5] dated March 1981, contains articles reporting the narrowing of labeled indications for Bendectin, cardiac problems associated with the use of disopyramide, a change in the recommended starting dose of chlorthalidone, a warning (to be included in official labeling) of potentially fatal fat accumulations in the lungs of premature and small-for-age infants receiving intravenous fat emulsions, and a revision in information that manufacturers provide health professionals on the role of aspirin in transient ischemic attacks. The *FDA Drug*

Bulletin, now in its eleventh year of publication, according to readership surveys, is both widely read and highly regarded by practitioners as a source of prescribing and related information.

Recalls

From time to time, experience in the use of a marketed product or a problem in its manufacture, packaging, distribution, or labeling makes it necessary to recall the product. This step is accomplished with the cooperation of the manufacturer who gets in touch with those to whom the product has been shipped, advising that further distribution and use are to be stopped. If necessary, the FDA issues a press release advising that a product is being recalled so that the risk of continued use will be held to a minimum. The FDA monitors recalls to be certain that they are carried out thoroughly and promptly. While the agency does not have the legal authority to order product recalls, manufacturers and others in the distribution chain—including prescribers—are usually eager to cooperate in preventing harm from the use of a product that has been recalled.

Conclusion

It is a continuing challenge to the thoughtful practitioner to sort out from available information—for example, continuing medical-education courses, the medical literature, advertising, and other sources—the prescribing information he or she judges to be the most authoritative and reliable. For its part, the FDA feels, and acts on, a responsibility to the professions to make certain that the information on which drug approval is based is presented fairly, accurately, and thoroughly wherever it is represented—in official labeling, in drug advertising and promotion, and in other endeavors that seek to influence prescribing practices. With essentially the same goal in mind, the FDA attempts to assemble and make available information on experience with marketed drugs so that prescribers are able to benefit from the collective experience of their colleagues and to minimize the risks that inevitably are associated with drug therapy. The FDA sees this function as part and parcel of its responsibility as a public-health, scientific regulatory agency.

The FDA believes that its activities—mandatory, such as evaluating drugs for safety and efficacy, and discretionary, such as informing the health professions through the *FDA Drug Bulletin*—are essential and that they complement, for the practicing physician, other information like that available in the medical literature.

Notes

1. *Federal Register,* 44 FR (June 26, 1979):37434.

2. *Federal Register,* 45 FR (November 18, 1980):76356.

3. *National Disease and Therapeutic Index* (Ambler, Pa.: IMS America, Ltd.; June 1978–1979).

4. "Tetracycline Pediatric Drug to be Withdrawn from the Market," *FDA Drug Bulletin* (May 1978):23–24.

5. "Pediatric Tetracycline Use," *FDA Drug Bulletin* (November 1979):29–30.

6 Can Improved Postmarketing Surveillance (Phase IV) Permit Earlier Drug Approval?

William M. Wardell

The Need for More-Efficient Drug Development

There is a close relationship between the way drugs are used and the process of drug development. If drug utilization—including the prompt detection of adverse effects—were perfect, then there would be little need for controls of drug development or introduction, and the patient would benefit both from improved therapy today and from the expeditious appearance of better medicines in the future. In this chapter, therefore, I consider postmarketing surveillance (or Phase IV) as it affects the drug-development process and, in particular, whether or not it would be possible to use postmarketing surveillance as a substitute for some of the late clinical premarketing studies (Phase III) that are required at present.

Why is it necessary to be concerned about the process of drug development, and why is postmarketing surveillance important in this regard? The future of drug development in the United States does not appear to me to have the rosy future that seems to be accorded to it currently, at least by the financial community.[1,2] Indeed, some of the measures that I believe foreshadow the future of research and innovation suggest that the U.S. pharmaceutical industry's research output is declining and that small firms in particular are coming to depend increasingly upon foreign innovations. This interpretation is supported in part by the following evidence, and although some of the values are based on preliminary analyses, the trends are clear cut. The causes of these trends are not yet explained but are probably complex.

The number of new chemical entities that the entire U.S.-owned industry is bringing to the stage of first human investigation declined abruptly—by nearly 50 percent—in 1975 after a decade of stability and has remained at the same low level since then.[3] This is the largest change since the precipitous decline of 1961–1963. While the reasons for the decline in the mid-1970s are not yet clear, the fact is striking, and its future implications (in terms of the availability of U.S.-originated compounds for approval in the mid-1980s and later) could be considerable. Of course, the patient stands to benefit from useful new drugs regardless of their origin, so that innovation should be welcomed and encouraged from all parts of the world. However, since the U.S. research-based pharmaceutical industry forms a large part of the total world effort, changes in the input or output of U.S. research are of worldwide concern.

At the investigational-new-drug (IND) stage, the percentage of U.S. firms' new-chemical-entities filings that represent self-originated molecules fell from approximately 80 percent in the mid-1970s to two-thirds in the latter 1970s. Thus, one-third of all U.S.-owned firms' investigational new drugs for new chemical entities are now filed on licensed and acquired compounds (of which over 80 percent are foreign innovations).[4] Small U.S. firms are affected particularly; in the last five years their dependence on licensed and acquired compounds for their new-chemical-entities investigational new drugs has risen to nearly 50 percent.

The average time required from investigational-new-drug filing to new-drug-application (NDA) approval of a successful drug sponsored by a U.S.-owned firm is now approximately eight years; the time from synthesis to approval is over twelve years. The effective patent life—that is, the time remaining from approval of the NDA to expiration of the main patent—has declined as the time required for development has increased. From an average of nearly fourteen years in 1966, effective patent life has fallen to less than ten years in 1979–1980. Most of this four-year decline is due to an increase in the clinical investigation time in the United States, while the remainder is due to an increased preclinical time and quicker issuance of the patent.[5]

While the causes of all these marked trends are probably complex and subject to disagreement, the trends are obvious and some of them give cause for concern about the future output of the pharmaceutical R&D effort in the U.S.

Postmarketing Surveillance and the Deregulation Programs

Partly because of general concern about the future of pharmaceutical innovation, there has been a new administrative initiative in the United States aimed at making the process of drug development more efficient by providing regulatory relief, or deregulation, provided this can be done without impairing safety.

Conversely, critics of deregulation express concern about the implications of deregulation, mainly on the grounds of safety; there are already signs of a reaction developing. These concerns should be taken seriously because maintaining safety obviously must be a primary consideration in any program of deregulation, as I have discussed in an earlier paper.[6] In this chapter I show why the tenuous position of postmarketing surveillance among the deregulation proposals should be strengthened and discuss how and whether or not it could be.

Substituting postmarketing surveillance for some of the currently required premarket clinical testing is one of the few drug-regulation proposals that appears to have lost favor in the current discussion despite its importance. The problem stems from the need to use postmarketing surveillance as a substitute for some of the currently required premarketing studies if the maximum improvement in efficiency is to result; otherwise, postmarketing surveillance simply would become an additional phase that would increase the regulatory burden further. It is important to examine the possible contribution of such surveillance in deregulation carefully because the six-year investigational-new-drug phase (which represents three-quarters of the eight-year clinical plus regulatory time in the United States is the only place where there is much opportunity for shortening the overall process of drug development. One of the major ways of doing this would be by trading off, or substituting, excessive premarketing requirements by postmarketing studies that confer equal (or greater) safety.

The idea of improving postmarketing surveillance and using it as a substitute has been considered a promising alternative for many years. It was, for example, under consideration in a joint evaluation study proposed in 1976 by the National Bureau of Standards' Experimental Technology Incentives Program (ETIP), in conjunction with the FDA, entitled "An Experiment in Post-Marketing Surveillance of New Drugs."[7] The work of this study was later merged with the work of the Joint Commission on Prescription Drug Use (JCPDU).[8] (The latter body did not specifically consider the trade-off question.) The ETIP study is still proceeding, in conjunction with the FDA, to explore how postmarketing surveillance can be linked with the drug-development and -approval processes. The general principle of trading off some premarketing studies for better postmarketing surveillance has been mentioned by several FDA commissioners, including Commissioner Schmidt.

However, the manner in which postmarketing surveillance currently is being implemented leaves no doubt that it is being added to most of the existing premarketing requirements. This obviously will tend to raise the barriers to drug development by lengthening the duration of the process and by increasing costs. Regulatory officials both in the United States and the United Kingdom have stated that they could not envisage as politically feasible any substitution that would involve even an apparent reduction in premarketing requirements. Furthermore, it is the stated aim of at least one consumer group that postmarketing surveillance specifically should be added to the existing premarket requirements, not substituted for them.

Potential Time Savings by Concurrent NDA Review and Substitution of Premarketing Studies by Postmarketing Surveillance

For the reasons given in the last section, I believe the concept of postmarketing surveillance as a substitute for premarketing studies should be pursued vigorously as one of the tools of deregulation—that is, it should be used explicitly as a clearly defined trade-off or substitute for currently required premarketing studies where equivalent safety can be ensured.

Although this idea has long been discussed, it has until now been a pipe dream with little chance of implementation so that it has not been analyzed in much detail to see what would be involved in practical terms. What exactly that currently is being done prior to marketing could be given up? What are the implications of substitution for the various parties involved—patient, physician, government, industry? One can soon see that the issues raised are quite complex and cannot be solved in a short presentation. However, in an initial discussion like this we at least can begin to define the issues in more-concrete terms to see where the opportunities and the problems lie.

Concurrent NDA Review. Before dealing with the substitution of any premarketing studies, it is worth noting that a substantial saving in time is available simply by having the NDA reviewed concurrently with these studies rather than consecutively as at present. This would require the NDA to be submitted at the end of early human studies rather than at the end of the late clinical premarketing studies. Since the average durations of NDA review and premarketing studies are now similar (two to three years each), the results of the late clinical premarketing studies (if written up and submitted promptly) would be available for considerations toward the end of the NDA review process. This proposal does not involve any reduction of premarket studies at all; it is essentially the same as the developing-NDA (review-by-stages) system proposed by the FDA in the mid-1970s. In this way at least two years could be eliminated from the development time without any change in the amount or type of evidence required for approval or in the standard of review. It is not clear to me why this idea—and indeed the whole of FDA's developing-NDA proposal—has not been supported enthusiastically by industry and the agency because the potential savings produced by efforts at this point are much greater than could be achieved by attempts to streamline the present NDA phase, which is where most of the attention of the deregulation efforts is being directed. Admittedly, it would require more staff work, but it would be a pity if such an apparently cost-effective increase in efficiency were to fall victim to budget stringencies.

Substitution of Postmarketing Surveillance for Late Clinical Premarketing Studies. Substitution of adequate postmarketing surveillance for all or part of the existing late clinical premarketing studies would require, for a start, even more-careful organization of the NDA submission and review. Not all drugs would be appropriate for this procedure. It would be necessary to identify a particularly suitable candidate early in human testing and also to submit at least the initial portions of the NDA at this time so that the review process could commence. The results of the remaining early human testing studies then would be submitted as they became available for the last portion of the review shortly after the study was completed. In this way all the data could be analyzed very soon after the end of early human testing.

The potential reduction in development time that these ideas could yield is substantial. Merely by beginning the NDA review earlier, at least two years could be cut from the present eight-year IND-NDA period without omitting any late clinical premarketing studies at all. Allowing, in addition, some or all of these studies to be substituted easily could bring the savings to four years, or half the present IND-NDA period. In no other part of the drug-development process could this much time be saved feasibly.

Barriers to Implementation

There do not seem to be any substantial barriers in principle to the idea of concurrent NDA review, because the amount of evidence required prior to marketing is not changed by this procedure. However, substitution of postmarketing surveillance for premarketing studies does involve some reduction in the amount of evidence required prior to marketing, and this in turn raises a number of problems or at least questions that need to be answered. These questions have not been analyzed widely. Some of the more-obvious ones are discussed in the following sections.

What Information Would Be Preserved? What Would Be Foregone? Current early human studies determine whether or not a drug has any efficacy at all in the condition under investigation and whether or not frequent adverse reactions occur in the relatively short durations of such studies. At a minimum, all this information still would be available. Later clinical premarketing studies explore in addition the efficacy and toxicity of the drug in greater numbers of patients with less closely standardized disease states, resembling real-world conditions of medical practice. As well as providing more knowledge of the drug itself, these premarketing studies give information about drug-disease and drug-drug interactions and about adverse reactions of lower (but still not rare) incidence. Obviously, some or all of this clinical premarketing information would have to be foregone if postmarketing surveillance were to be substituted for it. If the drug were reviewed as early as the end of early clinical studies, there already would be information about the drug's overall efficacy and its most common adverse reactions and necessary precautions. The fine details of its properties would be unknown. This could be more acceptable for some classes of drugs (for example, antibiotics) than for others. However, the differences involved in proceeding directly to postmarketing surveillance instead of to premarketing studies are quantitative, not qualitative. The main difference consists of conditions under which the next step is taken and not necessarily the nature of the step itself.

What Is Adequate Postmarketing Surveillance. In particular, can it substitute for part or most of the premarketing phase without risking the high standard of safety that we have now achieved in drug development? This is the most important issue.

Although examples do exist of the substitution of all of the premarketing phase by postmarketing surveillance (for example, in the case of the early NDA approval for levodopa in 1970), there is not yet enough experience with the idea to let us formulate rules by which equivalent safety can be assured; however, complete safety cannot be guaranteed with the present system, either. I believe the adequacy of any given postmarketing-surveillance-substituting plan could be judged fairly easily from the facts about the particular drug involved. It is not intrinsically hazardous to prescribe rather new drugs to patients who stand to benefit from them, provided the available information gives a reasonable description of the drug and that the drug's prescribing and the monitoring of the patient are performed to the highest existing standards of science and medicine. These conditions are being met every day in the phased system of drug research, with a degree of safety that is so great it is usually overlooked. There is no reason why the safety standards of postmarketing surveillance could not be made equal to, or even surpass, those of the present phased premarketing studies; when this is achieved, then postmarketing surveillance will be an adequate substitute for those studies. If fairly comparable safety cannot be achieved in a given case, then obviously that drug would not be a candidate for early approval under the particular postmarketing-surveillance plan proposed.

Special Precautions to Facilitate Substitution of the Late Clinical Premarketing Phase by Postmarketing Surveillance

At the outset, I shall assume that the particular drug will have been selected as a candidate for early approval and postmarketing surveillance because its efficacy and toxicity, as revealed during first and second phase studies, make it of particular therapeutic interest. (I have seen several instances that satisfy these criteria.)

Because of the implications associated with reducing marketing requirements, it is possible that special precautions might be deemed necessary in the case of some drugs, either for medical reasons or for reasons of legal liability. In such a case, the patient would need to be fully aware of the status of the drug, the available information on its efficacy and toxicity, and the degree of monitoring required for its safe use. The physician would need to understand clearly the status of the drug, the circumstances in which its use would be appropriate, and the side effects he or she should watch for in order to monitor the patient satisfactorily. In special cases, perhaps additional ideas are needed—for example, a method for highlighting the fact of a drug's early approval and thus the need for special surveillance. Such a method, employing a distinctive mark on the drug's package and promotional materials for a defined time after initial marketing, already has been implemented abroad. Although this may give a new drug the image of being not quite approved, it is one possible approach to the problem of increasing the awareness of physicians and patients to drugs that need special precautions. If all new drugs were marketed similarly, this need not necessarily be an unwelcome stigma.

One important point from these considerations is that the onus and initiative is squarely on the company to propose and implement—or at least to support—a postmarketing-surveillance method that will detect trouble in a drug early and that will allow rapid assessment of its real magnitude. In this respect, the company's needs are similar to those of the patient, the physician, and the regulator. The company needs to ensure that the drug is used properly and that all toxicity—both expected and unexpected—is detected, evaluated, and responded to promptly. The correct response to a problem may range all the way from changing the drug's labeling, advertising, and educational materials to restricting its promotion or even withdrawing it if the circumstances should warrant. Indeed, the onus always has been on the company to do this; deregulation simply would increase its responsibility.

Numerous other ideas have been suggested as a way of facilitating earlier approval. The idea of a regulatory category of restricted or limited initial release has been put forward as a way to handle situations of this type. While regulation-based restricted-release mechanisms do exist in some countries, I do not think these would be appropriate or feasible in the United States. Rather, an alternative already is available to any firm—namely, fine tuning of a drug's initial use by the firm's control of its own promotional activity. This would be a commonsense voluntary approach rather than one based on regulatory or legal controls to ensure that—where deemed necessary in the earliest stages—the particular surveillance system being used indeed is monitoring the drug properly. For example, in the case of a drug that was to be approved unusually early in its developmental history, if the firm could only perform the appropriate type and degree of surveillance in a restricted geographical area, then at its initial launch the full promotion of the drug (for example, detailing by sales representatives) could be restricted to that particular geographical area. Apart from this change in detailing, the distribution, prescribing, and dispensing could remain unchanged throughout the country.

Medicolegal Issues

The risk of litigation may prove to be a substantial disincentive to early approval of new drugs, particularly in the United States. If this risk were perceived to be large enough to require patients to give informed consent before receiving a drug that had early-release status, then it is doubtful that any company would be interested in proceeding. The medicolegal climate is an important determinant of whether or not any premarketing-studies-substitution plan will work. Therefore, public understanding of, and attitudes toward, the risks and benefits of both existing and new treatments is an equally important consideration.

Conclusions

Review of the NDA concurrently with the clinical studies and substitution of postmarketing surveillance for the premarketing studies are among the few feasible ways now available to increase the efficiency of the drug-development process to any large extent. Substitution cannot be achieved without full safeguards, however. I realize that some of the suggestions discussed here might seem unpalatable to those in government and industry involved in the process; even concomitant review of the NDA would involve considerably more work and time pressure at the sponsoring company in preparing the NDA and more staff or consultants at the agency to review the application. Certain of the other ideas and consequences may make the idea of substituting postmarketing surveillance for premarketing studies less feasible than it appears at first sight. Nevertheless, the potential rewards to all parties are very great—namely, a halving of the investigational-new-drug-NDA time now and higher incentives to innovation in the future. It is worth exploring every idea that might help us to achieve this end and being on the lookout for special drug or disease situations in which these and other ideas might be evaluated on a pilot scale.

If present trends continue, the drug-development system is in danger of grinding to a halt. I believe that concurrent NDA review plus a substitution of postmarketing surveillance for some of the premarketing phase could do much to restore research efficiency and incentives. However, formidable barriers exist to implementation of this model, and considerable work must be done by sponsors, regulators, researchers, and the public to determine whether or not and how these barriers can be reduced safely and practically.

Notes

1. M. Magnet, "The Scramble for the Next Superdrug," *Fortune* 104 (October 19, 1981):94–112;
2. P. Bornstein, "Follow the New Directions," *Forbes* (14 September 1981):55–58.
3. W.M. Wardell, J. DiRaddo, and A.G. Trimble, "Development of New Drugs Originated and Acquired by United States-Owned Pharmaceutical Firms, 1963–1976," *Clinical Pharmacology and Therapeutics* 28 (August 1980):270–277.
4. Unpublished analyses, Center for Study of Drug Development, Rochester, N.Y., 1982.
5. M.M. Eisman and W.M. Wardell, "The Decline in Effective Patent Life of New Drugs," *Research Management* 21 (January 1981):18–21.
6. W.M. Wardell, "Deregulation of Drug Development: If Effective, Can it Be Safe?" (Paper presented at the Fourth International Meeting of Pharmaceutical Physicians, Paris, 28–30 April 1981).
7. C. Chapman and V. Berlin (Experimental Technology Incentives Program, National Bureau of Standards) and M.J. Finkel and J.A. Halperin (Bureau of Drugs, Food and Drug Administration), "An Experiment in Post-Marketing Surveillance of New Drugs," March 1976.
8. Joint Commission on Prescription Drug Use, *Final Report* (Rockville, Md., January 1980).

7 Models of Postmarketing Surveillance: The Experience with Cimetidine

Thomas G. Davis

Because of SK&F's recent broad experience in the formal monitoring of cimetidine, my impressions are prefaced by informing you that cimetidine has been monitored via three mechanisms. One is the worldwide spontaneous reporting system,[1] and the other two are formal postmarketing-surveillance systems in the United States and the United Kingdom.[2] I direct most of my comments in this chapter to the formal surveillance study in the United States.

Our original goal was to collect a cohort of patients large enough to enable us to analyze the benefits of therapy as well as the adversities. Statistical analysis indicated that based on premarketing experience, 10,000 patients would provide a 90 percent probability of detecting an event with an incidence of 1 in 4,000. To establish this cohort, we recruited 1,200 physicians from various fields of specialty (table 7–1) to provide data on the first 10 patients to whom they prescribed cimetidine. These practitioners were in no way restricted in their use of the drug. For purposes of reporting adversity, we collected a total of 9,900 patients. For analysis of disease, this number decreased to 9,000, representing nearly a 90 percent respondence. The second phase of this study involved a follow-up report six months after the initial course of Tagamet®. This phase resulted in 7,248 patients, who had by that time experienced 9,763 courses of therapy with cimetidine.

Table 7–2 depicts the type of gastrointestinal disease that was treated in this cohort. The age distribution (table 7–3) was far greater than one would ever have in premarketing studies and is concentrated heavily in the 40–60-year age grouping. Table 7–4 depicts the number of reported adverse effects. These totaled 567 effects reported on 440 patients, an adversity percentage of 4.4 percent. Not all of these reactions have proved attributable to the drug, however. In the second phase, the percentage of adversity decreased to 1.8 percent, which is somewhat predictable since this group of patients would include chiefly those who were able to tolerate the drug.

Table 7-1
Patients Treated with Cimetidine, by Type of Practice

Type	*Number*	*Percent*
General practitioner/Family practice	4,951	54.9
Internists	2,405	26.6
Gastroenterologists	1,353	14.9
Internal medicine/Gastroenterology	179	1.9
Not shown	138	1.5

Source: L.M. Gifford et al., "Cimetidine Postmarket Surveillance Program, Interim Report on Phase I," *Journal of the American Medical Association* 243 (18 April 1980):1534. Copyright © 1980, American Medical Association.

Table 7-2
Conditions Treated with Cimetidine

Condition	*Number of Patients*
Duodenal disease	4,208
Peptic disease	1,407
Gastric disease	1,588
Esophageal disease	1,082
Other frequently reported gastrointestinal[a]	243
Zollinger-Ellison syndrome	18
Miscellaneous	480
Total	9,026

Source: L.M. Gifford et al., "Cimetidine Postmarket Surveillance Program, Interim Report on Phase I," *Journal of the American Medical Association* 243 (18 April 1980):1534. Copyright © 1980, American Medical Association.

[a]Twenty-five cases or more.

Table 7-3
Total Age/Sex Distribution

Age	*Number of Patients*	*Men*	*Women*	*Not Stated*
Under 16	216	102	100	14
16-19	182	81	99	2
20-29	942	479	446	17

Table 7–3 continued

Age	*Number of Patients*	*Men*	*Women*	*Not Stated*
30–39	1,369	691	655	23
40–49	1,609	781	796	32
50–59	1,992	1,019	921	52
60–69	1,511	733	752	26
70 and over	1,205	518	667	20
Not stated	—	—	—	—
Total	9,026	4,404	4,436	186

Source: L.M. Gifford et al., "Cimetidine Postmarket Surveillance Program, Interim Report on Phase I," *Journal of the American Medical Association* 243 (18 April 1980):1534. Copyright © 1980, American Medical Association.

Table 7–4
Adverse Effects

		Patients Reporting Adverse Effects	
Type	*Total Adverse Effects Reported*	*Number*	*Percent*
Gastrointestinal	247	208	2.1
Central nervous system	131	108	1.2
Allergic/Skin	54	46	0.5
Endocrine	25	25	0.3
Musculoskeletal	20	20	0.2
Urinary tract	18	18	0.2
Autonomic	15	14	0.2
Sensory organs	14	14	0.2
Cardiovascular	14	11	0.1
Blood	8	8	0.1
Miscellaneous	21	21	0.2
Total	567		

Source: L.M. Gifford et al., "Cimetidine Postmarket Surveillance Program, Interim Report on Phase I," *Journal of the American Medical Association* 243 (18 April 1980):1534. Copyright © 1980, American Medical Association.

Note: Adverse effects (567) reported by 440/9,907 patients (4.4 percent).

Table 7-5
Overall Efficacy

Efficacy	*Number of Patients*	*Percent*
Excellent	4,984	55.2
Good	2,845	31.5
Fair	404	4.5
Poor	252	2.8
Worse	35	0.4
Not shown	506	5.6
Total	9,026	

Source: L.M. Gifford et al., "Cimetidine Postmarket Surveillance Program, Interim Report on Phase I," *Journal of the American Medical Association* 243 (18 April 1980):1534. Copyright © 1980, American Medical Association.

Finally, we are of course interested in whether the drug is of benefit. Table 7-5 indicates that, in better than 80 percent of the patients, overall reported efficacy was very good indeed.

Detection of Adversity?

What are the advantages of carrying out such an intensive postmarketing-surveillance program? The original purpose that attracted the industry—namely to hasten drug approval by reducing some of the premarketing requirements—has gone by the wayside. What, then, could be expected? Surveillance might uncover adversity not revealed in the premarketing clinical studies. This did not occur. In fact, we maintained a structured spontaneous worldwide reporting system during the duration of this study, and this system first detected adversities not reported during the clinical evaluation. Study of this cohort of 10,000 patients did not reveal anything in terms of adversity that we did not already know from controlled study or that we did not pick up quickly through the spontaneous reporting system. However, this study did serve to confirm much of our premarketing experience, both in terms of safety as well as efficacy, and this confirmation is certainly of value. It also provided a cohort of patients not typical of those chosen for premarketing studies.

We looked carefully for new indications for the drug, but unfortunately, the cohort did not reveal any. I would not rule out finding new indications in other formal programs, however.

One might predict that conclusions concerning the attribution of adverse reactions in such a study would be more accurate than those in a spontaneous system, where follow-up is very difficult. I believe it is true in this case. Perhaps the most useful advantage from the study was the availability of the cohort for review. This review has been particularly useful in properly evaluating reported drug interactions. For example, cimetidine interferes with some of the microsomal systems in the liver responsible for the clearing of important benzodiazepines such as Valium and Librium. In fact, some studies have shown that cimetidine may extend the half-life of these drugs and increase the blood concentration. However, 500 patients in our cohort who took these drugs with cimetidine experienced no reported adversity.

In another example, recently reported in the *New England Journal of Medicine,*[3] an interaction between cimetidine and propranolol indicated that propranolol-caused bradycardia was aggravated and prolonged by cimetidine. An analysis of our cohort showed that 269 patients had taken both drugs concurrently, again with no report of adversity. If we extrapolate to worldwide patient use, we can presume that approximately 300,000 patients have taken cimetidine and propranolol concomitantly without a clinical problem.

Disadvantages do exist in mounting this kind of study. One, of course, is the cost, and it remains uncertain that the cost was justified. Additionally, if one were dependent upon such formal studies, there would be a built-in delay in the receipt and analysis of reports because of the complexity of this project. By contrast, the spontaneous reporting system is rapid. One spontaneous report clearly showed that a patient taking an oral anticoagulant had a significant prolongation of his prothrombin time while taking cimetidine. This was confirmed on rechallenge, and the information was incorporated into the data sheet immediately.

I emphasize again that the study did not reveal a single new adverse event. In fact, one of the disadvantages of overreliance on such a study is that regardless of the size of the cohort, it remains limited in scope and one may still miss important but rare events.

Conclusion

Formal postmarketing-surveillance programs can provide useful information and, in appropriate situations, are valuable despite their costs. However, it is not necessary to mandate this structure for many newly approved drugs. It may make more sense to monitor carefully a drug that will be used widely but that does not represent an important therapeutic advance because there is not a natural tendency to report adversity promptly. There is a much greater desire to report adverse effects in the medical literature in the case of a breakthrough drug. Beta-blockers are a good example of this phenomenon. Contrast the number of articles during the first two years of propranolol versus the second and third beta-blockers approved. There is no longer a rush for precedence, and it may be precisely in this instance where significant side effects could occur and not be reported promptly. Thus, based on this experience I would recommend formal postmarketing surveillance for drugs that are not breakthrough and for compounds that, although needed, are dangerous. I would not insist on formal cohort monitoring for important new drugs that are likely to revolutionize the therapeutic approach to specific disease entities because spontaneous reporting will fulfill our needs for uncovering adversity. This conclusion could, of course, be qualified by returning to some of the original goals of postmarketing surveillance in order to coordinate and expedite the flow of new drug discovery and development. I agree that a formal postmarketing mechanism still should be a tool for selectively easing the approval process.

Notes

1. T.G. Davis, D.L. Pickett, and J.H. Schlosser, "Evaluation of a Worldwide Spontaneous Reporting System with Cimetidine," *Journal of the American Medical Association* 243 (16 May 1980):1912–1914.
2. L.M. Gifford, M.E. Aeugle, R.M. Myerson, and P.J. Tannenbaum, "Cimetidine Postmarket Outpatient Surveillance Program, Interim Report on Phase I," *Journal of the American Medical Association* 243 (18 April 1980):1532–1535.
3. J. Feely, G.R. Wilkinson, and A.J.J. Wood, "Reduction of Liver Blood Flow and Propranolol Metabolism by Cimetidine," *New England Journal of Medicine* 304 (19 March 1981):692–695.

Part III
Pharmacy

8 The Evolving Clinical Role of Pharmacy

Robert L. Lantos

It is natural that any profession must respond to changes that affect its primary purpose if it is to continue to exist. Historically, the primary purpose of the pharmacist was to interpret the physician's prescription and to prepare the dosage form so as to make it suitable to dispense to the patient. This usually required compounding, a skill for which the pharmacist was educated and trained thoroughly. The advent of the prefabricated dosage form by the pharmaceutical industry, which grew to large proportions following World War II, diminished dramatically the compounding role of the pharmacist.

The success of the prefabricated standardized dosage form relieved the pharmacist of his compounding function but increased dramatically his dispensing capabilities. Potentially, the needs for the pharmacist's services changed from those of manipulative skills to advisory skills pertinent to a greater knowledge of the clinical aspect of drugs, their optimum dosage, their side effects, their adverse effects, their interactions, and their misuse.

Response to the changing character of the profession was slow, on the part of both the pharmacy practitioners and educators. An early attempt at clinical-pharmacy education was begun at the University of Washington during World War II. This innovation later was described in the following editorial appearing in *Drug Intelligence and Clinical Pharmacy:*

> One of the most dramatic events of recent years is the emergence of the concept of clinical pharmacy and its belated adoption by colleges of pharmacy as an educational tool. It is sad to have to say, however, that it was the narrow provincialism of pharmaceutical educators themselves which held back the development of the concept of clinical pharmacy for more than a quarter of a century. Clinical pharmacy as an educational tool was begun by Professor L. Wait Rising at the University of Washington in 1944 but was disapproved by resolution by both the American Association of Colleges of Pharmacy and the American Council on Pharmaceutical Education in 1946. This action abruptly terminated an imaginative research program in teaching methods without even giving the professor who originated it, the students taking the course, or the pharmacists participating in it an opportunity to be heard. The value of the clinical pharmacy experiment at the University of Washington was again brought to the attention of the pharmaceutical educators in 1953 by Professor H.W. Youngken, Jr., then at the University of Washington, but the idea lay dormant for many years until recently resurrected.[1]

What is clinical pharmacy and what constitutes its resurrection? It is best described as a concept of pharmacy practice in which the pharmacist utilizes judgment in the application of pharmaceutical sciences to foster the safe and appropriate use of drugs.[2] It places the emphasis of judgment on things clinical (patients) rather than on the product.

Although clinical pharmacy can be practiced in both the hospital and community pharmacy, its development began and flourished in the hospital. The medication-error studies by Barker and McConnell at the University of Florida in the early 1960s,[3] and later continued by Barker, Kimbrough, and Heller at the University of Arkansas,[4] identified the pharmacist as a contributor to patient care. The results of these studies signaled significant problems with traditional systems of drug distribution. The unit-dose method of drug distribution was evaluated and was found to reduce medication errors. Implementation of unit-dose drug-distribution systems required pharmacists to be placed in patient-care areas to plan and expedite the system, which resulted in increased pharmacist, physician, and patient interaction.[5, 6]

Another factor that influenced the evolution of clinical pharmacy was the establishment of drug-information centers during the 1960s. The pharmacist traditionally has provided information about prescriptions, but the drug-information center established this activity as an area of pharmacy specialization.[7]

The drug-distribution studies and the emergence of drug-information centers demanded that a pharmaceutical-curriculum revision occur to prepare pharmacists for involvement in patient care. The federal government's Bureau of Health Resources Development mandated clinical-pharmacy-education programs for all pharmacy students in 1971 through its capitation grant program.[8] Large numbers of pharmacy students began to receive a clinically oriented education.

As clinical-pharmacy-practice opportunities in both community and institutional setting were increasing, the National Center for Health Services Research and Development created an interdisciplinary task force in 1971 to develop specific working criteria to define new roles. Their criteria were based on professional functions currently being performed or likely to be performed by pharmacists. The classification included these tasks:[9]

Prescribing drugs,

Dispensing and administering drugs,

Documenting professional activities,

Contributing directly to patient care,

Reviewing drug utilization,

Educating physicians,

Consulting with physicians.

It is beyond the scope of this chapter to elaborate on each of these behaviors. However, because of current studies, pending legislation in some states, and the nationwide attention being given the role of the pharmacist in the prescribing of drugs, the remainder of this chapter focuses on this function (see chapter 11). In describing the role of the pharmacist in prescribing drugs, the task force stated that the physician determines if drug therapy is indicated and usually chooses the drug. Under certain circumstances, the pharmacist might assist in planning drug therapy and may at times prescribe at the request of the physician. The task force further states:[10]

> Pharmacists, in reissuing prescriptions designated to be refilled at the request of the patient, may be regarded as performing a prescribing function.
>
> Pharmacists, in complying with standing orders of the physician, may be performing an independent prescribing function. *Standing orders* refers to a prearranged plan of understanding between the physician and the pharmacist that permits the latter to dispense medications under certain circumstances without the immediate concurrence of the physician.
>
> Pharmacists and pharmacy residents often help medical students to plan drug regimens.
>
> Physicians may share responsibility for prescribing with the pharmacist when the latter has demonstrated competence. This may include the selection of drugs, dosage forms, and frequency of use based on the physician's diagnosis.
>
> Pharmacists prescribe OTC drugs. Also, by recommending against the purchase and/or use of OTC drugs, they perform a prescribing function.
>
> Pharmacists prescribe medications in emergency situations when they decide it is in the best interest of the patient.
>
> Pharmacists, after consultation with the prescriber, may select and dispense a drug other than the one prescribed by the physician, when they practice under the authority of the drug-formulary system.
>
> Pharmacists may be considered to be performing a prescribing function

when they reply to inquiries from patients about continued use of medications previously prescribed.

Since the task force outlined the role of the pharmacist in the prescribing of drugs a decade ago, several programs have been developed throughout the nation. The Indian Health Service implemented a pharmacist practitioner training program in 1973.[11] The objectives of this program were:

To develop, implement, and evaluate a prototype practice model in which the pharmacist provides acute medical-care services for ambulatory patients with many of the more commonly seen illnesses;

To develop, implement, and evaluate a prototype practice model in which the pharmacist, at the discretion of a physician, is responsible for the management of stabilized chronic ambulatory patients' care;

To develop a transferable training program utilized to train other pharmacists for similar roles.

The assumption was made that a clinically trained pharmacist possesses knowledge of disease entities and their therapy. To provide comprehensive primary patient care, the pharmacist needed training primarily in the area of history taking, physical examination, and assessment of health-care problems. The successful training program showed that the pharmacist practitioner could provide a broader scope of patient-service functions. The pharmacist practitioner can serve in a primary health-care role when and where needed, yet he or she can retain the ability to perform traditional pharmacy functions.

California became the first state directly to legislate prescribing authority to pharmacists. The California law (AB717) originated with nurse practitioners and physician assistants seeking to expand their scope of practice. Pharmacy became the third profession to be included in the legislation. A limited number of four-year pilot projects began in 1978, at the University of Southern California's (USC) School of Pharmacy, under the direction of Glenn Stimmel. Dr. Stimmel discovered when he assumed the role of project director that many of the pharmacists had been prescribing medications and modifying drug therapy for some time. He stated, "Because we had pharmacists with prescribing capabilities and experience, it made it easy to start the project. Most of the pharmacists joining the USC project needed only some additional physical assessment skills."[12]

Pharmacists at USC and at the University of California's School of Pharmacy, where a parallel exists, enter the study after passing a pathology-therapeutics examination and a twenty-to-thirty hour physical-assessment course. In both study groups, physicians supervise pharmacists' prescribing activities via established formularies and protocols usually developed with pharmacy input. The law prohibits pharmacists from prescribing narcotics. Most of the approximately fifty California pharmacists in the study will assume their prescribing roles in the practice settings where they worked previously. Study sites include hospital and ambulatory-care clinics, extended-care facilities, and community pharmacies.

The outcome of the AB717 pilot project is awaited not only by the California legislature but also by pharmacy groups in other states. The revised Pharmacy Practice Act in the state of Washington, passed in 1979, included the following definition of the practice of pharmacy:

> The practice of pharmacy includes the practice of and responsibility for . . . initiating or modifying of drug therapy in accordance with written guidelines or protocols previously established and approved for his or her practice by a practitioner authorized to prescribe drugs.[13]

In order to limit and prevent abuses of this authority by pharmacists, the Board of Pharmacy, in July 1980, enacted a regulation that stated:

> A pharmacist planning to exercise prescriptive authority . . . shall make application through and receive approval from the Board prior to commencement of this aspect of the practice of pharmacy.[14]

The Minnesota State Pharmaceutical Association, in responding to a state investigation of escalating health-care costs, proposed to the Commission on Health Care Costs of the Minnesota State Medical Association the desirability of legally authorizing pharmacists to dispense certain drugs without a physician's prescription.[15]

Pharmacists in Michigan may have the opportunity to prescribe. Although Michigan's legislature recently passed a new public-health code that implicitly allows pharmacists to prescribe, until the board revamps its rules and regulations, the legality of pharmacist prescribing remains uncertain.[16] In other states, including North Carolina, Tennessee, Georgia, Arizona, and West Virginia, legislative approval for pharmacist prescribing has been or is being pursued.

It should be recognized that these laws are a logical extension of those already enabling prescribing by nurse practitioners and physician assistants whose training in pharmacology falls short of the pharmacist's. Fred M. Eckel, professor of hospital pharmacy at the University of North Carolina and a member of his state's committee that is rewriting the state's pharmacy-practice act, has stated, "If society is going to give non-physicians the right to use drugs as North Carolina has given to optometrists, nurse practitioners and physician's assistants, the same right should be extended to pharmacists, the most widely distributed and readily available health professionals."[17] There is still physician disapproval of pharmacist prescribing; however, the public desire for decreasing health costs may most influence the state legislator. Pharmacists have an opportunity to utilize their education in this new approach to the treatment of patients. Certainly the added responsibility imposes a greater risk of liability. The question also arises as to how the pharmacist is to be paid for assuming this new prescribing role. The questions and risks should not deter the pharmacist from moving to prescribe; even more so than other paramedical prescribers, I believe, he or she is unusually qualified to do so.

Notes

1. D.E. Francke, "Drug Intelligence and Clinical Pharmacy," *Drug Intelligence and Clinical Pharmacy* 3 (1969):157.
2. G.N. Franck, "Evolvement of Clinical Pharmacy," *Drug Intelligence and Clinical Pharmacy* 3 (1969):353.
3. K.N. Barker and W.E. McConnell, "The Problem in Detecting Medication Errors in a Hospital," *American Journal of Hospital Pharmacy* 19 (1962):361.
4. K.N. Barker, W. Kimbrough, and W.M. Heller, *A Study of Medication Errors in a Hosptial* (Fayetteville: University of Arkansas, 1966).
5. K.N. Barker and W.M. Heller, "The Development of a Centralized Unit Dose Dispensing System: Part One, Description of University of Arkansas Medical Center Experimental Systems," *American Journal of Hospital Pharmacy* 20 (1963):568.
6. H.J. Black and W.W. Iester "Decentralized Pharmacy Operations Utilizing the Unit Dose Concept," *American Journal of Hospital Pharmacy* 25 (1968):381–382.
7. American Society of Hospital Pharmacists, "The Hospital Pharmacist and Drug Information Services," *American Journal of Hospital Pharmacy* 25 (1968):381–382.
8. Public Law 92-157, Comprehensive Health Manpower Training Act of 1971.
9. "Report of the Task Force on the Pharmacist's Clinical Role, *Journal of the American Pharmaceutical Association* NS11 (1971):482–485.
10. Ibid.
11. G.P. Copeland and D.A. Apgar, "The Pharmacist Practitioner Training Program," *Drug Intelligence and Clinical Pharmacy* 14 (1980): 114–119.
12. B. Eichelberger "Pharmacist Prescribing Being Pursued in State Legislature," *American Journal of Hospital Pharmacy* 36 (1979):258.

13. D.B. Christensen, "Pharmacist Perscriptive Authority: An Update," *Washington Pharmacist* (May-June 1981), p. 6.

14. Ibid.

15. D.A. Dee, "Expanding the Role of the Pharmacist in Improving Health Care: Some Proposals," *Minnesota Pharmacist* (March 1978), p. 14.

16. R.P. Hoffman, "Prescribing within One's Scope of Practice," *Hospital Pharmacy* 16 (1981):186.

17. R. Hershberger, "The Great American Health Show," *Medical World News* 21 (September 15, 1980):39.

9 The Impact of State Generic Drug Substitution Laws

Theodore Goldberg and *Carolee DeVito*

Many changes have occurred in the United States in attitudes and legislation concerning drug product selection by pharmacists. This chapter will review the evolution of state generic drug laws and the impact they have had on drug product substitution to date.

Prior to World War II, drug therapy was at a relatively primitive stage of development. Drug companies were growing slowly and showed only modest profits. Many of the drugs available were neither very helpful nor harmful, and even the limited number of drugs that was reasonably effective and potent was compounded by the pharmacist on an individual basis; that is, unlike today, drugs were not prefabricated or prepackaged. Thus, the potential for harm or mischief to be caused by unscrupulous or illegal drug counterfeiters was rather limited.

All this changed during and immediately following World War II. The discovery and synthesis of potent new drugs transformed drug manufacturing from little more than a cottage industry to a highly competitive and profitable one. However, as drugs became more effective, potent, and readily available, there was increasing concern among health professionals that these new agents be of high quality. Prescribers and pharmacists alike recognized that the new chemicals required manufacturing techniques far more sophisticated than those necessary for their predecessors. Substantially greater surveillance and monitoring would also be necessary in order to protect the public from potentially unsafe products and practices. These fears were soon borne out when a few unscrupulous manufacturers found that they could, at great profit, produce and distribute inferior drug substitutes.[1] These counterfeit substances were ineffective at best but often were potentially harmful, and they were difficult to detect and virtually impossible to control.

Evaluation of Generic Substitution Laws

In an effort to combat such deceptive and unsafe practices, major pharmaceutical manufacturers united to form the National Pharmaceutical Council (NPC), the purpose of which was to "promote optimal standards and assure the public of high-quality pharmaceutical products."[2] The NPC introduced several regulatory practices, including the designation of secret and difficult-to-copy product identifier codes. Counterfeit substances were sought out, and pharmacists who purchased and dispensed the bogus pharmaceutical products were identified and prosecuted.

Most important, and most effective, however, was the enactment by practically every state in the union of a law or regulation prohibiting pharmacists from substituting among drug products and requiring them to dispense only the product identified on the prescription form. This widespread adoption of antisubstitution requirements received overwhelming support from physicians and drug manufacturers as well as from pharmacists and consumers.

Universal antisubstitution sentiment continued largely unchallenged throughout the 1950s and 1960s. By the late 1960s and early 1970s, however, attitudes regarding drug manufacturing practices and government surveillance had changed considerably. The manufacture and distribution of counterfeit drugs was no longer a problem, and antisubstitution laws came under new scrutiny. Questions were raised about the existing legislation, and it was argued that granting near-exclusive monopolies to certain drug companies, even beyond the normal seventeen-year patent-protection limit, unnecessarily restricted competition and resulted in unnecessarily high costs to consumers. In addition, it was suggested that such restrictions infringed on the professional activities of pharmacists, who were trained as "drug experts" and thus were most competent to select, from among available alternatives, the particular product to be dispensed.

This renewed interest in the consequences of antisubstitution practices resulted in the coalition of three important groups: policymakers and legislators, professional pharmacists, and consumers. Each faction of this coalition believed that it had something to gain from the revision of antisubstitution legislation, and, once united, their power and influence were considerable. Thus, from the early 1970s to the present, this coalition managed almost completely to reverse public policy on drug substitution. Michigan was the first state to reverse its position on antisubstitution requirements, when, in 1974, it adopted legislation allowing pharmacists, under certain conditions, to dispense a product different from the one identified on the prescription form. Today, 49 out of 50 states have replaced their antisubstitution laws with ones that allow, encourage, or even require substitution of a less costly generic equivalent for a more expensive drug that may have been prescribed.

Basic Assumptions

Before we present our findings on the effect of these laws to date, it may be helpful to review some of the assumptions or concerns that were instrumental in the development and enactment of these laws. The first and perhaps most important consideration was that consumers wanted to save money by purchasing lower-priced generic equivalents. The second assumption was that pharmacists wished to expand their professional domain to include the right to select, from among alternatives, the product to be dispensed. (It was further expected that these professionals would actually and substantially exercise this option.) A third assumption was that there was, in fact, a significant proportion of prescriptions written for drugs that had two or more generically equivalent products with significantly different prices. This assumption was somewhat clouded, however, by confusing and imprecise terminology; that is, what exactly was meant by generics, brand name, or substitution. The final assumption (or perhaps it would be more accurate to label it "fear") affecting the development of generic substitution laws was that physicians would indiscriminately or excessively exercise their prerogatives to prohibit generic substitution. These concerns clearly affected the developing laws. The major components of these laws are summarized in figure 9–1.

What We Have Learned: A Selective Review of Research Results

Initial Survey

We began our research in the summer of 1974, just prior to the enactment of Michigan's drug product substitution (DPS) law.[3] The attitudes of pharmacists and physicians regarding this issue were sampled (87 percent response rate) with some interesting results.

Attitudes. Only 34 percent of the physicians surveyed, compared to over 50 percent of the pharmacists, favored a new DPS law, although 60 percent of both groups believed that the provisions of the law would result in consumer savings. More physicians than pharmacists believed that there were no significant differences in generically equivalent drugs. With regard to the technical competence of the pharmacist to select safely among generically equivalent products, the majority of both physicians and pharmacists considered the pharmacist to be technically qualified, although fewer physicians (60 percent) than pharmacists (82.5 percent) expressed this belief. Just over half (56 percent) of physicians said they would encourage substitution, either selectively or generally, and about 60 percent of physicians reported that they prescribed generically "whenever possible" or "sometimes."

Expertise. We also sought to determine how well physicians and pharmacists could identify "generically equivalent substitutes" for seven categories

Permissive vs. Mandatory. Some states (e.g. Vermont) *require* substitution of less costly products. However, even those states with mandatory substitution requirements limit the mandate to choices consistent with professional judgment and product availability. Hence, these regulations should be interpreted as a statement of legislative intent and not an attempt to limit professional decision-making or prerogatives.

Formulary and Formulary Development. Many states provide lists of acceptable (positive formulary) and unacceptable (negative formulary) product interchanges. In addition, some states specify or appoint individuals responsible for maintaining, distributing, and updating these lists. The formularies were expected to promote substitution by providing explicit guidelines for product choice.

Prohibition of Substitution by Physician. States give physicians the right to prohibit substitution of the product described. Allowable terminology varies: DAW (dispense as written), NS (no substitution), Medically Necessary, and so on. Other states require the equivalent of physician request before the pharmacist can substitute a less costly product. For example, in New York and Rhode Island, the physician must sign the prescription on either a "substitution allowed" or "substitution not allowed" line. The extent of prescriber prohibition of substitution seems to vary with the specific regulatory mechanism adopted.

Pass-on of Savings to Consumers. States seem to be consistent in their objective to save the consumer money. However, laws vary considerably with regard to calculation of savings and ultimate pass-on of savings to consumers. Since the price of the product prescribed is compared to the product dispensed, consumer savings are often dependent on the pharmacy stock and the pharmacist's purchase price, which is difficult to ascertain. There is some evidence that this component should be amended to provide the pharmacist with financial incentives to substitute; that is, to share in the savings from substitution. This has occurred in the state of Washington and in an experiment by Michigan Blue Cross/Blue Shield.

Consumer Request/Approval. Several states require the request or approval of the consumer before the pharmacist can substitute generically equivalent drugs. It was not clear, however, whether this provision prohibits the pharmacist from initiating or suggesting substitution. This consumer request requirement was repealed in Michigan less than a year after it was enacted. This had little effect on the rate of substitution.

Labeling. Additional labeling and/or record-keeping is required by many states.

Liability. Since the drug industry has challenged DPS laws with claims of product superiority and promises to share in liability, the question of additional liability to physician and pharmacist is specifically addressed. Some state laws stress that greater liability is not the intention of the substitution legislation, which seems to have an important psychological effect. Most states have not provided a specific exemption in their legislation.

Enforcement and Monitoring. Some states have developed guidelines for evaluation and enforcement mechanisms for DPS laws.

Figure 9–1. Major Components of State Generic-Drug Laws

of drugs. For each of seven products listed as "prescribed drugs" a second list of "possible substitutes" was provided. Physicians and pharmacists were asked to identify those products in the "possible substitutes" list that were "generically equivalent" to the designated "product prescribed." On the average, fewer than 30 percent of physicians correctly identified drugs that were, in fact, "generic equivalents." An average of 36.3 percent incorrectly identified as "possible substitutes those drugs that were not generically equivalent and therefore not substitutable. Pharmacists fared better in this area: 57 percent correctly identified drugs that were in fact "generic equivalents," but 36 percent incorrectly identified inequivalents.

This initial survey raised many questions about the soon-to-be-enacted legislation, such as how would pharmacists and physicians respond to these laws? Would the potentially substantial savings be passed along to the consumer when substitution took place? And, could the impact on quality be assessed, given claims by manufacturers of therapeutic inequivalence, some lack of confidence in the pharmacists competence, and the knowledge gaps of both physicians and pharmacists?

Subsequent Research

Subsequent research was conducted in Michigan, Wisconsin, Vermont, and Rhode Island.[4] Prescribing and dispensing patterns for drug orders filled in noninstitutional pharmacies were studied for periods prior to and subsequent to enactment of DPS laws in each of these states. Savings were computed based on actual prices charged, and only *written* records were used. In no case was "intention" or memory the basis for drawing conclusions. The data presented here provide the basis for evaluating the effectiveness of DPS laws in these states as well as conjecture about the possibility of modifying some of the provisions for the future. However, since our findings were extensive, they will be reported only selectively, with emphasis placed on the overall impact of DPS legislation in the state surveyed.

Are DPS Laws Effective?

Substitution Potential

In every state studied, over half of all new prescriptions were for multiple-source drugs; that is, more than one product is available for the generic class, strength, and dosage prescribed. For example, the most recent (April 1978–March 1979) data from Michigan show that 54.3 percent of prescriptions were multiple source, and over 18 percent of these were written generically. (For nonbranded generically written prescriptions, no specific product was identified and the pharmacist was therefore *required* to select the product to be dispensed.) Similar findings occurred for other states and study years. In fact, the potential for substitution, as defined by the percentage of multiple-source prescriptions, is closer to 60 percent in Wisconsin, Vermont, and Rhode Island. In addition, the need to include provisions for product choice for generically written prescriptions is highlighted by the fact that in Vermont, nearly 40 percent of multiple-source prescriptions are generically written.

Savings Potential

The potential impact in savings to the consumer seems unquestionably significant. The most recent national data report that expenditures for drugs and drug sundries are 7.9 percent of health care costs (higher than expenditures for dental care and close to expenditures for nursing home care). Since there are alternative products potentially available at reduced prices for more than half of all new prescriptions written, the public has an opportunity to save considerable money. However, the potential for consumer savings actually depends on several other factors, including the physician's permission to substitute and price variation among generically equivalent products.

Substitution Prohibition. Based on the results of our study, substitution is rarely prohibited in states that require a handwritten statement of prohibition: about 5 percent of multiple-source prescriptions in Michigan, about 1.5 percent in Wisconsin, and less than 1.5 percent in Vermont. However, in Rhode Island (and New York), where physicians sign prescriptions on either a "substitution prohibited" or "substitution allowed" line, substitution is prohibited more than 38 percent of the time.

When data were summarized for the first year's experience with Michigan and Wisconsin DPS laws, much interest was expressed in the intentions of physicians who prohibited substitution. Although the percentage of prescriptions that prohibited substitution in these states was not large, there was some suggestion that it might be very great in states with two-signature lines provisions. In New York and Rhode Island, where this provision is used, prescribers "prohibit" substitution for drugs ordered generically about as often as they do for those ordered by brand name. In addition, they often indicate "do not substitute" for single-source products. Does this prohibition of substitution reflect a conscious decision and serious concern over the safety of generic substitution, or is it a result of an inappropriately applied prohibition mechanism?

Price Variation. Wide price variation among generic equivalents—that is, evidence of additional potential savings—has been demonstrated by comparing prices of products prescribed with prices of products dispensed. Estimated savings are based on actual market price, market structure, incentives, and state laws. In the states studied to date, we calculate a savings of about 25 percent (about $1.00 to $1.25) per prescription when generic equivalents are substituted.

Savings also can occur as the result of dispensing lower cost products when filling generically written prescriptions. This is measured by comparing the price of the actual product dispensed for generically written prescriptions with the average price of all products within the same drug entity (and thus potentially dispensable). However, pharmacists do not select as low priced a product when filling generically written prescriptions as they do when generic *substitution* occurs.

Disappointing Results

Although the potential for substitution and savings appears to be great in the four states studied, the actual experience has been disappointing. The most current data show the rate of substitution for multiple-source prescriptions (excluding generically written prescriptions and prescriptions for which prescribers prohibited substitution) to be 8.6 percent in Vermont, 2.6 percent in Rhode Island, 7.4 percent in Michigan, and 5.1 percent in Wisconsin. Note the low percentages in all states, even though Vermont and Rhode Island have mandatory DPS laws, whereas Michigan and Wisconsin have "permissive" laws. Since Vermont, Rhode Island, and Wisconsin have positive formularies, the substitution rate for formulary entities is perhaps more legitimate to report. This rate is 14.4 percent for Vermont and 18.1 for Wisconsin, but only 6.6 percent for Rhode Island (which uses a two-signature-line method for prohibiting substitution). Similar findings have been reported in a limited study of DPS legislation in Florida, Delaware, and Illinois.

It may be impossible to attribute the success or failure of certain drug product selection laws to any one provision or assumption, but much can be learned from our four-state study; original assumptions, which were instrumental to the development and enactment of state generic drug laws, must now be reevaluated on the basis of experience.

Although consumer involvement and professional prerogatives seemed to be important factors when DPS laws were first conceived, the laws have, in fact, evoked little response. It may be a bit of an exaggeration, but it seems fair to conclude that *consumers generally do not request substitution, physicians generally do not prohibit substitution, and pharmacists generally do not substitute.* It seems apparent that relative apathy has prevailed on all sides.

The Future of DPS Laws

If policymakers, health care professionals, and consumers are not pleased with the results of the existing generic substitution laws, perhaps they would do well to reevaluate the original objectives and components and develop new and more successful drug laws, based on actual experience. This "second generation" of laws could then incorporate the *known incentives* to substitution as well as eliminate the *known barriers.* On the basis of our experience to date, the following guidelines would seem to be useful to the development of more effective legislation.

Elimination of the Two-Signature-Lines Provision

If the intent of DPS laws is to encourage substitution whenever possible without compromising quality, then the "two-signature-lines" provision should be avoided. Prescribers' control over the product dispensed can be protected with a "Dispense as Written" provision: that is, prescribers can prohibit substitution by indicating their wishes in their own handwriting at the time the prescription is written.

Use of Positive Formularies

Although negative formularies do provide a formal statement about questionable products, there is no evidence that any knowledge gap is filled by this type of guide. Positive formularies, on the other hand, have a known and significant effect on the rate of and savings from generic substitution. Pharmacists do not see positive formularies as restrictive, but, rather see these lists as guides to product selection and acceptable behavior.[5] In addition, positive formularies allow states to address explicitly questions of quality assurance in drug product selection. Thus, development, maintenance, and expansion of a positive formulary seems to be a worthwhile investment for those states wishing to promote drug product selection. Perhaps the best way to improve these positive formularies is to rest the responsibility for their development with a federal agency such as the FDA. The resources and expertise centralized in that organization would be difficult to copy on a state-by-state basis.

Improve Terminology

There is some real confusion and lack of clarity concerning terminology, such as generally equivalent, bioequivalent, therapeutically equivalent, etc. The FDA has shown strong leadership in defining the meaning of these terms as well as in making available lists of approved and questionable products.

Include Provisions for Generically Written Prescriptions

Since many multiple-source prescriptions are generically written, and since prescribers may expect these orders to be filled with relatively low-cost products, explicit regulations can be developed to guide product choice. If a drug product listed in the formulary is prescribed generically, the prescription could be filled with a drug-product equivalent having a cost not higher than the average wholesale cost of all equivalents. Pharmacists should choose the lowest priced product consistent with professional judgment.

Mandatory DPS Laws

Data from the states studied show that mandatory DPS laws result in higher substitution rates (nearly double in Vermont). Since greater substitution and savings can be achieved with this provision, it seems reasonable to support its inclusion in future legislation. Mandatory regulations obviously do not result in the substitution of all or even the majority of multiple-source prescriptions. Professional judgment is *always* protected (the pharmacist must substitute only when consistent with professional judgment), pharmacy inventories ultimately limit the choice of substitutes, and prescribers can always prohibit substitution. Thus, mandatory laws seem to pose no greater risk than in non-mandatory states, whereas they are effective stimulants to substitution.

Increase Consumer Education

Although consumer support was instrumental in the adoption of state DPS laws, this attitude has not translated into widespread or significant changes in consumer behavior. It is possible that the public needs more education in this area, especially at the time of drug purchase. Price posting of commonly prescribed drugs can help in some cases, but a more ambitious campaign of consumer education is needed if the consumer is ultimately to act in an intelligent and informed manner.

Increased Monitoring and Enforcement

The issue of monitoring and enforcing of generic substitution laws must be addressed. The public should have confidence in the ability of responsible government agencies to monitor quality in the drug industry, and members of the health profession must also have confidence in the comparative drug information available.

Share Savings with Pharmacists

Currently, most state laws require that all savings be passed on to the consumer. However, the low rate of substitution to date can be interpreted as evidence that the pharmacists do not feel inclined to pass on *all* savings at a time when they are incurring new administrative costs. The Federal Trade Commission (FTC) has suggested that pharmacists not be required to pass on savings at all, but instead, that market forces will provide the necessary inducement to lower consumer prices. We do not believe, however, that there is any evidence to support this "free-market" approach. Virtually no other state health care regulation has adopted a free-market approach; the regulation of reimbursement for drug costs under Medicaid and every other provider of health care is accepted as necessary. It seems rather risky, therefore, to rely on the type of approach suggested by the FTC.

Thus, a major consideration in the modification of DPS laws is the possibility of encouraging substitution by *sharing* savings between the pharmacist and the consumer. This could be accomplished with a regulatory provision that calls for the dispensing of the "lowest cost product in stock" when multiple-source prescriptions are filled. This mandatory provision could then be complemented with provisions requiring a pass-on of a substantial proportion of savings when substitution occurs. The 40/60 suggestion adopted in the state of Washington seems to be a reasonable way to encourage substitution by pharmacists while assuring that the majority (60 percent) of savings is passed on to the consumer.

In Conclusion

The goals of DPS legislation can be met only if both the rate of substitution and the resultant savings are substantial. Prescription records have consistently demonstrated that significant savings accrue *when substitution occurs.* Thus, the necessary change is an increase in the substitution rate.

Many states are now seriously reviewing the effectiveness of their generic drug laws. As a result, we anticipate that a new round of amended laws is in the offing. Although we cannot answer with certainty all of the questions concerning the effectiveness of the original DPS laws, we can document the fact that some of the components of these laws *specifically* affected their success (that is, mandatory drug product selection, positive formularies, prescriber prohibition of substitution by written directive on the prescription order). It is hoped that the knowledge and experience gained to date will be used to create new and effective drug substitution practices.

Notes

1. For a more detailed discussion of the background, circumstances, and reasons for the development of antisubstitution laws, see "A White Paper on . . . The Pharmacist's Role in Product Selection"; "An Overview of the Antisubstitution Laws and the American Pharmaceutical Association's Advocacy of This Amendment Relative to Drug Product Selection"; A Background and Position Paper Issued by the Board of Trustees American Pharmaceutical Association, March, 1971.

2. National Pharmaceutical Council, *Pharmaceutical Benefits under State Medical Assistance Programs* (Washington, D.C., no date).

3. The law, which took effect on 1 January 1975, Michigan Public Act 155, 1974.

4. Publications reporting on the methodology of the study as well as various aspects of the findings include T. Goldberg et al., "Evaluation of Impact on Drug Substitution Legislation," *Journal of the American Pharmaceutical Association* 16 (February 1976); Goldberg et al., "Impact of Drug Substitution Legislation: A Report of the First Year's Experience," *Journal of the American Pharmaceutical Association* 17 (April 1977):216–226, G.W. Aldridge et al., "Profile of the Doubters: Pharmacists Who Doubt That Members of Their Profession Can Safely Select among Drug Products," *Contemporary Pharmacy Practice* (Spring 1979):80–87; C.A. DeVito et al., "Framework and Development of a Comprehensive Drug Product Coding System," *Contemporary Pharmacy Practice* (Spring 1979): 62–65; T.A. Goldberg et al., "Evaluation of Economics Effects of Drug Product Selection Legislation," *Medical Care* 17 (April 1979):411–419; and T. Goldberg and C. DeVito, "The Impact of State Generic Drug Substitution Laws," *Drug Therapy* 11 (December 1981):75–80.

5. This impression confirms the earlier findings of the Federal Trade

Commission that, in a 1978 study, found that: ''An equally larger number of pharmacists [65.3 percent of those in the state studied] (particularly staff pharmacists) apparently prefer a positive formulary because of the guidance it provides in selecting drug products.'' Federal Trade Commissioner, Bureau of Consumer Protection, *Drug Product Selection: Staff Report to the Federal Trade Commission* (Washington, D.C., January 1979).

10 Why Providers and Consumers? What Happened to Physicians and Patients?

Leroy L. Schwartz

I am pleased that I am called a practicing physician rather than a vendor. Whereas not many years ago we used to have patients, today we deal with consumers, and we treat them, not in hospitals but in health-care facilities, staffed not by professionals such as pharmacists, nurses, and physical therapists but by providers. However, some would say: What is in a name? What is the difference what we are called? Will the health care provided the patient suffer if we are vendors and they are consumers? I believe that if health-care has not suffered yet, it inevitably must because the primary principle in the treatment of illness is more scientific than economic. The present debate on the generic substitution of one drug product for another is a good example of how our policymakers have attempted to cut health-care costs by placing the economic cart before the scientific horse regardless of the possible harmful effect on the patient. It also illustrates the difficulties encountered by practicing physicians, pharmacists, and the public because of the mixed signals they receive from the various sides in the controversy. These conflicting signals are the topic of this chapter.

Over the years, some segments of the media have taken the view that the issue of generic prescribing and substitution is, for all intents and purposes, simply a question of money and that physicians should prescribe generics in order to save money for the patient.

For example, *The New York Times* editorialized that the sole case against generic prescribing or generic substitution comes from the drug manufacturers and that it is clearly self-serving—that is, simply a question of profits.[1] Conversely, a considerable body of evidence exists upon which a number of equally credible organizations have presented a series of opinions and recommendations that do not square with *The New York Times* assessment that the issue is mainly economic and not scientific. In 1970, the American Pharmaceutical Association Academy of Pharmaceutical Sciences summarized its recommendations on drug-product quality, including the following:

> 1. Drug products from different sources may differ in quality in several respects. These differences, individually or collectively, may lead to substantial differences in therapeutic effect and/or safety.

> 2. In particular, differences in the rate and completeness of release of the active ingredient may result in varying therapeutic or adverse effects. This is true of a variety of products whose number is still uncertain, but potentially large.[2]

It appeared that the scientists had spoken and that practitioners had found the scientific backing for their reluctance to substitute one drug product for another or to prescribe generically. Not so long after this pronouncement, however, a burgeoning consumer movement began to influence health-care policy. In order to save money, a concerted effort was made to have the various states repeal their antisubstitution laws and to promote generic prescribing. Because of earlier concerns about health-care consequences of substitution and before any large-scale progeneric government programs were put into effect, Congress decided again to look at the possible medical problems that could arise from such programs. Thus, in 1974, the congressional Office of Technology Assessment (OTA) gathered a group of outstanding scientists and physicians to assess the scientific aspects of the issue and to furnish a report to Congress. This study focusing on drug bioequivalence endorsed the concept of generic substitution, but for a number of reasons, it signaled practicing physicians and pharmacists to exercise considerable caution. It maintained that:

> Current standards and regulatory practices do not insure bioequivalence for drug products. Variations in the bioavailability of drug products have been recognized as responsible for a few therapeutic failures. It is probable that other therapeutic failures (or toxicity) of a similar origin have escaped recognition.
>
> Present compendial standards and guidelines for current good manufacturing practice do not insure quality and uniform bioavailability for drug products. Not only may the products of different manufacturers vary, but the product of a single manufacturer may vary from batch to batch or may change during storage.[3]

The response of consumer groups to the report was to diminish problematic statements. An example appeared in *Consumer Reports:*

> After examining the OTA Panel Report *Consumer Reports* concluded that "The controversy over bioequivalence [has] at last [been] put into perspective. . . . ask your doctor to prescribe a drug by its generic name."[4]

Further, in a commentary on the topic, Anita Johnson and Sidney Wolfe of the Health Research Group pointed out that:

> "Bioequivalence" is a spurious issue for purposes of selecting the best drug buy. While there may be small differences in the rate of absorption between drug products, these differences rarely have medical importance. The FDA

> requires from all drug manufacturers proof that their drugs are effective in the body.[5]

The battle was joined. The signals were again conflicting as to how best to prescribe for the patient, and the practicing physician and pharmacist again were caught in the middle. Other parties now joined in the debate. The FDA, obviously believing that it was able to regulate effectively the quality of the various products, joined the side of the progeneric forces, noting in a 1978 issue of the *FDA Consumer* that:

> All drugs, whether they are sold under their brand names or their generic names, must meet the same FDA standards for safety, strength, purity, and effectiveness. And all drug manufacturers, big or small, are subject to FDA inspection and must follow the agency's current Good Manufacturing Practice Regulations. That is why FDA believes that there is no significant differences in quality between generic and brand name drugs.[6]

Nevertheless, in a 1981 address, the deputy director of the FDA Division of Biopharmaceutics noted in retrospect that:

> Digoxin was on the marketplace for many years, with physicians believing that they had high patient variability when in fact about 10% of the market had high drug product bioavailability variability. It was some several years before formulations that were as little as 10% bioavailable were discovered and removed from the marketplace.[7]

Even with present-day standards his contention is that:

> The compendial monographs . . . do not adequately test for all the necessary variables which would permit drugs to be marketed without FDA preclearance.[8]

Yet he indicated that his audience would find it:

> Perhaps somewhat surprising that only 45% of the total manufactured prescription drug products in the marketplace 2 years ago have been approved for both safety and efficacy.[9]

If so many products on the market do not have FDA approval, can the various manufacturers be relied upon to produce a product that is interchangeable with the brand-name product or, for that matter, a quality product at all in the absence of such approval? Former FDA Commissioner Donald Kennedy believed they could and did:

> We've maintained compliance records on all firms who make drugs. As far as our records are concerned, large and small firms, brand name and generic firms have indistinguishable records of performance.[10]

> FDA concurrence in the New York Drug list reflects the Agency's view that there is no consistent difference in quality between drug products sold by large and small firms or between drugs sold under a brand name or "generic" name. We have a single standard for drugs in this country.[11]

This was a clear signal to practitioners that they could rely on the FDA and the quality of generic-drug products. Other observers, however, were not convinced, and they produced a different message. For example, economist David Schwartzman, in his study of the pharmaceutical industry, claimed that:

> Small firms are unlikely to be able to develop adequate quality assurance programs, since they do not have required resources to undertake them. Policymakers who are concerned with the problem of the quality of drugs must therefore be prepared to accept the elimination of small firms from the industry as a result of regulations which are intended to provide quality assurance.[12]

In a later study, pharmacologist Lawrence Block seemed to underline Schwartzman's contention. His research indicated that smaller firms tend to have disproportionately greater incidences of quality problems. Block arrived at this conclusion after discovering that, of questionable products, 85% with potentially impaired bioavailability were manufactured by firms whose volume of sales was less than $5 million in 1978. Further, nearly 90% of the slippage in quality control was detected *after* distribution of the drug had begun.[13]

This signal, if noted, might have caused practitioners to ask, with patient care and liability in mind, whether it was ever prudent to prescribe generically or to encourage substitution. Could it be that seriously ill patients were the subjects of uncontrolled substitution experiments. If their clinical condition worsened, their physician might worry that the substitution was the cause of the problem, despite the FDA's assurance that the products involved were therapeutically equivalent. For example, some patients go back into depression after substitution of a generic tricyclic antidepressant, and said substitution could be unbeknownst to the physician. The authors of one report found that:

> There is substantial evidence that a minimum plasma level of a tricyclic compound is essential to therapeutic response. If the bioequivalence of tricyclics varies from manufacturer to manufacturer for the same compound, or from batch to batch produced by one manufacturer, then patients will achieve different plasma levels even though they are being given identical amounts of the active ingredient. . . . The case we have reported suggests that, like digitalis preparations, tricyclics should be prescribed by brand name.[14]

Is it possible to find out the comparative bioavailability or therapeutic equivalence of product versions the practitioner may wish to prescribe or the pharmacist may wish to substitute? Although with the enactment of product-substitution laws in forty-nine states, it would be expected that such information would be available, yet there is evidence to the contrary. A recent study at the Georgia University Pharmacy School tried to find out just how reliable and available is the drug-bioavailability information from both brand-name and generic manufacturers. The researchers found:

> A net decrease in the quantity of bioavailability information available to our study population in 1978 relative to 1976. . . . and . . . that the effort by the FDA to expand and implement bioavailability studies has had little or no effect on the availability of this information to pharmacy students and, perhaps, to other elements of this community.[15]

Thus, the practitioner may not be able to find the necessary information to prescribe properly generically, and the pharmacist would not have the information upon which to substitute prudently. This may pose a particular dilemma for those who deal with special population groups such as infants and children or the elderly where special pharmacokinetic problems exist and where prior drug testing is often inadequate. For example, although many physicians prescribing for infants and children may not know it, the Committee on Drugs of the American Academy of Pediatrics feel strongly that:

> Cost alone should not receive the highest priority in the choice of drug or drug product. Drug disposition in the sick infant and child has not been adequately investigated at this time; and the data which would allow the pediatrician to prescribe generically and expect consistent therapeutic results does not exist. Therefore the pediatrician must acquaint himself with dose-response relationships of known entities and not prescribe products with which he has no familiarity.[16]

Now what was the practitioner to do? When three out of four New York State physicians refused to permit generic substitution, an assistant attorney general called for changes in the current law that would require physicians to write "medically necessary" if prescribing by brand name. In addition, the state attorney general and the New York City consumer-affairs commissioner urged that the generic-drug law be amended to permit criminal prosecution against violators of the statute. Thus, even though there is considerable evidence to the contrary, under such circumstances practicing physicians and pharmacists may feel constrained to practice according to official policy guidelines that may have more of a political than medical basis. Yet, in 1974, Professor Jan Koch-Weser of Harvard Medical School warned that:

> No amount of wishful thinking or administrative fiat can change the present state of affairs in which differences in drug bioavailability from different products are very common and therapeutic inequivalence because of such differences is a potentially serious threat to patient welfare.[17]

Given the mixed signals reaching the practitioners, perhaps the best they can do is be professionals and inform the patient about the cost-benefits trade-off, if they can, and let the patients decide whether they would like to save the money and take the possible risks. Or they can react as vendors toward consumers and leave it to caveat emptor.

Notes

1. "Rx Against Brand-Name Medicine," *The New York Times,* 9 June 1977, p. A20.
2. Academy of Pharmaceutical Sciences, "Drug Product Quality," *Journal of the American Pharmaceutical Associates* NSIO (1970):107–116.
3. Office of Technology Assessment Drug Bioequivalence Study Panel, *Drug Bioequivalence* (Washington, D.C.: Government Printing Office, 1974), pp. 1–2.
4. "How to Pay Less for Prescription Drugs," *Consumer Reports* 40 (January, 1975):50, 53.
5. A. Johnson and S. Wolf, Letter from Health Research Group to the FDA, 14 February 1975.
6. A. Hecht, "Generic Drugs: How Good Are They?" *FDA Consumer* (February 1978):1–4.
7. J.P. Skelly, "Preclearance of Generics—Yes or No? An FDA Perspective," (Presented at the Twentieth Annual International Pharmacy Conference, Austin, Texas, 23–26 February 1981).
8. Ibid.
9. Ibid.
10. D. Kennedy, Interview on the "Today Show," 24 January 1978.
11. DHEW, "New York Drug List," Press release (Washington, D.C., 23 January 1978).
12. D. Schwartzman, *Innovation in the Pharmaceutical Industry* (Baltimore: Johns Hopkins University Press, 1976), p. 248.
13. L.H. Block, "An Evaluation of Drug Product Citations in the FDA Weekly Reports between 1970 and 1978," *Contemporary Pharmacy Practice* 3 (1980):171–179.
14. R.B. Ostroff and J.P. Doherty, "Tricyclics, Bioequivalence and Clinical Response," *American Journal of Psychiatry* 135 (1978):1560–1561.

15. A.C. Capomacchia et al., "Drug Bioavailability Data: (Un)Available," *American Journal of Pharmacy Education* 43 (1979):231–233.

16. Committee on Drugs, "Generic Prescribing," *Pediatrics* 57 (1976): 275–277.

17. J. Koch-Wesser, "Bioavailability of Drugs (Part 2)," *New England Journal of Medicine* 291 (1974):503–506.

11 The Pharmacist as Prescriber

William F. McGhan and
Glen L. Stimmel

During the last decade, clinically trained pharmacists have expanded their patient-care responsibilities significanctly to include assessing drug response, identifying drug-induced adverse effects and drug interactions, and maximizing drug compliance through patient education. The nature of this care has been advisory since drug prescribing remained the sole responsibility of the physician. On 15 September 1977, however, California law AB717 was approved, allowing pharmacists to prescribe drugs when engaged in an experimental health manpower project authorized by the California State Department of Health.

Background

Because pharmacists have not been able to prescribe drugs legally, except in a special Indian Health Service Program, little of the literature directly addresses the evaluation of pharmacist prescribing. Significant literature exists, however, that suggests the positive impact clinically trained pharmacists have on the quality and economy of drug prescribing and even more supportive literature evaluating the adequacy of nurse practitioners' and physician assistants' drug prescribing.

In 1974 Cheung and Kayne reported on their study carried out in four skilled-nursing facilities, one of which served as a control. The data demonstrated that clinical-pharmacy services resulted in a savings estimated at $80,000 per year for 300 patients (73¢ per patient per day) through a reduction in the use of inappropriate or unnecessary drugs and prevention of adverse drug reactions.[1]

Brands and others have described pharmacist practitioners in the Indian Health Service who were trained to diagnose and treat acute self-limiting diseases and to treat chronic diseases of ambulatory patients.[2] Results showed that in a one-year period, 70 percent seen were completely cared for by the pharmacist, that the time required to see patients was essentially the same for pharmacists versus physicians, that the quality of care determined by physician chart review was satisfactory, and that acceptance by patients was excellent. Erickson, in describing the same Indian Health Service Program, found that the pharmacist was able to provide patient monitoring between physician visits and that this monitoring extended the interval between physician visits.[3]

McKenney and associates studied the effect of clinical-pharmacist services on a group of hypertensive patients compared to a group randomized to normal physician care.[4] Results for the pharmacist group showed significant improvement in the patients' knowledge of hypertension and its treatment, in drug compliance, and a significant increase in the number of patients whose blood pressures were within the normal range when compared to the physician-treated group. Physician time was reduced greatly in the population monitored by the pharmacist.

Rosen and Holmes evaluated the impact of a clinically trained pharmacist upon the treatment of chronic psychiatric outpatients being maintained within their communities.[5] The cost of a pharmacist providing medication-monitoring services was 40 percent of the cost of providing that service by a psychiatrist. The pharmacists' patients were found to be functioning in the community as well or better than other patients, and their satisfaction with treatment provided was at least equal to other psychiatric outpatients sampled.

Helling and associates studied patient attitudes toward their general quality of health care received from family-practice offices.[6] Patients were assigned randomly to a control group that received no clinical-pharmacy services and to an experimental group in which patients received direct clinical-pharmacy services. The experimental group was found to be significantly more satisfied with health care than the control group. These findings suggest that patient acceptance of medical services can be increased markedly with direct pharmacist-patient encounters.

There have been many studies of nurse practitioners' contributions to quality and economy of patient care. Best known is the Burlington randomized trial of nurse practitioners with family physicians that showed that both groups of patients had similar mortality rates.[7] No differences were found in physical, social, or emotional functioning. The quality of care rendered was similar as assessed by indicator conditions. Satisfaction was high among both patients and professional personnel. Yankauer and associates studied pediatric nurse practitioners in the Boston area.[8] Of seventy-three nurses studied, employment was divided equally between agency and private practice. The pediatricians using nurse practitioners were found to have greater time to devote to selected patients, and the quality of care provided by these nurses was evaluated as good.

Greenfield and associates studied a nurse and physician assistant protocol system to a nonprotocol physician-only system in an HMO.[9] This prospective randomized study found that physician time per patient was reduced 92 percent and that cost per patient visit, including practitioner time, lab tests, and medication was reduced 20 percent by utilizing these assistants. Kane and associates have shown that patients treated by a trained-assistant tend to fare about as well as those seen by a physician in regaining their usual functional status[10] and that these patients achieve good results while faculty physician patients achieve poor results in an examination of estimated levels of function and earliest data of recovery in a family-practice clinic.[11] The number of articles on the quality of care by nonphysician providers continues to increase.[12, 13, 14, 15]

These studies of pharmacists, nurse practitioners, and physician assistants suggest that a significant amount of patient care can be provided by other health-care practitioners and that pharmacists in particular can contribute to improved quality and economy of drug prescribing for patients.

The Law

AB717 allows two pilot projects in which pharmacists prescribe and administer drugs under the supervision of a physician. One of these two projects was awarded to the USC School of Pharmacy in October 1978. The pilot projects will continue until 31 December 1982 when all projects will terminate, perhaps to be replaced by more-permanent and improved legislation. In addition to pharmacists, AB717 allows drug-prescribing projects for nurses and physician assistants.[16]

Each trainee prescriber must complete a training program and successfully pass a written certifying examination before prescribing begins. Each trainee must have an identified supervising physician, and supervisory meetings must occur a minimum of once every two weeks. Every prescription written must be reviewed by the supervising physician to assess safety and quality of prescribing. Trainees are restricted to the project's formulary and must use a special triplicate prescription form that includes additional information for evaluation purposes, such as patient age, weight, diagnosis, other medication, and other medical diagnoses. Each project is responsible for developing its own training program, examination, and formulary.

Formulary

The projects were required to submit a formulary for approval by the state Department of Health Services. Drugs are approved either for renewal only or initiation and renewal or disapproved by a state committee of physicians and pharmacists. The USC project formulary currently contains approximately 300 drugs, and the major drug categories are shown in the following list.

- Anthelmintics,
- Antimicrobials,
- Anticoagulants,
- Anticonvulsants,
- Antihistamine/decongestants,
- Antiinflammatory,
- Antineoplastic,
- Antiparkinson
- Antispasmodics,
- Biologicals
- Bronchodilators,
- Cardiovascular,
- Contraceptives,
- Dermatologicals,
- Diagnostic agents,
- Endocrine,
- Gastrointestinal,
- Gynecological,
- Muscle relaxants,
- Ophthalmologic,
- Otic,
- Psychotropics,
- Vitamins/minerals.

All narcotic drugs and some other frequently misused drugs are prohibited from the AB717 formularies by law. From this project formulary, the pharmacist prescriber and his or her supervising physician develop the formulary for their particular site. While some pharmacists have the entire project formulary available for their use, many pharmacist prescribers have restricted their formulary since their patient population is limited to certain disease states—for example, an anticoagulation clinic.

A very broad project formulary was felt to be necessary in order to evaluate a pharmacist's ability to prescribe drugs competently for a variety of disease states. For example, to evaluate a pharmacist's ability to treat hypertensive patients, the pharmacist could not be restricted to thiazide diuretics alone. Although previously used, project or statewide prescribing protocols or algorithms are not encouraged because it is felt that protocols are too inflexible to allow a valid assessment of a prescriber's decision making.

Prescription Form

A standardized triplicate prescription form must be used by all AB717 prescribers. Copy A (white) is a typical prescription form that is given to the patient to be filled by a drug dispenser (figure 11–1). The bottom half of copies B (blue) and C (yellow) contain additional information useful for evaluation purposes (figure 11–2). With each prescription the prescriber records the patient's chart number, age, weight, and sex. Also recorded is the indication for the prescription, which includes the diagnosis and other descriptive information when appropriate (for example, hypertension, BP 150/90; akathisia, dose increased from 2 mg. BID). The abbreviations under prescriber activity allow the prescriber to indicate whether or not the

PATIENT NAME (PRINT)

ADDRESS

81411

SIGNATURE

DATE ______

PRINTED NAME

HMPP PRESCRIBER NO ______

REFILL ______ DEA NO. ______

Figure 11-1. Prescription Form Given to Patient

81411

SIGNATURE

DATE ______________

PRINTED NAME

HMPP PRESCRIBER NO. ______________

REFILL ______________ DEA NO. ______________

CHART NO.: _______ AGE: _______ WEIGHT: ____ lbs ____ oz SEX: M F

INDICATION FOR PRESCRIPTION:

PRESCRIBER ACTIVITY

IN RE DI MD PH LA

OTHER MEDICATIONS IN USE:

OTHER HEALTH CONDITIONS:
(Including allergies)

Figure 11-2. Prescription Copy B and C for Evaluation

drug is new or a refill, the prescriber also dispensed the drug, a physician was consulted, and lab tests were ordered. Other drugs and other health conditions of the patient also are recorded. Copy B remains at the prescribing site, while copy C is mailed to the USC project office. The patient's name and address do not appear on copy C to protect the patient confidentiality.

Training

Because the USC project began with pharmacists who were practicing already in clinical areas, a new comprehensive training program was not necessary. The only formal training required for these pharmacists to prescribe and evaluate drug therapy was a physical-assessment-skills course. The content of such a course is shown in the following list:

General Approach to Examination

Head, ears, eyes, nose, and throat (HEENT):

Examination of the mouth and throat,
Eyes,
Ears,
Nose,
Head and neck;

Pulmonary/Chest:

Review of anatomy, posterior-anterior chest,
General approach and examination,
Posterior Chest:
  Inspection,
  Palpation,
  Percussion,
  Auscultation,
Anterior chest wall;

Cardiac:

Review of anatomy,
Cardiac-cycle sounds,
Inspection and palpation,
Percussion,
Auscultation,
Arterial pulses,
Venous pulse;

Neurology:

Cranial nerves 1–12,
Deep tendon reflexes,
Motor system (cerebellar function),
Sensory system;

Miscellaneous:
Skin,
Abdomen,
Musculoskeletal system.

This thirty-hour course, organized by physicians, provides clinical information and practical experience for the pharmacist prescriber. The focus of the course is not on differential diagnosis but on the assessment of change in disease state as a function of drug response and drug-induced adverse effects. The course serves only as an introduction to physical assessment, with an expectation that refinement of skills would occur in the practice setting with the supervising physician. All other prescribing competencies presently are taught in California's schools of pharmacy as well as in continuing-education courses readily available to practicing pharmacists.

Competencies

The general competencies the trainee pharmacist must meet before entering the prescribing phase include the following:

The ability to select an appropriate drug based upon the diagnosis established by the physician;

Extensive knowledge of drugs included in the basic formulary, including classification, therapeutic use, dose, dosage schedules, modes of administration, adverse effects and toxicity, drug interactions, and contraindications;

The ability to educate the patient about the drugs being prescribed;

Knowledge of reliable sources of current drug information;

Knowledge of appropriate state and federal laws and regulations and limitations under AB717 regarding legal prescribing;

Knowledge of evaluation processes developed by the sponsoring project and the state department of health;

Physical-assessment skills necessary to assess drug-caused disease-state change and drug-induced adverse effects of drugs present in the project's basic formulary.

Certification

Each project is experimenting with various testing mechanisms for certifying their pharmacists, nurses, or physician assistants for prescribing. The USC examination covers competencies in three areas—clinical therapeutics, physical assessment, and AB717 prescribing regulations. Although some pharmacists practice in specialty areas, a comprehensive exam for all pharmacists was administered. The first exam developed consisted of over 200 items in multiple-choice format.

Item analysis was utilized to discard or improve the test questions that were written in a confusing manner or poor discriminators for scoring. The cut-off for discrimination occurred when there was a negative phi correlation and less than 20 percent of the subjects selected the correct answer. The intent was to obtain an overall average item difficulty of 70 percent for this five-response multiple-choice test. The reliability of the exam is reasonably high with an overall Kuder-Richardson (Formula 20) test reliability of .89. The three sections of the exam and their reliability were clinical therapeutics (KR 20 = .836), physical assessment (KR 20 = .883), and law (KR 20 = .840).[17]

The passing score was determined after considering a minimally acceptable percentage of possible points (absolute standard approach) and examining the distribution of scores (normative approach).[18] The project staff decided an acceptable grade was correct answers to 60 percent or more of the total questions. This level of attainment was equivalent to one standard deviation (equal to 14) below the mean (mean = 136). Of the thirty pharmacists initially taking this exam, twenty-five achieved passing scores.

In order to assess further the validity of the exam, we gave the test to a group of thirteen physicians in an internal-medicine residency program. The residents were administered the two parts of the exam dealing with clinical therapeutics and physical assessment. Table 11–1 displays the means, standard deviation, and *T*-test results, and *P*-values, comparing the physicians to the original pharmacist test results.

Pharmacists averaged slightly better than physicians on clinical therapeutics, but pharmacists had a significantly lower average score than physicians on physical assessment. For the total score there was no significant difference. These results tend to validate that the 60 percent correct level was reasonable. If anything, we were a little too strict with our passing score since, on this basis, two of the thirteen physicians failed the exam. We felt, however, that pharmacists who passed this exam would be good prescribers.

Table 11–1
A Comparison of AB717 Examination Results between Physicians and Pharmacists

	Physicians[a]	*Pharmacists*[b]		
Test Area	*Mean and Standard Deviation*	*Mean and Standard Deviation*	*t-value*	*P-value (p =)*
Clinical therapeutics	78.2 ± 9.4	83.9 ± 9.4	1.83	NS
Physical assessment	49.5 ± 4.3	41.4 ± 6.08	4.89	.01
Total Test	127.7 ± 12	125.4 ± 14	.51	NS

Note: NS means not significant.
[a] $N = 11$.
[b] $N = 30$.

Assessing Prescription Completeness

To evaluate the prescriptions as the copies arrive at the USC project office, two different forms have been developed. The first form is the prescription audit form (figure 11–3). This form primarily assesses the process component of the prescription by determining if the prescription is completely filled out and what steps were involved in processing the prescription (for example, Was a lab test ordered? Was a physician consulted?). This basic completion audit form is utilized by pharmacy students who serve as research assistants.

We learned some interesting facts from surveying the audit forms. For example, at a mental-health clinic, refill prescriptions accounted for one-third of prescriptions while two-thirds constituted new therapy for the patients. Physician consultation was necessary for about 20 percent of the pharmacists' prescriptions that involved primarily initiation of a new drug class for new patients.

Pharmacists ordered laboratory tests with nearly 10 percent of prescriptions, most of which were baseline tests ordered with new drugs. In this particular mental-health center, pharmacists dispensed their own prescriptions about two-thirds of the time.

Assessing Prescribing Appropriateness

The second monitoring device is the prescription evaluation form (figure 11–4) and this form is designed to assess the overall appropriateness of the

Required Data		Yes	No
a. Age	a		
b. Sex	b		
c. Indication for prescription	c		
d. Other health cond. (including allergies)	d		
e. Other medications in use	e		
f. Initial prescription	f		
g. Refilled prescription	g		
h. MD consulted	h		
i. Pharmacist consulted	i		
j. Signature	j		
k. License classification (i.e., PA-C)	k		
l. Registration number	l		
m. Date of prescription	m		
n. Lab test ordered	n		
o. Dispense	o		

Figure 11-3. Prescription Audit Form

pharmacists' prescriptions. Because the USC project formulary contains over 300 drugs, it has not been possible to develop explicit criteria to evaluate each drug. We normally use tracer drug groups that have explicit appropriateness criteria. The prescriptions are evaluated by clinical-pharmacy faculty and physicians. The practitioners who evaluate the prescriptions are not involved as AB717 prescribers because we hoped to reduce biases by separating prescribers and evaluators. We usually used evaluations from both physicians and pharmacists. This made it possible to examine inter-rater reliability between the pharmacist and physician evaluators.

The evaluation thus far has a reasonable amount of internal consistency (coefficient alpha of .884). We have found no consistently significant correlation between scores on the completion audit form and the evaluation form.

We now briefly discuss results on two studies using psychotropic and hypertensive drugs as tracers to assess the appropriateness of prescribing by pharmacists and physicians.

	DEFINITELY YES	PROBABLY YES	UNCERTAIN	PROBABLY NO	DEFINITELY NO
1. Is drug therapy necessary?	1	2	3	4	5
2. Is chosen drug appropriate for diagnosis?	1	2	3	4	5
3. Is drug interaction absent? (drug-drug, drug-disease, drug lab)? *	1	2	3	4	5
4. Is quantity (and refills)* appropriate?	1	2	3	4	5
5. Is dose appropriate? (for age, diagnosis)*	1	2	3	4	5
6. Are patient directions (sig)* appropriate?	1	2	3	4	5
7. Will prescription have positive effect on patients' health?	1	2	3	4	5

Comments:

Was generic drug [ ] or brand name drug [ ] prescribed?

* Circle for clarification if problem

Prescription reviewed by ________ (initials)

Figure 11-4. Prescription Evaluation Form

Comparing Pharmacists and Physicians on Prescribing Psychotropic Medications

For the study reported here, three pharmacist prescribers' orders were compared to two psychiatrists' psychotropic-drug orders to assess the safety and quality of prescribing. Sixty prescriptions were selected randomly from each prescriber, twenty for each of the following drug classes: neuroleptic drugs, antiparkinson drugs, and antidepressants. Two psychiatrist judges and two psychiatric pharmacist judges, independent of the project and blind to the identity of the prescribers, evaluated each prescription. A reproducible scoring system with a five-point scale was used to assess (1) whether or not drug therapy was necessary, (2) the appropriateness of the drug for the diagnosis, (3) the potential for drug interaction, (4) the appropriateness of dose and dosage schedule, (5) directions, and (6) whether or not the prescription would have a positive effect on the patient's health. The explicit standards for scoring the prescriptions were based on criteria of the American Psychiatric Association. The null hypothesis implies that there would be no difference in the quality of prescribing between psychiatrists and pharmacists for hospitalized psychiatric patients. The inter-rater reliability coefficient for the judges was about .80 using the *Statistical Package for the Social Sciences* reliability analysis.[19]

For neuroleptic drugs, there was no difference on scales 1, 2, 4, and 6, but pharmacists scored better than psychiatrists on scales 3 and 5 ($P < .05$). For antiparkinson drugs, there was no difference on all scales except scale 5, in which pharmacists were rated better ($P < .05$). For antidepressants, there was no difference on scales 3, 4, and 5, but pharmacists were rated better on scales 1, 2, and 6 ($P < .05$). There were no scales for any drug class in which psychiatrists were rated better than pharmacists. For neuroleptic and antiparkinson drugs, the total mean scores were not different, but for antidepressants the total mean score was better for pharmacists than psychiatrists ($P < .05$). Total mean scores for all drugs combined showed that pharmacist prescriptions were rated significantly better than those of psychiatrists ($P < .05$). Although statistical differences did occur in various areas mentioned earlier, the mean scores on the five-point scales of both prescriber groups suggested that these pharmacists and psychiatrists were prescribing drugs appropriately.

Comparing Pharmacists and Physicians on Prescribing Hypertensive Medications.

The null hypothesis implies that there would be no difference between pharmacists and physicians as to the quality of drug prescribing for patients with hypertension. Over 150 prescriptions were selected randomly from two project pharmacists and three physicians in an ambulatory-care clinic. Demographic data indicated that the patient groups were similar. One physician and one pharmacist were used as judges to score the prescriptions on seven different scales related to appropriate therapy. For scoring, the judges used explicit, national criteria for appropriate treatment of high blood pressure and were blinded as to the prescription writer by transforming the prescription data to computer printouts.[20] The inter-rater reliability between the two judges was acceptable with a coefficient of .65.

There was no difference between the physician and pharmacist prescriptions on the scoring for presence of potential drug interactions, appropriateness of quantities, dose, and patient directions. Pharmacist prescribers did significantly better, however, than physicians on choosing the appropriate drug, prescribing for a positive effect on the patient's health, and overall appropriateness from combining all the scales ($P < .05$).

Conclusion

California was the first state to legislate prescribing authority for pharmacists directly. AB717 originated with nurse practitioners and physician assistants seeking to expand the scope of their practice. Since they may by law examine patients and initiate some treatment, they sought through AB717 to include drug prescribing. For a variety of reasons, drug-prescribing authorization requires legislation rather than regulation changes. Pharmacy became the third new profession to be included in legislation permitting pilot prescribing projects. The current AB717 law also allows dispensing by nurse practioners and physician assistants. AB717 thus represents a significant opportunity to determine if pharmacists can prescribe drugs safely and effectively.

During the life of this project, it will be possible to determine the advantages prescribing authority offers to pharmacy and to the health-care system and what limitations should exist. It must be decided what limitations are necessary to accompany prescribing authority, what additional training and certification is necessary, what type of physician-pharmacist relationship is advisable, how to answer concerns of conflict of interest if the pharmacist prescriber also is the dispenser, and which drugs the pharmacists may prescribe. The data reported here indicate that the project pharmacists can prescribe medications appropriately, and we expect pharmacist-prescriber projects to emerge in many other states in the future.

Notes

1. A. Cheung and R. Kayne, "An Application of Clinical Pharmacy Services in Extended Care Facilities," *California Pharmacist* 25 (1978): 22–28.

2. A.J. Brands, "Treating Ambulatory Patients," *U.S. Pharmacist* 2 (1977):70–74.

3. S.H. Erickson, "Primary Care by a Pharmacist in an Outpatient Clinic," *American Journal of Hospital Pharmacy* 34 (1977):1086–1090.

4. J.M. McKenney et al., "The Effect of Clinical Pharmacy Services on Patients with Essential Hypertension," *Circulation* 48 (1973):1104–1111.

5. C.E. Rosen and S. Holmes, "Pharmacist's Impact on Chronic Psychiatric Outpatients in Community Mental Health," *American Journal of Hospital Pharmacy* 35 (1978):704–708.

6. D.K. Helling, C.D. Helper, and M.E. Jones, "Effect of Direct Clinical Pharmaceutical Services on Patients. Prescriptions of Health Care Quality," *American Journal of Hospital Pharmacy* 36 (1979):325–329.

7. W.O. Spitzer et al., "The Burlington Randomized Trial of the Nurse Practitioner," *New England Journal of Medicine* 290 (1974): 251–256.

8. A. Yankauer, S. Tripp, and P. Andrews, "The Outcomes of Service Impact of a Pediatric Nurse Practitioner Training Program—Nurse Practitioner Training Outcomes," *American Journal of Public Health* 62 (1972):347–353.

9. S. Greenfield et al., "Efficiency and Cost of Primary Care by Nurses and Physician Assistants," *New England Journal of Medicine* 298 (1978):305–309.

10. R.L. Kane, D.M. Olsen, and C.H. Castle, "Medex and Their Physician Preceptors: Quality of Care," *Journal of the American Medical Association* 236 (1976):2509–2512.

11. R.L. Kane et al., "Differences in the Outcomes of Acute Episodes of Care Provided by Various Types of Family Practitioners," *Journal of Family Practice* 6 (1978):133–139.

12. G.L. Stimmel and W.F. McGhan, "Pharmacists Prescribe Drugs in Pilot Project," *Forum on Medicine* 3 (1980):404–405.

13. J.M. McKenney et al., "Effect of Pharmacist Drug Monitoring and Patient Evaluation on Hypertensive Patients," *Contemporary Pharmacy Practice* (Fall 1978):50–56.

14. D.W. Hawkins et al., "Evaluation of a Clinical Pharmacist in Caring for Hypertensive and Diabetic Patients," *American Journal of Hospital Pharmacy* 36 (1979):1321–1325.

15. H.C. Sox, "Quality of Patient Care by Nurse Practitioners and Physician's Assistants: A Ten Year Perspective," *Annals of Internal Medicine* 91 (1979):459–468.

16. Stimmel and McGhan, "Pharmacists Prescribe Drugs."

17. J.C. Nunally, *Psychometric Theory* (New York: McGraw-Hill, 1978).

18. C.G. Schoon, C.M. Guillion, and P. Ferrara, "Bayesian Statistics, Credentialing Examinations and the Determination of Passing Points," *Evaluation and the Health Professions* 2 (June 1979):181–202.

19. G.H. Hull and N.H. Nie, *Statistical Package for the Social Sciences—Update* (New York: McGraw-Hill, 1979).

20. Anonymous, *The 1980 Report of the Joint National Committee on Detection, Evaluation, and Treatment of High Blood Pressure* (Bethesda, Md.: National Institute of Health, June 1980).

Part IV
Psychoactive Issues

12 Psychotherapeutic Drugs: A Current Assessment of Prevalence and Patterns of Use

Glen D. Mellinger and
Mitchell B. Balter

This chapter presents data from the 1979 National Survey of Psychotherapeutic Drug Use. The data were obtained from a rigorous cross-section probability sample of noninstitutionalized American adults, ages 18–79. Persons 60–79 years of age were oversampled at a ratio of 1.67:1. We completed interviews with 3,161 persons. The overall completion rate was 76 percent of all persons designated as eligible for the sample.

Interviews lasted an average of seventy-five minutes and covered a wide range of topics including prevalence and patterns of using psychotherapeutic drugs; emotional, physical, and situational factors that may be associated with such use; and attitudes toward using psychotherapeutic drugs (specifically, the anti-anxiety agents). This chapter focuses on prevalence of use, sources from which the drugs were obtained, and patterns—that is, frequency and regularity—of use.

The 1979 study was the latest in a series of community-based surveys, including an earlier national survey in 1970–1971.[1] The household surveys have been part of a broader National Institute of Mental Health (NIMH) program of research on the medical use of psychotherapeutic drugs. Most of these surveys have been conducted by the Institute for Research in Social Behavior (Oakland, California) in close collaboration with the staff of NIMH. The 1970 survey was conducted jointly with the Social Research Group of the George Washington University (Washington, D.C.).[2]

The continuing objective of the NIMH research program is to obtain rigorous empirical evidence regarding the nature and extent of psychotherapeutic-drug use, a topic that, in the United States, is controversial and emotionally charged. In addition to the household-survey data, the NIMH program also has obtained and analyzed nationally representative data on the volume of prescriptions filled in drug stores,[3] on prescribing practices of

G.O. Mellinger and M.B. Balter, "Prevalence and Patterns of Use of Psychotherapeutic Drugs: Results from a 1979 National Survey of American Adults," in *Epidemiological Impact of Psychotropic Drugs: Proceedings of International Seminar on Epidemiological Impact of Psychotropic Drugs,* eds. G. Tognoni, C. Bellantuono, and M. Lader (Amsterdam: Elsevier/North-Holland Biomedical Press, 1981). Reprinted with permission.

physicians,[4] and on the diagnostic and therapeutic activities of private medical practitioners.[5] One of the authors (Balter) and his colleagues at NIMH currently are analyzing national mortality data based on all 1975 and 1978 death certificates for which the International Classification of Diseases cause-of-death code (as assigned by the National Center for Health Statistics) indicated the involvement of a psychotropic drug or related drugs of interest—namely, narcotics and alcohol.

In addition to the national and other household surveys conducted in the United States, comparative cross-national data on prevalence of anti-anxiety/sedative drug use also were obtained in nine Western European countries in 1971.[6] The cross-national surveys are being repeated in Europe now.

Finally, this long-range research program also has included two rigorous validation studies—one in 1971 to test the validity of the procedures we use to obtain data on prevalence of psychotherapeutic-drug use, the other in 1978 to assess our survey methods of obtaining data on emotional distress, especially anxiety and depression.[7]

The household surveys make an especially important contribution to this program of research in the United States because we have no nationally centralized records that cover outpatient medical care. Without household surveys, there would be no way to obtain person-based data on the complex processes of acquiring and using psychotherapeutic drugs that may have been prescribed by more than one physician, filled in more than one drugstore, and for that matter, acquired outside conventional medical channels.[8] The survey data, combined with data from the other sources mentioned, thus provide a unique and comprehensive source of information encompassing the therapeutic practices of physicians, drugstore outflow, and the behavior, attitudes, and other characteristics of patients, former patients, and nonpatients in the general population.

Previous Findings on Psychotherapeutic-Drug Use

In general, the empirical evidence from these various sources has helped to dispel many popular misconceptions regarding the prescribing practices of physicians and the use of psychotherapeutic drugs by outpatients. On the basis of drugstore prescribing and household survey data, some major conclusions about psychotherapeutic-drug consumption are as follows:

> The annual volume of psychotherapeutic prescriptions filled in drugstores in the United States rose from 122.5 million in 1964 to a peak of 214.7 million in 1973—an overall increase of 75 percent. Anti-anxiety agents and antidepressants mainly were responsible for the increase.[9]

Since that time there has been a sharp reversal of the trend observed earlier. In fact, the total volume of prescriptions for psychotherapeutic drugs declined 28 percent from 1973 to 1979, so that the number of prescriptions filled in 1979 was approximately equal to the figure a decade earlier.[10]

Patterns of prescribing by physicians in office-based private practice usually were found to be conservative with respect to daily dosage, number of refills permitted, and similar indicators. More-recent data indicate that prescribing patterns are becoming even more conservative.[11]

The most widely used psychotherapeutic drugs often were found to be prescribed in cases where the physician had diagnosed and was treating some physical condition that may have originated in, been further aggravated by, or resulted in emotional distress. We found, for example, that new therapy with anti-anxiety agents was at least as likely to be directed to patients with a primary diagnosis of a physical disorder as to those with a primary diagnosis of a mental disorder.[12]

The bulk of the prescribing of psychotherapeutic drugs to outpatients was found to be in the hands of general practitioners and internists rather than psychiatrists.[13]

In the 1970 national household survey, we found the following:

The U.S. public typically was conservative in its attitudes toward medically prescribed psychotherapeutic drugs (as typified by the anti-anxiety agents) and tended to regard use of these drugs as appropriate only under conditions of relatively extreme distress and/or impairment of social functioning.[14]

Precisely under these conditions of distress or impairment was use of psychotherapeutic drugs (especially regular and prolonged use) found typically to occur, that is, the majority of psychotherapeutic-drug users, in contrast to nonusers, reported high levels of psychic distress and/or life crisis.[15]

Further evidence of public conservatism with respect to psychotherapeutic drug use was reflected in two additional findings:

Among persons who reported both a high level of life crisis and a high level of psychic distress, a substantial majority (more than two-thirds) had not used medically prescribed psychotherapeutic drugs during the year prior to interview.[16]

Persons who had used these drugs were disproportionately middle-aged and older and typically used them intermittently or for relatively short periods of time.[17]

Thus, the observed patterns of medical use were not consistent with either an abuse or self-indulgent-consumer model of drug consumption but conformed to an illness model in which treatment is associated with brief or intermittent episodes of distress and is discontinued when the treatment produces its desired effect or when the conditions producing the symptoms subside.

Data from the cross-national studies conducted in 1971 lent further perspective to the result obtained in the national survey. The comparative data demonstrated that the United States ranked only slightly above the middle among the nine European countries with respect to prevalence of using medically prescribed anti-anxiety sedative drugs.[18]

Concepts and Methods

Classification of Drugs

The outcome of any survey of psychotherapeutic-drug use obviously depends upon which drugs are included. The rationale for including or excluding particular drugs or classes of drugs is very important, as are the underlying principles of classification. Differences in drug classifications can lead to very different conclusions about the character, extent, and appropriateness of drug prescribing and use. To take an obvious but important example, one would expect quite different underlying clinical conditions and patterns of use associated with hypnotic medications as compared with antidepressants. Too many investigators in the field of drug utilization appear to be unaware of the clinical significance of these classification distinctions vis-a-vis drug use.

Our research proceeds from a therapeutic model of drug use that focuses on clusters of psychic symptoms associated with anxiety and depression, on somatic and situational conditions that often occur in combination with such symptoms, and on the psychotherapeutic medications commonly used in treating these symptoms and conditions.

From this point of view, primary classification based on chemical structure or pharmacological action are inapplicable. The former tend to group drugs with different clinical uses; the latter tend to create large heterogeneous groupings with little relationship to clinical practice.

A classification scheme based on clinical applications in medicine is clearly most appropriate for this research. Only by applying clinical and therapeutic principles of drug classification can we begin to assess the extent to which drugs have been used appropriately or inappropriately.

It clearly would be misleading, for example, to include a medication such as prochlorperazine (Compazine) (which, in the United States, is used primarily as an anti-emetic) in the general class of psychotherapeutic drugs, even though as a phenothiazine it is structurally similar to many of the antipsychotic drugs. It would be equally misleading to include amphetamine or the narcotic analgesics, even though their pharmacological actions have direct and powerful effects on mood.

In short, this research is concerned with the prescription drugs that have a primary or principal effect on mood, emotions, mental processes, or behavior and that are commonly used by clinicians to treat mental or emotional disorders or to alleviate overt symptoms of psychic and emotional distress.

Medicines that meet these two definitional criteria have been categorized further according to therapeutic class on the basis of their use in clinical practice—the principal purposes for which they are prescribed. We thus define five major therapeutic classes of drugs: (1) anti-anxiety agents, (2) hypnotics, (3) daytime sedatives, (4) antidepressants (including lithium), and (5) antipsychotics. Within each major therapeutic class, we have subcategorized drugs on the basis of chemical structure. The classification system appears in table 12–1. Our interest centers on prescription drugs that are obtained via a physician, but we will also present data on the use of such drugs obtained from nonmedical sources and the use of OTC drugs marketed as tranquilizers—for example, Cope and Compoz or sleeping pills such as Nytol, Sleepeze, and Sominex.

Collection of Data on Psychotherapeutic-Drug Use

Prior to the first national survey in 1970, we spent a great deal of time and effort developing and testing the methods we use to obtain data on drug use. Our approach is health oriented and is designed to establish and maintain good rapport with respondents.

The questioning strategy is designed specifically to help respondents to recall and identify, by name of drug and class, the drugs they have used. We use three aids to memory: (1) for each class of psychotherapeutic drug, a description of the function that class is intended to serve (for example, to calm down, to relax, or to reduce nervous tension); (2) the name of the drug class (for example, tranquilizers or sedatives); and (3) a drug-recognition chart that depicts, life sized and in color, more than 250 different psychotherapeutic drugs in their various forms and strengths. The drug chart provides still another aid to recall by listing the name (for example, Valium) of each drug pictured.

The questioning procedure may be illustrated for the hypnotic class. While showing a respondent the chart for drugs in this class, the interviewer says: "Here are some pictures of pills or medicines that people take to help

Table 12-1
Classification of Prescription Psychotherapeutic Drugs

Drug Class	*Examples: Generic Names*	*Examples: Trade Names*
Anti-anxiety agents		
Benzodiazepines	Diazepam, chlordiazepoxide, clorazepate, lorazepam, oxazepam	Valium, Librium, Tranxene, Ativan, Serax
Substituted diols	Meprobamate, tybamate	Equanil and Miltown, Tybatran
Miscellaneous	Hydroxyzine	Atarax, Vistaril
Hypnotics		
Barbiturates (short acting)	Secobarbital, pentobarbital, secobarbital/amobarbital	Seconal, Nembutal, Tuinal
Others	Flurazepam, chloral hydrate, ethchlorvynol, glutethimide	Dalmane, Noctec, Placidyl, Doriden
Daytime sedatives		
Barbiturates (long acting and intermediate acting)	Phenobarbital, butabarbital	Luminal, Butisol
Others	Bromisovalum	Bromural
Antidepressants		
Tricyclics	Amitriptyline, imipramine, desipramine	Elavil, Tofranil, Norpramin
Monoamine oxidase (MAO) inhibitors	Phenelzine, tranylcypromine, isocarboxazid	Nardil, Parnate, Marplan
Others	Amitriptyline, perphenazine, amitriptyline, chlordia-zepoxide, doxepin, lithium	Triavil and Etrafon, Limbitrol, Sinequan, Eskalith
Antipsychotics		
Phenothiazines	Thioridazine, chlorproma-zine, trifluoperazine	Mellaril, Thorazine, Stelazine
Butyrophenones	Haloperidol	Haldol
Thioxanthenes	Thiothixene, chlorprothixene	Navane, Taractan

them get to sleep at night or to stay asleep—I mean the ones that are often called sleeping pills. Have your ever taken any of these—or any pills or medicines like them—for any reason?''

In the 1970 survey, about 5 percent of the respondents who had used psychotherapeutic drugs were not able to identify the name of one or more drugs they had used. Less difficulty was experienced in identifying drugs used recently, of course, than in identifying those used in the distant past. By 1979, the percentage of persons who could not identify the name of a drug had declined to 0.4 percent.

Prior to the first national survey, we conducted a large-scale and systematic validation study to test these methods for collecting data on psychotherapeutic-drug use. The validity study found some underreporting of psychotherapeutic-drug use, but the level of underreporting was not high enough to alter any major conclusions. For example, the percentage of accurate responses was 83 percent for anti-anxiety agents, which account for the major share of psychotherapeutic-drug use.[19] Thus, an observed prevalence of 11 percent is probably closer to 13 percent.

Sampling

In both national surveys, data were obtained in personal interviews with respondents selected by rigorous probability-sampling methods to represent a cross section of American adults living in households. As defined, both samples excluded persons who were institutionalized at the time of the surveys. One person per household was designated randomly for interview, and no replacements were allowed.

Because of the growing interest in (and concern about) the use of medications by older persons, we oversampled persons in the 60–79 age range. Specifically, we selected such persons with a probability 1.67 greater than that of persons 18–59.[20] In the following analyses, we have compensated for this inequality in the probability of selection by weighting each respondent's data by the inverse of the selection probability.[21]

As in most large surveys, we used cluster sampling that, together with disproportionate sampling and other design considerations, typically produces larger variances than those implied by simple random-sampling models. The sampling design of the survey also made it possible to calculate the magnitude of design effects on sampling variances. From these calculations one should assume that clustering and other aspects of the sample design increased sampling variations by 50 percent and standard errors (SE) by about 22.5 percent. Thus, the 95 percent confidence interval (CI) for a percentage (p) reported here should be estimated by the following:

$$\mathrm{CI} = p \pm 1.96\mathrm{SE}_p \times 1.225,$$

where

$$\mathrm{SE}_p = \left[\frac{p(1-p)}{N} \right]^{1/2}.$$

It can be assumed that all differences referred to in the text have been tested for statistical significance, using the t-test of differences between proportions:

$$t = \frac{(p_1 - p_2)}{\sqrt{(p_1 q_1)n_1 + (p_2 q_2)n_2}}$$

We have used a t-value of 2.40 (1.96 × 1.225) as the criterion of statistical significance. In the text, NS signifies not significant.

Results

The plan in this section is to present results from the 1979 survey on the past-year prevalence of using medically prescribed psychotherapeutic drugs and on the patterns of using these drugs in terms of frequency and regularity of use.

Medically Prescribed Drugs. From the data in table 12–2, we draw the following conclusions about the prevalence of using medically prescribed psychotherapeutic drugs:

> As is well known, anti-anxiety agents are much more widely used than any of the other five classes of psychotherapeutic drugs, and use of this class of medications is almost two times more prevalent among women than it is among men. Thus, 14.1 percent of the women and 7.5 percent of the men reported using a medically prescribed anti-anxiety agent one or more times during the year prior to interview.
>
> For the next most widely used class, hypnotics, 3 percent of the women and 2.1 percent of the men (NS) reported use during the past year. It should be noted that use of antipsychotics and antidepressants is underrepresented in these data to the extent that these medications are used among hospitalized patients, who were not included in the sample.
>
> Overall, 20.2 percent of the women and 11 percent of the men (16 percent of the men and women combined) had used one or more drugs in these classes during the past year.
>
> In general, prevalence of use was higher among older persons than among younger persons, but the precise relation of age to prevalence differed from class to class. For the anti-anxiety agents, for example, use was most common among persons 50–64 years of age and, if anything, declined slightly beyond that age. Use of hypnotics was most common among the 65–79-year olds. Use of antipsychotics was not clearly or consistently related to age.

Patterns of Use. As defined previously, prevalence of use encompasses a broad range of patterns of using psychotherapeutic drugs—that is, from use on only one or two occasions to regular daily use over long periods of time. Frequency, regularity, and duration of use are obviously important with respect to the therapeutic intent of the physician, as well as the psycholog-

Table 12-2
Prevalence of Past-Year Use of Medically Prescribed Psychotherapeutic Drugs, by Drug Class, Age, and Sex

	Percent Using during Past Twelve Months in Age Group				
Drug Class and Sex	*18–34*	*35–49*	*50–64*	*65–79*	*All*
Anti-anxiety agents					
Men	4.1	8.1	12.4	9.1	7.5
Women	7.9	16.6	19.5	18.7	14.1
Hypnotics					
Men	0.8	0.7	4.1	5.3	2.1
Women	1.7	2.4	3.5	6.5	3
Daytime sedatives					
Men	0.5	0.4	1.3	0.8	0.7
Women	1.5	1.4	2.4	2.6	1.9
Antidepressants					
Men	0.3	1.8	1.9	2.8	1.3
Women	2.1	1.1	4.7	4.1	2.8
Antipsychotics					
Men	0.8	0.4	2	1.1	1
Women	1.8	2.1	0.6	1.2	1.5
Any of the five classes					
Men	6.1	9.7	18.3	16.2	11
Women	13.3	21.4	26.5	27.5	20.2
Number of Persons, (unweighted)					
Men	(452)	(257)	(340)	(285)	(1,334)
Women	(577)	(310)	(427)	(513)	(1,827)

Note: Figures refer to use of medications obtained through conventional medical channels, excluding hospital use.

ical and physical well-being of the patient. With respect to the hypnotics and minor tranquilizers, long-term continuous use raises important questions about potential for physical dependence as well as efficacy. These concerns sometimes overshadow the fact that, under some conditions, underuse of psychotherapeutic drugs can pose health risks that are no less serious than overuse. The self-initiated discontinuation or underuse of antidepressants by a suicidal patient illustrates the point.

In table 12-3, therefore, we present data on patterns of using medically prescribed psychotherapeutic drugs. We have defined these patterns in terms of two characteristics of use: (1) longest period (duration) of regular daily use and (2) frequency of use—that is total number of days used during the past year.

Table 12–3
Past-Year Pattern of Use of Medically Prescribed Psychotherapeutic Drugs, by Drug Class

	Percent Distributions for Drug Class				
Daily Use[a] *Total Days*[b]	*Anti-anxiety Agents*	*Hypnotics*	*Daytime Sedatives*	*Anti-depressants*	*Anti-psychotics*
Daily use < 7 consecutive days					
Total < 30 days	4.7	1.6	0.4	0.2	0.4
Total ≥ 30 days	1.3	0.2	0	0.1	0
Daily use 7–13 consecutive days					
Total < 30 days	0.5	c	0.1	0.1	0.1
Total ≥ 30 days	0.3	0.1	0	0	0
Consecutive daily use ≥ 2 < 4 weeks					
Total < 30 days	0.3	0	c	0.1	0.1
Total ≥ 30 days	0.2	0.1	c	c	0
Consecutive daily use ≥ 1 < 4 months	1.4	0.1	0.1	0.5	0.2
Consecutive daily use ≥ 4 < 12 months	0.6	0.2	0.1	0.2	0.1
Consecutive daily use ≥ 12 months	1.6	0.3	0.5	0.8	0.3
Pattern not ascertained	0.2	c	c	c	c
Did not use drug in class in past year	88.9	97.4	98.7	97.90	98.7
Number of persons (unweighted)	(3,161)	(3,161)	(3,161)	(3,161)	(3,161)

Note: Figures refer to use of medications obtained through conventional medical channels, excluding hospital use.

[a] Longest period of daily use. (See text for definition.)

[b] Total number of days on which drug was used during the past year.

[c] Less than 0.05 percent.

Several features of the classification should be noted. First, it applies only to people who had used a medication in a specified class during the previous twelve months. Second, the patterns themselves apply to use during the past year. This comment is obvious as it applies to number of days of use during the past twelve months; it is less obvious with respect to longest period of continuous use, which could have begun more than twelve months prior to the interview and was so counted if it did. Third, in calculating longest period of daily use, we included medications that were last used more than twelve months ago, provided that those medications had been used on a regular daily basis and that last use either coincided with or overlapped the first use of another medication in the same class that was used daily for a period that continued into the present year.[22]

These classification rules are somewhat arbitrary, of course, and they are deliberately conservative in that they recognize long periods of regular use of one or more medications with similar clinical action, even though some of that use may have occurred outside the current year. In this respect, the classification system gives priority to daily use of long duration because of the potential clinical and pharmacological significance of such use.

The patterns of use described in table 12–3 thus differentiate, first, on the basis of longest period of daily use. Then, for each of the three periods involving use for less than four weeks, we further distinguish according to use on less than thirty days during the past twelve months versus use on thirty or more days. Notice, of course, that daily use for one month or longer implies (generally) a frequency of thirty or more days.

We call attention to the following results in table 12–3:

> Although the figures shown in this table are small, it is clear that for medically prescribed anti-anxiety agents and hypnotics, short-term and infrequent use is more common than long-term daily use. For example, 4.7 percent of the persons in the sample used anti-anxiety agents for less than thirty days during the year before interview and never used these medications for as many as seven days in a row. Another 0.8 percent used drugs in this class for more than six days in a row but less than thirty days in all. Altogether then, we estimate that 5.5 percent of the persons in the general population used anti-anxiety agents for a total of less than thirty days during the past year. These persons constitute almost exactly half of the users of anti-anxiety agents.[23]
>
> At the other end of the scale, 1.6 percent of the persons in this national sample (14.8 percent of the users) reported a period of longest daily use of anti-anxiety agents that was twelve months or longer. These persons, together with the 0.6 percent of the sample who had used daily more than four and less than twelve months constitute about twenty percent of the users and represent a group about which one might be concerned. More on this later.
>
> As one might expect, patterns of hypnotic use are weighted even more heavily in the direction of short-term and infrequent use. A total of 1.6 percent of the sample (61.2 percent of the users) had used hypnotics

on fewer than thirty days during the past year and had not used them as many as seven days in a row.

Again, however, we found some persons using hypnotics regularly for longer periods of time than current medical opinion would deem advisable in ordinary circumstances. In particular, 0.6 percent reported using these medications daily for a month or longer, and 0.3 percent reported daily use for twelve or more months. The former constitute 22.2 percent of the hypnotics users and the latter, 10.5 percent.

Patterns of using antidepressants are in striking contrast to those found for the anti-anxiety agents and especially the hypnotics. Typically, the antidepressants are used regularly for rather extended periods of time. Among the users of this class of medications, 71.4 percent used daily for a month or longer, and 38.3 percent reported using daily for at least a year. Use for periods as long as these undoubtedly denotes a substantial period of illness and is consistent with prevailing standards of medical practice.

Use of Medications from Other Sources. Thus far, we have focused on use of psychotherapeutic drugs that were prescribed medically and obtained in conventional fashion. In table 12–4, we turn to use of prescription-type drugs that were obtained through nonmedical channels—that is, by borrowing from a friend, relative, or spouse. We use the shorthand term, NRx, to refer to prescription-type drugs obtained in this manner.[24] Table 12–4 also shows prevalence of use of OTC sleeping pills and tranquilizers. The major findings are as follows:

During the year prior to interview, 3.6 percent of the women and 2.5 percent of the men (NS) reported using a prescription-type medication they had obtained from a nonmedical source. For all persons the figure is 3.1 percent.

Of the five classes, anti-anxiety agents were most likely to have been obtained outside medical channels (2.3 percent of the women, 2 percent of the men), followed by hypnotics (0.9 percent of the women, 0.4 percent of the men). The differences are not statistically significant. The prevalence of NRx use of the other classes of drugs was even smaller and is not shown here.

Whereas use of medically prescribed psychotherapeutic drugs tends to be related positively to age, NRx use is found more often among younger persons than older persons.

OTC drugs (those marketed as sleeping pills or tranquilizers) are used somewhat more widely than the NRx drugs—3.9 percent versus 2.5

Table 12-4
Prevalence of Past-Year Use of Psychotherapeutic Drugs that Were Obtained without a Prescription or OTC, by Drug Class, Age, and Sex

Source, Drug Class, and Sex	*Percent Using during Past Twelve Months in Age Group*				
	18–34	*35–49*	*50–64*	*65–79*	*All*
Nonprescription source[a]					
Anti-anxiety agents					
Men	2.8	1.9	1.1	1.1	2
Women	3.6	1.2	1.8	1.3	2.3
Hypnotics					
Men	0.8	0	0	0.4	0.4
Women	1.9	0	0.6	0.3	0.9
Any of the five classes					
Men	3.6	1.9	1.1	1.9	2.5
Women	6.3	1.5	2.3	1.6	3.6
OTC source[b]					
Sleeping pills					
Men	5.1	3	0.3	2.1	3.2
Women	5	1.2	1.6	2	2.9
Tranquilizers					
Men	1	1.4	0.2	0	0.8
Women	1.1	1.2	1.8	1.3	1.3
Either					
Men	6.1	4.4	0.5	2.1	3.9
Women	6.1	2.4	3.4	3	4.2
Number of persons (unweighted)					
Men	(452)	(257)	(340)	(285)	(1,334)
Women	(577)	(310)	(427)	(513)	(1,827)

[a]Nonprescription refers to any of the five classes of prescription-type medications that were obtained through nonmedical channels—for example, by borrowing from a friend or relative.
[b]OTC denotes medications that are marketed as sleeping pills or tranquilizers and that can be purchased over the counter at a drug store or other store.

percent for men (NS) and 4.2 percent versus 3.6 percent for women (NS). Among OTC drugs, use of sleeping pills is more prevalent than use of tranquilizers.

Like the NRx drugs, we found use of OTC drugs to be more common among younger persons than older persons. Unlike the NRx drugs, however, prevalence of OTC use is about as high among men as it is among women.

Table 12–5 presents data on patterns of use for two of the five classes of NRx drugs, as well as any NRx, and for any OTC drug. Data for the remaining specific classes are based on too few cases to justify showing separately. From these data we draw the conclusion that, typically, NRx and OTC drugs are used infrequently and seldom on a daily basis for as long as a week at a time. We found 0.1 percent of the persons in the national survey reporting daily use of an NRx drug for a period of one to four months. These persons constituted about 3 percent of all NRx users. No one reported daily use for more than four months. Similarly, about 8 percent of the OTC users (0.3 percent of the total sample) reported using these drugs daily for a month or longer. About 3 percent of the OTC users said they had used OTC drugs daily for a year or longer. These persons were 0.1 percent of the total sample.

Discussion

Early in this chapter we reported a number of broad conclusions based on analysis of data from various sources prior to the 1979 National Survey of Psychotherapeutic Drug Use. In general, our examination of the earlier data supported the view that the prescribing practices of physicians, as well as the attitudes and drug-using behavior of the general public, tend to be moderate or conservative. Our criterion for this judgment was a reasonably good fit of data from the earlier survey and other sources to an implicit therapeutic model defining reasonable use of these medications in general medical practice. One might quarrel with that therapeutic model, if only to argue that clinical indications and treatment standards for the use of psychotherapeutic drugs in outpatients are not as clearly formulated or as normally agreed upon as one might wish. Nevertheless, the fact remains that the survey and other data on outpatient medical use seemed to be consistent with prevailing standards of reasonable medical practice.

Data from the 1979 survey reported here and in two other recent papers continue to support that general view.[25] In this chapter, for example, we have shown that psychotherapeutic drugs typically are used infrequently and for short periods of time, except in the case of two classes (antidepressants and antipsychotics) for which regular use for longer periods of time usually is deemed advisable. We have found that some use of prescription drugs are obtained outside medical channels. The prevalence of such use was low, however, and patterns of use (as in the case of OTC drugs) were infrequent and of short duration in the great majority of cases.

In a recent paper we compared the prevalence of use in 1979 with that in 1970. Overall, we found essentially no differences in prevalence, except for small but statistically significant declines in the prevalence of using hyp-

Table 12–5
Past-Year Patterns of Use of Psychotherapeutic Drugs that Were Obtained without a Prescription or OTC, by Drug Class

	Nonprescription[a] *(Percent)*			
Daily Use Total Days	*Anti-anxiety Agents*	*Hypnotics*	*Any*	*OTC*[b] *(Percent)*
Daily use < 7 days				
Total < 30 days	1.9	0.5	2.6	3.4
Total ≥ 30 days	0.1	0	0.1	0.2
Daily use 7–13 days	[c]	0	0.1	0.1
Daily use ≥ 2 < 4 weeks	0	0	0	[c]
Daily use ≥ 1 < 4 months	0.1	0	0.1	0.2
Daily use ≥ 4 < 12 months	0	0	0	[c]
Daily use ≥ 12 months	0	0	0	0.1
Pattern not ascertained	0.1	0.1	0.1	0.1
Did not use drug in class in past year	97.8	99.3	96.9	95.9
Number of persons (unweighted)	(3,161)	(3,161)	(3,161)	(3,161)

[a] Nonprescription denotes prescription type medications that were obtained through nonmedical channels—for example, borrowed from a friend or relative.

[b] OTC denotes medications that are marketed as sleeping pills or tranquilizers and that can be purchased over the counter at a drugstore or other store.

[c] Less than 0.05 percent.

notics and daytime sedatives. In the same paper, we reported evidence of increasing conservatism on the part of physicians in their prescribing practices. In another recent paper, we have reported that the attitudes of the U.S. public toward use of minor tranquilizers were much more negative in certain respects than they were nine years earlier.[26]

Although the picture that emerges from our current research is more comforting than alarming, there are potential trouble spots. We reported, for example, that 1.6 percent of the persons in the 1979 sample (about 15 percent of the anti-anxiety-agent users) had used these medications daily for a year or longer. Similarly, we found a minority of users of hypnotics who reported daily use of those medications for periods of time longer than empirical evidence or present clinical standards would seem to justify. More-searching questions about appropriateness of use might well be focused on these users. For example, what are the age, sex, and other demographic characteristics of these long-term users? What types and levels of emotional distress and situational stress do they exhibit? From what physical disorders do they suffer? Are these disorders incompatible with psychotherapeutic-drug treatment? Are they chronic illnesses, and do they occur in combination with high levels of distress? Have these persons experienced any adverse effects from using the medications? Has medical surveillance been adequate? To what extent is long-term regular use of these medications associated with the heavy and frequent use of alcohol or other medications?

In short, what is the clinical, pharmacological, and demographic context within which long-term regular use of anti-anxiety agents or hypnotics occurs? The 1979 survey was designed specifically with these and similar questions in mind. In the near future, therefore, it should be possible to provide data in greater detail that will enable us to draw more-refined evaluations regarding the use of psychotherapeutic drugs in the United States.

Notes

1. G.D. Mellinger, M.B. Balter, and D.I. Manheimer, "Patterns of Psychotherapeutic Drug Use among Adults in San Francisco," *Archives of General Psychiatry* 25 (1971):385–394; D.I. Manheimer et al., "Popular Attitudes and Beliefs about Tranquilizers," *American Journal of Psychiatry* 130 (1973):1246–1253; H.J. Parry et al., "National Patterns of Psychotherapeutic Drug Use," *Archives of General Psychiatry* 28 (1973):769–784; G.D. Mellinger et al., "An Overview of Psychotherapeutic Drug Use in the United States," *Drug Use: Epidemiological and Sociological Approaches,* eds. E. Josephson and E.E. Carroll (New York: Wiley & Sons, 1974) pp. 333–366; E.H. Uhlenhuth et al., "Symptom Intensity and Life Stress in the City," *Archives of General Psychiatry* 31 (1974):759–764; G.D. Mellinger et al. "Psychic Distress, Life Crisis, and Use of Psychotherapeutic Medications: National Drug Survey Data," *Archives of General Psychiatry* 35 (1978):1045–1052; E.H. Uhlenhuth, M.B. Balter, and R.S. Lipman, "Minor Tranquilizers: Clinical Correlates of Use in an Urban Population," *Archives of General Psychiatry* 35 (1978):650–655; and C.L. Huffine et al., *Structural Stress and Psychological Health: Testing Gove's Thesis* (Submitted for publication).

2. This research was supported by Public Health Service grants MH-12590, MH-12591, and MH-29819.

3. *National Prescription Audit* (Ambler, Pa.: IMS America, Ltd.) (formerly Gosselin & Co.).

4. Audatrex, IMS America, Ltd., special analyses by M.B. Balter.

5. *National Disease & Therapeutic Index* (NDTI), IMS America, Ltd. (formerly Lea & Associates), special analyses by M.B. Balter. See also M.B. Balter and J. Levine, "Character and Extent of Psychotherapeutic Drug

Usage in the United States, *Proceedings of the Fifth World Congress of Psychiatry, Mexico, 1971* (Amsterdam: Excerpta Medica, 1973); M.B. Balter, "An Analysis of Psychotherapeutic Drug Consumption in the United States," *Proceedings of the Anglo-American Conference on Drug Abuse* (London: Royal Society of Medicine, 1973), pp. 58–68; M.B. Balter "Coping with Illness: Choices, Alternatives and Consequences," in *Drug Development and Marketing,* ed. R.B. Helms (Washington, D.C.: American Enterprise Institute Center for Health Research, 1974); and M.B. Balter and M.L. Bauer, "Patterns of Prescribing and Use of Hypnotic Drugs in the United States," in *Sleep Disturbance and Hypnotic Drug Dependence,* ed. A.D. Clift (Amsterdam: Excerpta Medica, 1975).

6. M.B. Balter, J. Levine, and D.I. Manheimer, "Cross-national Study of the Extent of Anti-anxiety/Sedative Drug Use," *New England Journal of Medicine* 390 (1974):769–774.

7. H.J. Parry, M.B. Balter, and I.H. Cisin, "Primary Levels of Under-reporting of Psychotropic Drug Use," *Public Opinion Quarterly* 34 (1970–1971):582–592; and G.D. Mellinger, M.B. Balter, and E.H. Uhlenhuth "Evaluating a Household Survey Measure of Psychic Distress: I. Methods and Basic Findings of the Philadelphia Survey-Clinic Study. II. Improving Levels of Agreement between Survey and Clinical Measures" (In preparation, 1981).

8. Balter, "Coping with Illness," pp. 30–31.

9. G.D. Mellinger, M.B. Balter, and I.H. Cisin, "Changes in Medical Use of Psychotherapeutic Drugs: Results from National Surveys in 1970 and 1979" (In preparation).

10. Ibid., pp. 12–14.

11. Balter and Levine, "Character and Extent," pp. 87–88; Balter, "Analysis of Psychotherapeutic Drug Consumption," pp. 62–63, 65; Balter and Bauer, "Patterns of Prescribing," pp. 276–288, 291; and Mellinger, Balter, and Cisin, "Changes in Medical Use," pp. 25–26.

12. Parry, et al., "National Patterns," p. 774; Balter and Levine, "Character and Extent," p. 85; Balter, "Analysis of Psychotherapeutic Drug Consumption," p. 63; and M.B. Balter and J. Levine, "The Nature and Extent of Psychotropic Drug Usage in the United States," *Psychopharmacology Bulletin* 4 (1969):10.

13. Balter and Levine, "Character and Extent," pp. 84–85; Balter, "Analysis of Psychotherapeutic Drug Consumption," p. 62; and Balter and Levine, "Nature and Extent," p. 84.

14. Manheimer et al., "Popular Attitudes," p. 1249.

15. Mellinger et al., "Psychic Distress," pp. 1050–1051.

16. Ibid., p. 1051.

17. Mellinger et al., "Overview of Psychotherapeutic Drug Use," pp. 345–349.

18. Balter, Levine, and Manheimer, "Cross-national Study," p. 7.

19. Parry, Balter, and Cisin, "Primary Levels of Under-reporting," p. 587.

20. This oversampling was made possible with supplemental funding from the Center for Studies of the Mental Health of the Aging, NIMH.

21. The data also are weighted to compensate for two other inequalities in selection probability: (1) Only one respondent was selected per household; thus (since all households had an equal probability of selection), each person in a large household was less likely to be selected than each person in a smaller household. (2) A few listing areas were selected at a lower rate than others.

22. An example may help. Mr. A. first used chlordiazepoxide eighteen months ago and used it daily until fourteen months ago. Mr. A also reported first using diazepam fourteen months ago and used it daily until eleven months ago. We gave Mr. A. credit for a total of seven (eighteen to eleven) months of daily use.

23. Examination of more-detailed tabulations than those shown here reveals that 63 percent of the users of anti-anxiety agents reported using them on fewer than sixty days during the previous twelve months—that is, an average of less than once a week.

24. We defined as NRx users persons who said either they usually obtain these drugs from nonmedical sources or the last time they obtained such a drug it was from a nonmedical source. Of the NRx drugs, about 49 percent were obtained from a friend, 16 percent from the person's spouse, 27 percent from a relative, and the remainder from other sources. Men were more likely than women to obtain NRx drugs from a friend or wife; women were more likely to obtain them from a relative.

25. Mellinger, Balter, and Cisin, "Changes in Medical Use," p. 5; and J. Clinthorne et al., "Changes in Popular Attitudes and Beliefs about Tranquilizers: 1970–1979" Presented at the American College of Neuropsychopharmacology, 20th Annual Meeting, San Diago, Dec. 15 1981.

26. Clinthorne, "Changes in Popular Attitudes," p. 9.

13 Some Comments on the Clinical Appropriateness of Prescribing Psychoactive Drugs

Ruth Cooperstock

As a preface to this chapter on the clinical appropriateness of current psychotropic-drug use, I would like to share some remarks I heard recently on a radio program called "Cross Country Check-up." This is a two-hour long Canadian Broadcasting Corporation national program in which the audience phones in comments on the week's topic following its introduction by a guest expert. The topic under discussion was whether or not we use too many tranquilizers, and the studio guest was Dr. Heinz Lehmann, a noted psychopharmacologist.

Dr. Lehmann took the position that any psychic discomfort or suffering is undesirable and should always be minimized, with pharmacological agents as the cheapest and most practical means. For example, if flying creates anxiety, one should not hesitate to take diazepam prior to boarding a plane. Later on in the program he suggested that if there were appropriate consumer education over the next fifteen years or so, then it would be perfectly acceptable to permit diazepam to be sold OTC. Dr. Lehmann cited the work of John Marks extensively, particularly Marks's data on dependence that suggest that dependence is a phenomenon of such rare incidence as to be startling when it does occur.[1]

What may be of most interest here is the response Dr. Lehmann's remarks generated. There were calls from medical students, consumers of drugs, relatives of consumers, and practicing physicians. These people were reporting on their own experiences and, particularly in the case of the physicians and relatives, on their observations of dependence. Out of the more than twenty phone calls, only one supported Dr. Lehmann's position. If one can accept the clinical assessments of the general practitioners and psychiatrists who called in reporting their own observations and experiences, dependence is a more-common phenomenon than has been reported in the literature. Although neither benzodiazepine dependence nor phone-in programs are the subject under discussion, this anecdote at least illustrates some of the issues involved in a consideration of clinical appropriateness.

I find myself as a sociologist in the curious position of criticizing others

This commentary is not a specific rejoinder to chapter 12. That work was not available to this author at the time her article was prepared.

for relying on the tools of my own discipline to assess prevalence, patterns of use, and particularly, clinical appropriateness of use. Drs. Mellinger and Balter,[2] among others, have studied consistently psychotherapeutic-drug use through the use of large-scale surveys that utilize self-reports of life stress and drug use. Such surveys may be valuable in the measurement of consumption, especially when used in conjunction with prescription data and other sources of information like sales data to validate their findings. Another means of external validation is comparison with the findings of other investigators. Such cross checks and comparisons are desirable because there is good indication from the field of alcohol research that high consumers of alcohol underreport their use by approximately 50 percent in surveys and self-report studies when contrasted with sales figures.[3] These data suggest that serious validity problems may exist in relation to studies of any substances where stigma may be attached to use by some or many segments of the population.

In the case of psychoactive substance users, an additional problem related to the use of survey techniques is that of memory loss. Because of the demonstrated poor recall for major health events like a hospitalization, other researchers have established two weeks as the optimal period of recall in order to avoid underreporting.[4] Canadian and U.K. data, whether based on prescriptions or surveys, have identified the elderly as the highest consumers of anxiolytics, sedatives, and hypnotics.[5] Because of their higher levels of chronic illness and problems associated with aging, the elderly are also significantly higher consumers of prescription drugs overall, thus leading to the expectation of greater recall problems. Perhaps the most compelling argument for limiting questions to a short time period is the experimental and clinical findings of memory impairment resulting from normal doses of benzodiazepines, the most commonly prescribed anxiolytics and hypnotics.[6]

Clearly, there are many valuable and important uses of sedative/hypnotic drugs. There is general agreement that the basic uses should include in-hospital use for pre-anaesthesia and as hypnotics, for treatment of neuromuscular disorders, in acute anxiety, and to break the pattern of severe insomnia. However, I think we have to examine what is meant by clinical appropriateness, particularly as related to long-term use of sedative/hypnotics.

Perhaps many means exist, other than large-scale national surveys, by which clinical appropriateness can be measured. Studies that utilize an individual's medical records and that link these data with intensive inverviews are to my mind more likely to result in meaningful assessments of clinical appropriateness of physician's prescribing practices. Examples of some of the preliminary questions and issues that could be assessed within this context include the following: When was the last time you saw your doctor?

What drug(s) are you currently using? (This question permits an examination of total drug use and does not limit reporting to discrete classes or individual drugs.) For how long have you been using it (them)?

We are all familiar with the data that demonstrate that the established period of effectiveness of many sedative/hypnotics, particularly anti-anxiety agents, is not more than about two to four weeks.[7] Thus, the question of the length of time the substance has been consumed becomes quite critical in any assessment of clinical appropriateness. A recent study by Anderson found that more than half (56 percent) of psychotropic drugs used by a sample of adults in the United Kingdom initially had been prescribed more than one year previously and that almost half (48 percent) had been prescribed first two or more years earlier.[8] Fourteen percent of all people aged 55 and over were taking psychotropic drugs (primarily sedatives and hypnotics) that had been prescribed more than a year previously. Nearly three-fifths of all repeat prescriptions for this class of drug had been obtained without seeing the prescribing physician. Another recent study in the United Kingdom demonstrated that the older the individual the longer she or he was likely to have used a continuous prescription for psychotropics.[9] Conversely, with increasing age the likelihood of seeing a physician when receiving the prescription was diminished.

An Ontario study of preparations dispensed through an insuring agency found that almost half of all those receiving a prescription for a psychotropic in one year were likely to receive another such prescription three years later.[10] Thus, for the United Kingdom and Canada, at least, we see patterns of use extending over many years and a direct correlation between increasing age and rates of use. If physicians' assessments are accepted as an important component in the evaluation of the clinical appropriateness of prescription-drug use, then this lack of regular physician-patient contact would render such assessment difficult.

Although the efficacy of many sedative/hypnotics as anti-anxiety agents has not been proven for longer than a few weeks, one might argue that these drugs are acceptable for long-term use because of their possible placebo effect. If that is the case, is there any reason for concern? Can one of the acceptable criteria for clinical appropriateness be long-term use? Data suggest that attendant problems may exist that are frequently not evident to users and that will not be elicited via survey techniques. I am referring here to the problem of dependence and the possibilities of cognitive, memory, and motor impairment.

Data on dependence emerge from clinical case studies, controlled clinical trials, and intensive natural-history studies. We may become aware of the potential extent of dependence from surveys such as Anderson's cited earlier or that of Uhlenhuth, Balter, and Lipman, but its actual nature and gravity can be discerned only through the use of other methods.[11] Tyrer,

Rutherford, and Huggett conducted a controlled double-blind study of withdrawal among long-term, normal-dose users of benzodiazepines.[12] Depending upon the criteria applied, either 27 percent or 45 percent were found to be physically dependent on these drugs. Both Tyrer and associates and Petursson and Lader,[13] who also found marked withdrawal reactions in low-dose, long-term users of benzodiazepines, claimed that their data suggest a true withdrawal syndrome as distinct from the reemergence of the original symptoms for which the drug was prescribed. Both sets of investigators reported that many of the symptoms seen were not typical of anxiety, thus further supporting their thesis of pharmacological dependence.

Another area of knowledge that would appear relevant to an assessment of clinical appropriateness is information on the concurrent use of other prescribed or OTC drugs or of other substances used by the individual that affect the central nervous system. The most obvious concern is with the use of alcohol. Between 33 and 40 percent of patients attending two large treatment centers in Ontario for treatment of alcohol-related problems are reported to be users of and frequently dependent upon benzodiazepines.[14]

Because of the numbers of individuals in any developed nation who are using sedative/hypnotics on any given day, it is of special importance to investigate cognitive, memory, and learning impairment in judging clinical appropriateness. If such impairment is evident in an individual, then a risk-benefit analysis of his or her drug use would appear to be in order. Reviewing only controlled studies, Wittenborn found that both memory and learning are impaired by normal doses of benzodiazepines.[15] The deficit was particularly evident with regard to material learned during the period of drug use. While these studies were largely experimental in nature, Petursson and Lader found learning deficits in a population of long-term users of benzodiazepines.[16] These data are consistent with the responses of current and former benzodiazepine users studied at the Addiction Research Foundation of Ontario.[17] Almost all of these informants had acquired their drugs via prescriptions and had used them at normal dose levels.

Significantly, it was those individuals who used the benzodiazepines intermittently or had ceased use who commented on their learning and memory deficits. In some cases, informants quoted statements of family members regarding changes the users had not observed in themselves. An intermittent user said:

> [W]hile I was off the drug I was much more alert mentally, could think more rapidly and efficiently, and respond more actively to all stimuli.

Another ex-user commented that her school grades improved, while yet another said:

> I've also noticed over the period of half a year being off them that gradually month by month my thinking has gotten clearer and clearer. And my

> bridge playing has improved 2000%. And I'm much better at work. In every way my thinking is better.

In total, 26 percent of informants reported some cognitive or perceptual disturbance or deficit while on the drug, with the most frequent being an inability to concentrate and memory deficits. One-quarter of the informants reported impaired motor skills; driving performance and poorer coordination were the most frequent problems of this type mentioned.

More distressing to some of the informants than any of these problems was the effect of the drugs in dulling their emotional responses and the lethargic feelings that accompanied use. It is interesting that while 3 percent of those interviewed welcomed the masking effect, over one-third found the lethargy and dulling effect distressing. Many of these individuals reported feeling unmotivated to act—for example, to play with children after a day's work, to find a part-time job, and so forth. In many people this lethargy appeared to lower an already low self-esteem.

The primary social effect we found was that people saw the continued use of these drugs as a means of maintaining themselves in uncomfortable or conflict-laden social roles.[18] The female informants, especially, quickly ceased discussing their general health or emotional state and went on to relate their continued use of tranquilizers to problems within their marriages or family life. The drugs were described as substances that kept their anger from exploding, that permitted these women to behave like the compliant and loving wives they felt they should be. Among the male informants, use was identified commonly as a means of reducing tensions and anxieties generated by their work situations. Rather than functioning to hold a poor marriage together, as was the case for many women, continued drug use by the men served as a means of holding down an onerous job. These group interviews were striking for the awareness displayed by the informants of the structural problems in their lives. Many individuals recognized that their continued use of tranquilizers (as opposed to initial use) related less to their level of anxiety or general physical health than to unsatisfactory aspects of their life situations.

In many cases, those who had ceased using drugs had made a variety of changes in their lives. They talked of initiating marital counseling with their spouses, of changing jobs, of moving into the labor force, of joining support groups such as Al-Anon, or of planning for child care so that exercise or other classes were possible. There was little talk of substituting alcohol or other substances as coping modalities. One would hope that future studies of sedative/hypnotic-drug use would examine the full range of chemical and nonchemical coping modalities. Studies might explore the range and variety of means used to handle the high levels of psychological distress found in self-reported studies. In addition to visiting their general practitioners, do people first go, for example, to friends, family, counselors, consciousness-raising groups, or join new support networks? Is there differential utilization of such activities by the sexes and by different age, socioeconomic, and ethnic groups? If so, are such activities related to long-term psychotropic-drug use in these populations?

The survey data that continue to be cited widely in articles on psychotropic-drug use cannot by themselves be used to address many of the issues raised here. One would have to believe in an existential, nearly nonsocial, free-floating anxiety as etiologically significant in order to accept the survey method alone as a valid means of assessing appropriateness of prescribing. Instead, I would suggest that only careful, open-ended interview situations handled with great skill can, in fact, elicit the social and interpersonal causes of the tensions and anxieties that we are discussing. These are very real problems, they exist in a real world, and they may be addressed more successfully and humanely by nonchemical means, with short-term sedative/hypnotic-drug use only one of many possible modalities used to effect change.

Notes

1. J. Marks, *The Benzodiazepines—Use, Overuse, Misuse, Abuse* (Lancaster, England, MTP Press, 1978), p. 45.
2. G.D. Mellinger and M.B. Balter, "Psychotherapeutic Drugs: A Current Assessment," this volume.
3. R.E. Popham, and W. Schmidt, "Words and Deeds: The Validity of Self-Report Data on Alcohol Consumption," *Journal of Studies on Alcohol* 42 (March 1981):355–368.
4. U.S. DHEW, "Prescribed and Nonprescribed Medicines: Type and Use of Medicines, United States, July 1964–June 1965," *Vital and Health Statistics,* Series 10, no. 39 (1967), p. 2.
5. Canada Health Survey, *The Health of Canadians: Report of the Canada Health Survey,* Catalogue 82-538E (Ottowa: Health and Welfare Canada and Statistics Canada, June 1981); Saskatchewan Joint Committee of Drug Utilization, *Utilization of Mood-Modifying Drugs in Saskatchewan: 1977,* Report no. 3, (Regina, Saskatchewan, October 1979); R.M. Anderson, "The Use of Repeatedly Prescribed Medicines," *Journal of the Royal College of General Practitioners* 30 (October 1980):609–613; and K. Dunnell and A. Cartwright, *Medicine Takers, Prescribers and Hoarders* (London: Routledge & Kegan Paul, 1972).
6. R.A. Kleinknecht and D. Donaldson, "A Review of the Effects of Diazepam on Cognitive and Psychomotor Performance," *Journal of Nervous and Mental Disease* 161 (1975):399–411.

7. E.M. Sellers, "Clinical Pharmacology and Therapeutics of Benzodiazepines," *Canadian Medical Association Journal* 118 (24 June 1978): 1533–1538.

8. Anderson, "Use of Repeatedly Prescribed Medicines."

9. P.J. Dennis, "Monitoring of Psychotropic Drug Prescribing in General Practice," *British Medical Journal* 2 (1979):1115–1116.

10. R. Cooperstock, "Sex Differences in Psychotropic Drug Use," *Social Science and Medicine* 12B (1978):179–186.

11. E.H. Uhlenhuth, M.B. Balter, and R.S. Lipman, "Minor Tranquilizers: Clinical Correlates of Use in an Urban Population," *Archives of General Psychiatry* 35 (May 1978):650–655.

12. P. Tyrer, D. Rutherford, and T. Huggett, "Benzodiazepine Withdrawal Symptoms and Propranolol," *Lancet* (7 March 1981), pp. 520–522.

13. H. Petursson, and M.H. Lader, "Benzodiazepine Dependence," *British Journal of Addiction* 76 (June 1981):133–145.

14. U. Busto et al., "Benzodiazepine Use and Abuse in Alcoholics," *Clinical Pharmacology and Therapeutics* 31 (February 1982):207–208. See also personal communication, Dr. D. Macdonald, Donwood Institute, Toronto.

15. J.R. Wittenborn, "Effects of Benzodiazepines on Psychomotor Performance," *British Journal of Clinical Pharmacology* (Supplement 1) 7 (1979):61–67.

16. H. Petursson and M.H. Lader, "Withdrawal from Long-Term Benzodiazepine Treatment," *British Medical Journal* 283 (5 September 1981):643–645.

17. For a description of the sample and the nature of the study, see R. Cooperstock and H. Lennard, "Some Social Meanings of Tranquilizer Use," *Sociology of Health and Illness* 1 (December 1979):331–347.

18. For a fuller discussion of this point, see ibid.

14 The Regulation of Dangerous Psychoactive Drugs

James C. Anthony

This chapter develops some epidemiological ideas on psychoactive-drug-hazard reduction through regulation. Its focus is on the prescription drugs that are relatively potent influences on human mental life as it can be observed or described. Examples of these drugs include amphetamine, morphine, dextropropoxyphene, diazepam, methaqualone, and the barbiturates.

The term *drug hazard* refers to risks of loss or harm caused by drug activity after ingestion. Here, loss and harm include death, disease, disorder, disability, and their social and economic consequences. In this context, to say that a loss or harm is caused by drug activity means that, all else being equal, the risk of loss or harm falls when the drug is not taken and the risk rises when the drug is taken.

The epidemiological ideas developed in this chapter derive from some basic concepts of communicable-disease and injury epidemiology. These ideas are extensions from work by Gordon and Haddon on the epidemiology of injuries generally,[1] from work done at the University of Minnesota College of Pharmacy on modeling the drug flow from supply sources to an ultimate consumer and the consequences for the consumer and society,[2] and from ideas suggested by others.[3]

The Psychoactive-Drug Reservoir

Several concepts of communicable-disease epidemiology help to show where and when psychoactive-drug-hazard reduction through regulation might be helpful. One of these concepts is the reservoir of an infectious agent. Fox, Hall, and Elveback define the reservoir as "the total mechanism responsible for the perpetuation of the microbial species."[4] They note the utility of drawing analogies between the reservoirs for microbial agents of disease and the reservoirs for inanimate agents. The agents in their examples

This work developed from work with Albert Wertheimer, Tim Church, Chick Ahlgren, and Marc Kurzman and was aided by the teaching of Dr. Leonard Schuman and Mrs. Susan Baker. Of course, I am responsible for any errors.

for such analogies are toxic vapors and the physical force conveyed by a drill press.

These analogies seem to be most useful when they increase understanding of the means by which an inanimate agent is made available for interaction with a susceptible human. As in communicable-disease epidemiology, this increased understanding can lead to suggestions for practical measures to reduce hazards.

If psychoactive drugs are the analogues for the microbial agents in communicable-disease epidemiology, then the reservoir for a psychoactive drug may be defined roughly as the means by which the drug becomes available for consumption and through which availability is sustained. Figure 14–1 is a simplified, general representation of a psychoactive-drug reservoir within the United States. It is not as complex as drug-flow models developed previously[5]; it gives few details on the drug R&D process and other important aspects of the psychoactive-drug reservoir. Nevertheless, this figure, with additions given in the following paragraphs, is adequate for the present discussion of psychoactive-drug regulation.

The upper half of the figure represents the legally authorized channels of drug R&D, supply, and distribution to authorized consumers of the psychoactive drug. The open arrow between the drug R&D unit and the supply and manufacturing units illustrates that there is relatively little flow of drug product between these units; the flow is primarily one of ideas and techniques.

In this representation, the supply of the drug begins with a succession of manufacturing, importation, and storage steps and proceeds to wholesale-distribution and storage steps. The figure shows distribution flowing from the wholesaling unit to a retail unit (for example, pharmacy, clinic) where the drug is stored until it is dispensed to an authorized consumer, who may dispose of it at once or keep it in storage with releases over time.

Of course, some of the legally imported and manufactured drug supplies move through unauthorized channels of distribution to unauthorized consumers or move directly from an authorized consumer to an unauthorized consumer. This diversion may occur throughout the reservoir, with and without the cooperation of the authorized manufacturer, broker, or consumer (that is, through unauthorized gifts and sales or through theft and forged order forms or prescriptions).

The unauthorized channels of R&D, supply, and distribution are represented in the bottom half of figure 14–1. Diversion from authorized channels to unauthorized channels is shown by means of arrows crossing a line of diversion. The possibility for unauthorized supply through bootlegging and smuggling is represented in the lower half of the figure also.

Figure 14–1 can be used as a more-specific representation of the U.S. reservoir for amphetamine in the late 1960s and early 1970s, somewhat like

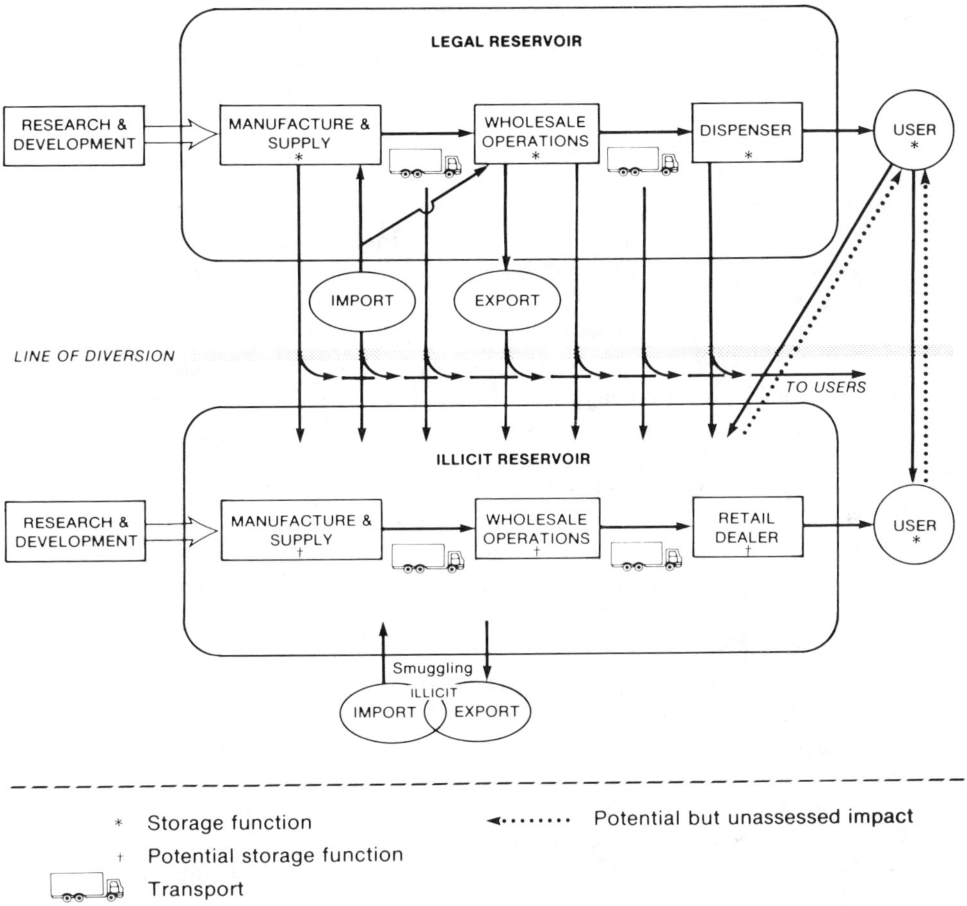

Figure 14–1. Simplified Representation of Psychoactive-Drug Reservoir in the United States, 1982

one drafted by Smith and Wesson.[6] This figure shows we know something of the degree of involvement of specific lines of diversion and unauthorized channels, and others comment on it.[7]

Bootlegging, smuggling, and unauthorized distribution, as well as diversion from authorized manufacturers, have been emphasized. Diversion from authorized wholesalers and dispensers and from authorized common carriers who transport the drug products is mentioned in the reports but seems to have been less prominent. Diversion from authorized consumers also is mentioned in the reports but does not appear to have been of major significance in terms of volume. Diversion of amphetamines from authorized R&D units is not mentioned in the literature.

Vectors, Vehicles, and an Interactive Model

Agents of infectious diseases are taken from reservoir to a host by means of a vector or vehicle, which are animate and inanimate conveyances respectively. However, the distinction between reservoir and vector or vehicle is not always clear cut. For example, the *Aedes aegypti* mosquito is part of the reservoir for the yellow-fever virus and is also a biological vector for transmission to humans. The reservoir for *Clostridium tetani,* the tetanus bacilli, includes soil, which may also be the vehicle for transmission.

In figure 14–1 drug distributors, prescribers, dispensers, and consumers were included as elements of the drug reservoir. Consumers were included because they may be a means of drug availability to others. Consumers also might be regarded as vectors who carry batches of the drug away from the manufacturers toward ultimate consumers. Either view is compatible with the development of epidemiological ideas on psychoactive-drug-hazard reduction through regulation.

It is important to notice the involvement of inanimate material in the storage and conveyance of drugs through and from the reservoir. These include screened and locked areas within factories; drums, boxes, and other containers for shipping between factories and distributors; the unit-dose or other pill containers in which medicines are dispensed; and the nonpsychoactive portion of the drug-product formulation (other therapeutic ingredients, fillers, and so on). Viewing the pill containers, fillers, and so on as vehicles draws attention to them as modifiable aspects of agent transmission to a host.

Once the psychoactive drug reaches the ultimate consumer and is ingested, there begins an interaction of this drug agent, the human host, and their environment. In psychopharmacology as in communicable-disease epidemiology, the results of human exposure to an agent cannot be understood fully without a consideration of this interaction. Drug-caused losses and harms are no exception to this rule.[8]

Figure 14–2 is a revision of figure 14–1 and takes note of inanimate means of conveyance within the reservoir and between the reservoir and consumer. It also depicts a traditional agent, host, and environment-interaction model, as well as some consequences of the interaction. This figure contains lines that go from the consequences on the right back toward the reservoir to indicate feedback to the suppliers, prescribers, and other distributors in the form of demand for new and existing psychoactive-drug products. To illustrate, one potential result of psychoactive-drug-taking

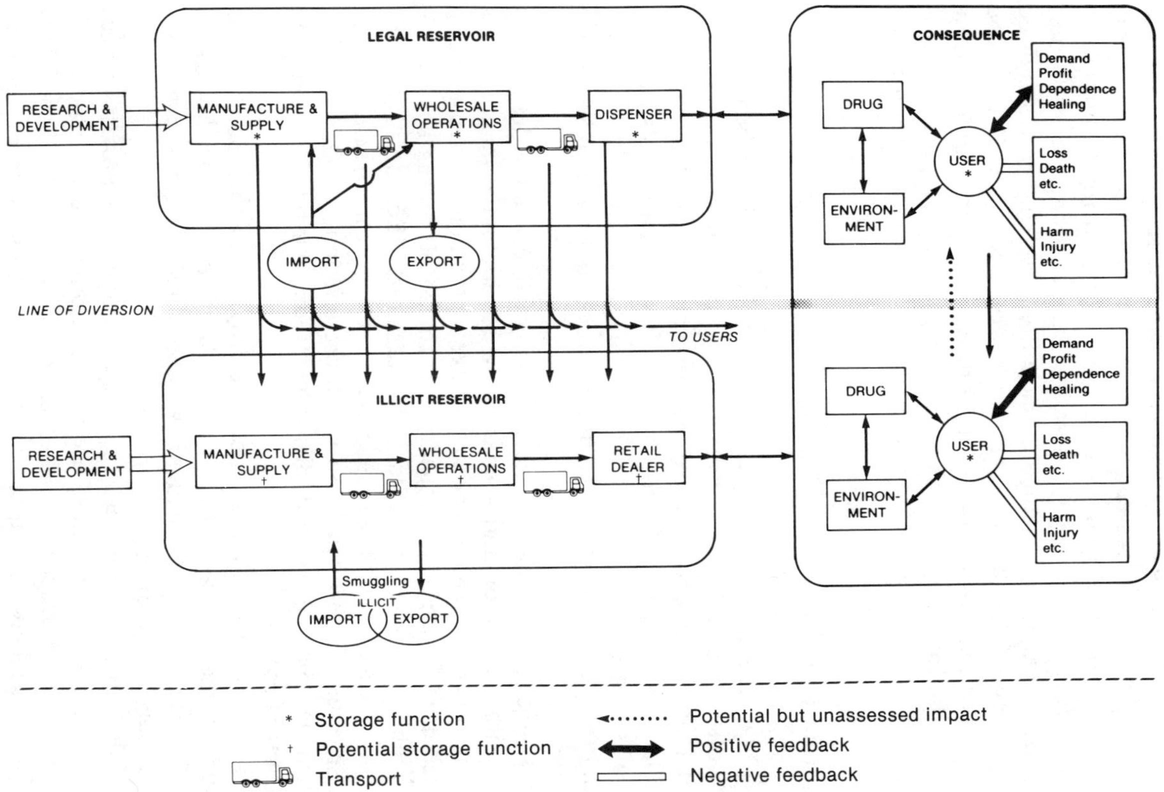

Figure 14-2. Simplified Representation of Psychoactive-Drug Reservoir in the United States, Showing Agent-Host-Environment Interaction and Examples of Its Consequences, 1982

is drug dependence, which entails continued drug use and implied demand for the drug. This demand for the drug affects the reservoir by helping to sustain the availability of the drug.

In summary, figure 14–2 represents a generalized reservoir for psychoactive drugs, showing various channels and elements in the flow of drug supplies to consumers. Appended to the reservoir is a representation of interaction between a drug agent, a host, and their environment, with some of the consequences of this interaction, including losses and harms as listed at the beginning of the chapter. The figure takes note of R&D units and demand from consumers as sources of influence within and upon the drug reservoir. In the following sections of this chapter, this graphic display is applied in a review of present federal regulation of psychoactive drugs.

The Controlled Substances Act of 1970

Excepting the federal Food, Drug and Cosmetic Act and its amendments, the Controlled Substances Act of 1970 (CSA 1970) is now the primary source of federal regulations on psychoactive drugs in the United States. CSA 1970 authorizes special federal controls over the supply, distribution, and use of any drug with a potential for abuse (excluding alcoholic beverages and tobacco specifically). To impose these controls is to schedule a drug.

CSA 1970 empowers the U.S. attorney general to consult with the secretary of Health, Education and Welfare [now Health and Human Services (DHHS)] in order to decide which drugs have a potential for abuse and to assign each drug to one of five schedules of control. If a drug has no safe and acceptable use in the United States, it is assigned to Schedule I and may be used only in government-approved research. Of more interest in this context are Schedules II through V, to which prescription and OTC psychoactive medicines may be assigned, depending upon their relative safety and potential for abuse.

Schedule II is reserved for psychoactive drugs with a high potential for abuse, and it is the most restrictive of these four medicine schedules. Of the many differences between Schedule II and the three less-restrictive schedules, the following are of prime importance.

Schedule II drugs are subject to production and import quotas, whereas medicines in the other schedules are not. Schedule II drug-import-and-export activities require special government permission, and all Schedule II drug transactions between suppliers and distributors must be reported routinely to the government; only the narcotic drugs in the other schedules are subject to these regulations. Special security measures like vault storage and special order forms are required for Schedule II drugs; less-intensive measures apply to the medicines in the other schedules. A new written prescription is required each time a Schedule II drug is dispensed, and no prescription refills are permitted. Prescriptions for Schedule III and IV medicines may be written or oral, and they may be refilled up to five times within six months of original issuance or renewal by the prescriber. Finally, the maximum criminal penalties for unauthorized trafficking (manufacture or distribution) in Schedule II narcotics are greater than those for trafficking in other scheduled drugs.

These major differences between Schedule II and the other medicine schedules should not obscure a basic similarity of the restrictions throughout. Sustaining the tradition of the Harrison Narcotic Act of 1914, CSA 1970 requires special government registration before the supply, distribution, prescribing, or dispensing of any scheduled drug is authorized. In addition, records on the supply and distribution of all these drugs must be kept available for government review. Any international transaction of a scheduled drug by a supplier or distributor must be reported to the government. The security required for the physical storage of these drugs is greater than that required for ordinary prescription products, with suppliers and distributors through the wholesale level required to maintain guards and alarm systems, keeping under constant surveillance areas that are dedicated to storage of the scheduled drugs. The regulations require that the government registration numbers must be checked whenever any of these drugs is distributed prior to dispensing to a consumer. Schedule II, III, and IV drugs may not be issued to a consumer without a valid prescription from a registered prescriber, while the nonprescription products of Schedule V may not be dispensed unless the dispensing party vouchsafes that the purchaser meets specified standards (for example, age and intention to use the product for a legitimate medical purpose). Criminal penalties for simple possession and use of these drugs do not vary by schedule.[9]

The preceding paragraphs indicate that the regulation of psychoactive drugs through CSA 1970 is pervasive. If one were to map the specific CSA 1970 control measures onto the graphic display of the drug reservoir in figure 14–2, there would be only a few unregulated or relatively unregulated elements and transactions. The shippers of scheduled drugs between supply and distribution points are relatively unregulated; the elaborate security systems of the manufacturing plant or permanent storage areas are difficult to reproduce in a portable form. The authorized consumers are also relatively unregulated: Criminal penalties for drug trafficking and Schedule V rules on drugs available without prescription are the only formal CSA 1970 restrictions on individuals in this role. Of course, diversion from consumers does not receive as high a federal drug-law-enforcement priority as unauthorized manufacturers and distributors of scheduled drugs because authorized consumers typically account for only a small proportion of the total volume of drug diversion.

Regulation throughout the reservoir would seem to be highly appropriate when the demand for a drug is relatively high, when drug hazards are at high levels, and when the psychoactive-drug reservoir is like that of amphetamine in the late 1960s and early 1970s. However, is the same true when these conditions do not hold? A review of the dextropropoxyphene situation in the late 1970s will help to clarify the issues raised by this question.

The Dextropropoxyphene Situation

Dextropropoxyphene is an analgesic drug. Since 1957, it has been marketed widely as a prescription-drug product under the name Darvon, a trademark of Eli Lilly and Company. Until 1976, the federal government regulated dextropropoxyphene as a prescription product. It was assigned to CSA 1970 Schedule IV in 1976. The government formally acknowledged its pharmacologic activity and classified it as a narcotic in 1980. This ruling followed a series of regulatory meetings and decisions prompted by two petitions from the Health Research Group, a consumer-advocacy organization. One petition argued that the drug should be declared an imminent hazard and removed from the drug market under the federal Food, Drug and Cosmetic Act. The other petition argued that, if this action were not taken, dextropropoxyphene should be assigned to Schedule II of CSA 1970. Despite the government ruling on dextropropoxyphene as a narcotic, both petitions were denied. However, in April 1980, the secretary-general of the United Nations (UN) advised the U.S. secretary of state of a UN Commission on Narcotic Drugs decision to control dextropropoxyphene as a Schedule II drug under the Single Convention on Narcotic Drugs, a convention that the United States has accepted formally. The Single Convention's Schedule II has some of the features of CSA 1970 Schedule II, such as manufacturing quotas.[10]

There is considerable demand for dextropropoxyphene in the authorized marketplace, as indicated by the number of prescriptions filled annually. In 1977, for example, the National Prescription Audit of IMS America, Ltd., reported that U.S. retail pharmacies filled an estimated 33.5 million dextropropoxyphene prescriptions.[11] Demand in the unauthorized marketplace is indicated by a unit street price several times the unit price in retail pharmacies.[12]

Dextropropoxyphene hazard exists. This drug is mentioned frequently in reports from those who provide the government with statistics on emergency-room visits and deaths involving drugs. For example, the DAWN panel of eighty-five geographically distributed medical examiners' offices reported 2985 drug-induced deaths in calendar year 1979, including suicides. Dextropropoxyphene was mentioned in 353 (12 percent) of these reports.[13]

For decedents who were using the drug just prior to death, it seems that medical examiners judge some 10 to 30 percent of their deaths to be due to dextropropoxyphene by itself. This estimate is important because the 12 percent prevalence of such use among those whose deaths were induced by drugs might simply reflect the prevalence of dextropropoxyphene use by this group just before death, with no implication that it caused any of the deaths.[14] It is important to mention that these medical-consumer reports were not usually accompanied by an analysis of body fluid for the drug.

For the sake of discussion, assume that dextropropoxyphene demand and hazard in the 1970s were at levels at least as high as amphetamine demand and hazard levels in the late 1960s and early 1970s (though this assumption is probably not true). Then, turn to the question of whether CSA 1970's pervasive control measures were suitable for dextropropoxyphene-hazard reduction. Refer again to figure 14–2 while I discuss the dextropropoxyphene reservoir for the United States in the 1970s, as garnered from the scientific and official literature.[15]

There was little diversion from sources of supply and higher-level distribution. There has been some diversion from dispensers via forged prescriptions, theft, and sale, as well as some from consumers via theft, gifts, and sale. There seems to have been very little, if any, supply by unauthorized individuals, though the drug has been available through unauthorized retail dealers. (This representation of the dextropropoxyphene reservoir seems to hold for the entire period of the drug's marketing, including the period from 1957 through 1975 when it was subject to federal prescription-drug controls only.)

Given such a reservoir that apparently would call for regulation targeted toward its specific problems of diversion near the end of the authorized supply and distribution channels, one legitimately may ask why the U.S. government has chosen to control it as a Schedule IV drug, why the U.S. government is considering seriously Schedule II controls, and whether or not alternatives exist to the pervasive tactics of CSA 1970 when a drug reservoir suggests that a more-refined approach is needed?

Why Schedule IV Regulation of Dextropropoxyphene?

By 1976, the regulators had reached a consensus: dextropropoxyphene had a potential for abuse at least in the sense that there was evidence that "individuals [were] taking the drug or drugs containing [dextropropoxyphene] in amounts sufficient to create a hazard to their health or to the safety of other individuals or of the community."[16] In the words of one participant in the decision: "The drug was in fact killing people."[17]

The U.S. attorney general is empowered to apply CSA 1970 controls to any prescription drug having that characteristic of potential for abuse.[18]

Though not required by law, Schedule V traditionally has been reserved for nonprescription products.[19]

Federal law provides for imposing some, but not all, of the regulations of individual CSA 1970 schedules, only if the product is a nonprescription nonnarcotic product, or contains one or more of certain Schedule III, IV, or V depressant or stimulant substances and is compounded with active medicinal ingredients having no depressant or stimulant effects on the central nervous system in order to vitiate the product's potential for abuse.[20]

Why Consider Schedule II Regulation of Dextropropoxyphene?

The Health Research Group petitioned the government to consider Schedule II regulation on the basis of an interpretation that clinical studies "fail to show that dextropropoxyphene is any more effective than aspirin and many show it to be less effective than aspirin, or, in some cases, no more effective than placebo";[21] a judgment that dextropropoxyphene was being prescribed indiscriminately and in situations when other products posing less hazard could be prescribed; a judgment that the many associated deaths outweigh the limited effectiveness of dextropropoxyphene; and a judgment that the Schedule II tactics, especially a manufacturing quota and a prohibition of prescription refills, would be needed to bring about a reduction in the number of dextropropoxyphene prescriptions written, which is the means by which dextropropoxyphene hazards would be reduced.[22] The government could not ignore this petition.

In 1967, the United States made the 1961 Single Convention on Narcotic Drugs part of its treaty obligations and agreed to conform to the rulings of the UN Commission on Narcotic Drugs. As noted previously, the commission has assigned dextropropoxyphene to Schedule II of the convention. To conform, the United States either must assign dextropropoxyphene to the CSA 1970 Schedule II or must impose regulation like a manufacturing quota in Schedule IV.

Do Alternatives Exist to CSA 1970 Regulation?

The U.S. attorney general may control drugs having a potential for abuse under CSA 1970. However, the legislation does not compel the attorney general to do so. Faced with a potential drug hazard or an increasing drug hazard, the attorney general may seek other remedies, with or without the assistance of other agencies of the government (for example, the State Department, the secretary of the DHHS, the FDA, the Center for Disease Control, or the National Institute on Drug Abuse).

The need for other remedies and increased flexibility in applying federal drug-hazard-reduction tactics seems clear. The breadth of CSA 1970 is so great that needed drug-hazard-reduction regulation at some points in the drug reservoir is blocked because strong opposition to irrelevant regulation exists at other points. This seems to have been the case with dextropropoxyphene, as well as other drugs.[23] Moreover, regulation through CSA 1970 adds cost at all levels of supply and distribution. The cost is passed on to the consumer or third-party payers, including the government.[24] The cost of these psychoactive-drug regulations could be much less if the attorney general considered some of the other available remedies.

Appeal for Specific Voluntary Tactics. For example, the FDA Drug Abuse Advisory Committee sought and obtained Eli Lilly and Company's agreement to develop and field an educational campaign for dextropropoxyphene-hazard reduction, directed toward prescribers, dispensers, and consumers.[25]

Drug-Epidemic-Intelligence Service. The attorney general could ask the Center for Disease Control for the assistance of an epidemic-intelligence-service officer in understanding the nature of potential or growing drug hazards involving specific psychoactive drugs. Such an officer's epidemiologic perspective would complement the law-enforcement perspectives of the Drug Enforcement Administration and might suggest alternatives to CSA 1970 regulation for control of the drug hazards. If the intelligence service cannot assist in this way, the National Institute on Drug Abuse might be able to do so.

Local and State Drug-Hazard-Reduction Tactics. Prior to imposing federal regulation via CSA 1970, the attorney general should consider whether or not local or state tactics would be effective. For example, most of the states have controlled-substances legislation analogous to CSA 1970, though few have included specific CSA 1970 tactics such as manufacturing quotas and import-export controls that are more national in focus. If the states' regulations had been used in the early waves of tactics to reduce dextropropoxyphene's hazards, control under CSA 1970 might have been unnecessary. Moreover, it might be unnecessary to apply the state controls if state and local associations and government agencies worked out standards of practice to follow when prescribing and dispensing psychoactive drugs that are diverted only at that level of distribution.

Three points are worth noting in relation to the suggestion to try local and state tactics as the early wave of a formal response to a growing or present psychoactive-drug hazard. First, states and localities with low hazard levels for a specific drug can postpone costly regulations until surveillance suggests that they are due. When CSA 1970 regulation takes effect, there is no possibility for this geopolitical variation in hazard-reduction tactics. Second, the Drug Enforcement Administration, the FDA, and the National Institute on Drug Abuse could work together to evaluate the effects of specific drug-hazard-reduction tactics (like prescription-refill prohibitions) by encouraging the states to stage the introduction of these tactics and employing what Donald Campbell calls an "interrupted time series design" to assess the drug-hazard levels in the first stage of states against the drug-hazard levels in the states staged later.[26] Third, by staging the states properly, one might assess the relative efficacy of certain states' special drug-hazard-reduction tactics such as requirements for triplicate prescription forms with a copy to a state headquarters and limits on the rate at which dosage units may be prescribed or dispensed.

CSA 1970 Exception Provisions. CSA 1970 permits the attorney general to except depressant and stimulant drugs from all or part of the Schedule III, IV, and V controls under the conditions described in the foregoing section. If this excepting power has been used to gain greater flexibility in applying CSA 1970 controls, references to it are well hidden. Nevertheless, it is an option should the proper situation arise.

International Psychoactive-Drug Control. As noted with respect to the Commission on Narcotic Drugs' dextropropoxyphene ruling, the United States is bound by international agreement to regulate the drug by manufacturing quotas. This obligation can be met without assigning it to Schedule II of CSA 1970. In the future, the U.S. government could request control of specific psychoactive drugs under the narcotic- and psychotropic-drug conventions in order to secure the internationally mandated regulations without the full trappings of CSA 1970. (It is somewhat ironic that, in some cases, the U.S. government can achieve greater drug-hazard-reduction flexibility through an international body than it can through its own federal legislation.)

Legislative Action. Greater flexibility in psychoactive-drug regulation could be achieved through new legislation that either rewrites CSA 1970 for greater flexibility or imposes specifically targeted tactics for a specific psychoactive drug, taking into account its reservoir and the consequences of its use including its hazards.

May Dextropropoxyphene Be Assigned to Schedule II?

Even if the just-mentioned alternative remedies were employed, it might be necessary to impose Schedule II controls on dextropropoxyphene (and on other psychoactive drugs with similar reservoirs). The reason for this is that the other remedies might not reduce the levels of drug hazard effectively. Moreover, it appears the Schedule II controls sometimes may be able to reduce the rate at which drugs are supplied to the population through authorized retail dispensing, as measured in terms of dosage units dispensed per unit of time. Occasionally, effects like this one are judged as politically acceptable alternatives to a demonstration that drug-hazard reduction has been achieved.[27]

Psychoactive-Drug Regulation: A Possibility for Change

In the foregoing, I have made implicit and explicit suggestions for change in the present approach to federal psychoactive-drug regulation. Namely, when confronted with a new psychoactive drug or with an existing or impending increase in psychoactive-drug-hazard levels, attempt to characterize the new situation, particularly in terms of the drug reservoir or other analogies, to increase understanding of the means of drug availability. Before selecting federal regulation from among the tactics, review a broad variety of hazard-reduction options including regulation at local, state, and international levels. Seriously consider options other than federal regulation that might achieve comparable results with more precision.

A review of drug-hazard-reduction options might be made easier if it were guided by a general strategy. Haddon recently has formulated a general approach to reducing damage from hazards in general, with the term *hazard* referring to agent, not risk of loss or harm as in this chapter. Though this approach was developed in the course of Haddon's work on the prevention and control of damage due to abnormal energy transfers, it is generally applicable to drug-hazard reduction as I have described it here.[28]

Haddon's ten general principles for hazard reduction are presented in the following list, along with examples of drug-hazard-reduction tactics based upon these principles.

Principle 1:	Prevent the initial marshaling of the agent.
Tactic:	Ban production of the drug worldwide.
Principle 2:	Reduce the amount of the agent marshaled.
Tactic:	Limit production of the drug (for example, through production quotas).
Principle 3:	Prevent release of the agent.
Tactic:	Ban marketing and dispensing of the drug.

Principle 4:	Modify the rate or spatial distribution of the agent's release from its source.
Tactics:	a. Impose annual distribution quotas. b. Restrict dispensing to specially controlled facilities (for example, restrict methadone dispensing to special clinics). c. Prescribe drugs according to a regimen that has a low probability of inducing dependence.
Principle 5:	Separate, in space or time, the agent from the susceptible person or population.
Tactics:	a. Ban importation and ban production within a state's borders. b. Restrict the movement of persons who distribute drugs in an unauthorized manner.
Principle 6:	Impose a material barrier between the agent and the susceptible person or population.
Tactics:	a. Store drugs in locked facilities. b. Store drugs in child-proof containers.
Principle 7:	Modify the agent's characteristics to reduce damage.
Tactic:	Formulate narcotics with small doses of narcotic antagonists to limit unwanted effects.
Principle 8:	Strengthen the susceptible person or population to reduce damage.
Tactic:	Modify cultural norms that support use of drugs in hazardous ways.
Principle 9:	Move rapidly to detect, evaluate, and counter the continuation and extension of damage.
Tactics:	a. Maintain drug-hazard surveillance. b. Develop a drug-hazard-epidemic intelligence service.
Principle 10:	Repair damage caused by the agent's interaction with susceptibles, and rehabilitate.
Tactic:	Offer rehabilitation services.[29]

Reviewing these, one finds that many of the principles already are represented in federal regulations on psychoactive drugs. Further, they can be mapped onto the graphic display of the drug flow and its consequences in figure 14–1. For example, principles 1 and 2 clearly relate to drug R&D and manufacture. Principles 3, 4, 5, and 6 relate to drug distribution, up to and including the vehicles by which drugs reach the ultimate consumer. Principle 7 relates to the drug R&D process and calls for a basic manipulation of the drug agent along the lines suggested by the attorney general's power to except depressant and stimulant drugs from CSA 1970 control measures. Principle 8 calls for a change in the host depicted in figure 14–2 while principles 9 and 10 call for attention to the consequences of agent-host-environment interaction and to the need for investigations of diversion and curtailment actions once diversion has occurred. Future work on the development of new tactics based upon these principles should prove fruitful.

Conclusion

One of the most important objectives for regulation of psychoactive drugs is the reduction of risks of loss and harm caused by drug activity after ingestion. Nevertheless, regulation—especially pervasive federal control via CSA 1970—comprises but one set of options for drug-hazard reduction. Other options are suggested by the epidemiologic idea of a reservoir for psychoactive drugs and by a review of William Haddon's general principles for hazard reduction. The chapter proposes that a timely but careful review of a broad variety of options should precede future decisions to regulate psychoactive drugs that pose increasingly great or otherwise intolerable hazards.

Notes

1. J.E. Gordon, "The Epidemiology of Accidents," *American Journal of Health* 39 (1949):504–515; and W. Haddon, "Advances in the Epidemiology of Injuries as a Basis for Public Policy," *Public Health Reports* 95 (1980):411–421.

2. A.I. Wertheimer et al., "A Provisional Drug Control Evaluation System," Phase One Report for DEA-74-31 (Unpublished Project Report, University of Minnesota College of Pharmacy, 1974), pp. D1–D55; and L.C. Weaver et al., "Evaluation of the Impact of Drug Control Scheduling," Final Report for DEA-74-31 (Unpublished Project Report, University of Minnesota College of Pharmacy, 1975).

3. J.P. Fox, C.E. Hall, and L.R. Elveback, *Epidemiology: Man and Disease* (New York: Macmillan, 1970), pp. 58–65; D.E. Smith and D.R. Wesson, "Legitimate and Illegitimate Distribution of Amphetamines and Barbiturates," *Journal of Psychedelic Drugs* 5 (1972):177–181; and E.H. Ellinwood, "The Epidemiology of Stimulant Abuse," in *Drug Use—Epidemiological and Sociological Approaches,* eds. E. Josephson and E.E. Carroll (Washington, D.C.: Hemisphere Publishing Corporation, 1974), pp. 303–329.

4. Fox, Hall, and Elveback, *Epidemiology.*

5. R.C. Smith "Traffic in Amphetamines: Patterns of Illegal Manufacture and Distribution," *Journal of Psychedelic Drugs* 2 (1969):20–24.

6. Smith and Wesson, Figure 16–1, this volume.

7. J.C. Kramer and R. Pinco, "Amphetamine Use and Misuse: A Medico-Legal View," in *Uppers and Downers,* eds. D.E. Smith and D.R. Wesson (Englewood Cliffs, N.J.: Prentice-Hall, 1973), pp. 9–22; J.P. Morgan and D. Kagan, "Street Amphetamine Quality and the Controlled Substances Act of 1970," *Journal of Psychedelic Drugs* 10 (1978):303–317; D.W. Byles, "Abuse Control Laws and the Drug Industry," in *Amphetamine Abuse,* ed. J.R. Russo (Springfield, Ill.: CC Thomas, 1968); W.H. McGlothlin, *Amphetamines, Barbiturates and Hallucinogens: An Analysis of Use, Distribution and Control,* SCID-TR-9 Report (Washington, D.C.: Drug Enforcement Administration, 1973); U.S., Congress, Senate, Committee on the Judiciary, Subcommittee to Investigate Juvenile Delinquency, *Hearings on S. Res. 32, Section 12, Amphetamine Legislation 1971,* and *Diet Pill (Amphetamines) Traffic, Abuse and Regulation,* 92nd Cong., 2d sess., 1971; K.A. Durrin, "Diversion as a Factor in Illicit Drug Traffic," *Drug and Cosmetic Industry* 107 (1970):28–30, 126–127, and U.S. Bureau of Narcotics and Dangerous Drugs, *Efforts to Prevent Dangerous Drugs from Reaching the Public* (Washington, D.C., 1972).

8. K. Rickels, ed., *Non-specific Factors in Drug Therapy* (Springfield, Ill.: CC Thomas, 1968), pp. 3–26; and see, for example, Z.J. Lipowski, *Delirium: Acute Brain Failure in Man* (Springfield, Ill.: CC Thomas, 1980), chapter 9.

9. Controlled Substances Act, 84 Stat. 1242, Public Law 91–513 (1970), Title II, Section 101.

10. U.S. Department of Justice, Bureau of Narcotics and Dangerous Drugs, "A Study of the Abuse Potential of Dextropropoxyphene with Control Recommendations" (Unpublished Drug Control Division document, Washington, D.C., 1973); Public Citizen's Health Research Group, Petition to Secretary of Health, Education, and Welfare, 21 November 1978; U.S., Congress, Senate, Select Committee on Small Business, Subcommittee on Monopoly and Anticompetitive Activities, *Propoxyphene,* 31 January, 1 February, and 5 February 1979; U.S. DHEW, Office of the Secretary, Order of the Secretary Denying Petition to Suspend New Drug Applications for Propoxyphene (Washington, D.C., 15 February 1979); Public Citizen's Health Research Group, Testimony of Sidney Wolfe, M.D., before FDA Drug Abuse Advisory Committee Hearing on Darvon, 17 April 1979 (Unpublished document, Washington, D.C., 1979); U.S. DHEW, FDA, Commissioner Donald Kennedy, "Propoxyphene," *Federal Register* 44 (2 March 1979):11837–11849; U.S. Department of Justice, Drug Enforcement Administration, Administrator Peter B. Bensinger. "Clas-

sification of Dextropropoxyphene as a Narcotic Drug in Schedule IV of the Controlled Substances Act," *Federal Register* 45 (24 June 1980):42264–42265 (to be codified at 21 C.F.R. pt. 1308); and J.P. Swazey, Medicine in the Public Interest, *Drug Abuse, Data Systems, and Regulatory Decisions* (Washington, D.C., 1977).

11. IMS America, Ltd., *National Prescription Audit,* Ambler, Pa. 1977.

12. U.S. Department of Justice, Abuse Potential of Dextropropoxyphene, and U.S. DHEW, Commissioner Donald Kennedy, "Propoxyphene."

13. IMS America, Ltd., *Drug Abuse Warning Network. 1979 DAWN Annual Report.* DEA Contract No 79-15. Washington, D.C.: U.S. Government Printing Office, 1980.

14. U.S. DHEW Commissioner Donald Kennedy and B.S. Finkle et al., "A National Assessment of Propoxyphene in Postmortem Medicolegal Investigation, 1972–75," *Journal of Forensic Science* 21 (1976):706–742.

15. Reference sources covered in notes 10 and 14. See also D.C. Chambers, A.D. Moffett, and W.R. Cuskey, "Five Patterns of Darvon Abuse," *International Journal of Addiction* 6 (1971):173–189.

16. U.S., Congress, House, Committee on Interstate and Foreign Commerce, House Rept. 91–1444, pt. 1, p. 34.

17. Medicine in the Public Interest, *Drug Abuse,* p. 20.

18. Controlled Substances Act, 1970.

19. U.S. DHEW, Office of the Secretary, Office of the General Counsel, Food and Drug Division, Attorney William W. Vodra, Summary of the Controlled Substances Act (Undated Memorandum to the FDA Controlled Substances Advisory Committee, Washington, D.C.).

20. Controlled Substances Act, 1970.

21. Public Citizen's Health Research Group, Petition.

22. Public Citizen's Health Research, Hearing.

23. U.S. DHEW, FDA, Drug Abuse Advisory Committee, "Transcript of Public Hearing on Darvon," 17 April 1979; and John Pekkanen, *The American Connection* (New York: Follett, 1974).

24. U.S., Congress, Senate, Committee on the Judiciary, Subcommittee to Investigate Juvenile Delinquency, "Testimony of D.O. Fedder, " *Hearings on S. Res. 255, Sect. 12., Drug Abuse: The Pharmacist,* 93rd. Cong., 2d sess., 28 March 1974, pp. 131–136.

25. Robert H. Furman, Vice-president, Eli Lilly and Company, Corporate Medical Affairs, Correspondence on Darvon informational program to James C. Anthony, 20 May 1981.

26. D.T. Campbell, "Reforms as Experiments" in *Handbook of Evaluation Research, vol. 1,* eds. E.J. Streuning and M. Guttentag (Beverly Hills: Sage Publications, 1975), pp. 781–789; and Campbell, "From

Description to Experimentation: Interpreting Trends as Quasi-Experiments," in *Problems of Measuring Change,* ed. C.W. Harris (Milwaukee: University of Wisconsin Press, 1967), pp. 212–253.

27. J.C. Anthony, *The Impact of Drug Scheduling: An Assessment of the Controlled Substances Act of 1970* (Ann Arbor, Mich.: University Microfilms, 1977).

28. W. Haddon, Jr., "Energy Damage and the Ten Countermeasure Strategies," *Journal of Trauma* 13 (1973):321–331.

29. Ibid.

15 Prescribing Hypnotic Drugs: A Reassuring Conservatism

Michael Weintraub, Andrew A. Sorensen, and *John P. Morgan*

In 1979, the Institute of Medicine of the National Academy of Sciences sponsored a report on hypnotic drugs, sleep disorders, and medical practice.[1] Their sources indicate that patients more than 60 years of age receive a disproportionately large number of prescriptions for hypnotics. The report favored prescribing "only very limited numbers of sleeping pills for use for a few nights at a time" and indicated the need for special caution if hypnotics were ever prescribed for elderly patients. The report also stressed the need for more research on the specific sleep problems of the elderly and their treatment. Since much of the information in the Institute of Medicine report came from unreferenced sources and from one-time surveys (not experiments) focused on hypnotic prescribing, some bias might emerge. Therefore, we decided to learn how a group of physicians whose prescribing of all drugs was monitored prescribed hypnotic drugs, particularly for patients over the age of 60 years.

Methods

Prescriptions collected between May 1974 and May 1975 in the course of a large-scale computerized study of prescribing by family-medicine practitioners were reviewed to obtain the data presented here. The prescribers, patient population, and method of monitoring have been described before.[2,3] Briefly, prescriptions are coded for patient identification, age, sex, diagnosis, and other prescription features (drug, dose, directions, volume of medication, and refills). All data on prescriptions for standard hypnotics and the antihistamine diphenhydramine hydrochloride to be taken at bedtime were obtained from the computerized data base.

Results

Of all adult prescriptions written by the monitored physicians, 1.6 percent were for hypnotic drugs (1.8 percent if diphenhydramine, taken at bedtime, is included). For patients 61 years of age or over, 3.4 percent of the prescriptions were for hypnotics (3.8 percent for hypnotics plus diphenhydramine). The breakdown of hypnotic prescriptions by age of recipient is given in table 15-1.

Most of the hypnotic prescriptions were written for flurazepam (77 percent of usual hypnotics, 69 percent if diphenhydramine is included). The drugs prescribed and the relationship to age are shown in table 15-2. Only a small number of prescriptions were written for barbiturates.

More than three-fourths of the prescriptions for flurazepam written for patients 61 years of age and over contained an order for thirty or fewer capsules. Younger patients also received relatively small prescriptions (see table

Table 15-1
Number of Hypnotic Prescriptions, by Age of Recipient

		Percent of Prescriptions	
Age (Years)	*Total Number of Prescriptions*[a]	*For Standard Hypnotics*[b]	*Including Bedtime Benadryl*
21-30	6,071	0.5	0.7
31-40	3,325	1.1	1.2
41-50	2,872	2.2	2.4
51-60	2,544	1.8	1,8
61-70	1,633	2.4	2.8
71-80	971	5	5.4
Over 80	508	3.3	3.9

[a]Prescriptions in data base.

[b]Chloral hydrate, flurazepam (Dalmane), glutethimide (Doriden), phenobarbital sodium (at bedtime only), and secobarbital sodium.

Table 15-2
Number of Hypnotic Prescriptions, by Drug and Age

	Age (Years)						
Drug	*21-30*	*31-40*	*41-50*	*51-60*	*61-70*	*71-80*	*Over 80*
Chloral hydrate	3	2	11	12	2	8	4
Flurazepam (Dalmane)	26	32	48	30	34	36	11
Glutethimide (Doriden)	0	0	0	4	3	3	1
Phenobarbital sodium (bedtime only)	1	0	3	0	1	1	1
Secobarbital sodium	0	2	2	0	0	1	0
Diphenhydramine hydrochloride (Benadryl) (bedtime only)	11	5	4	1	6	3	3
Total	41	41	68	47	46	52	20

15–3). Of prescriptions for patients 61 and over, one-third allowed no refills. The other two-thirds provided for one or two refills (mean, 1.75). Thirty-four percent of the small prescriptions (thirty or fewer capsules) allowed no refills. Table 15–4 summarizes refill and prescription-size data.

Table 15–3
Percentage of Flurazepam (Dalmane) Prescriptions, by Number of Capsules Ordered

	Flurazepam Prescriptions	
Number of Capsules Ordered	*60 Years and Under*	*61 Years and Over*
10	8.1	2.5
12	2.9	1.2
15	10.3	4.9
20	12.5	7.4
25	0.7	—
28	0.7	—
30	50	60.4
35	—	2.5
40	2.2	1.2
45	0.7	—
50	7.4	13.6
60	4.4	2.5
100	—	3.7

Table 15–4
Flurazepam Refills Allowed, by Number of Capsules Prescribed, for Patients Aged 61 and over

	Number of Refills Allowed							
Number of Capsules Ordered	*0*	*1*	*2*	*3*	*4*	*5*	*6*	*7*
10	1		1					
12	1							
15	2		2					
20	1	3	1	1				
30	16	13	3	5		9		3
35	1		1					
40		1						
50	3	1	1	1	2	3		
60	1			1				
100	1					1	1	
Total refills	27	18	9	8	2	13	1	3

No refills were written on 31.7 percent of all monitored hypnotic prescriptions, and more than one-half allowed two or fewer refills.

Prescribers did not decrease flurazepam dosage for older patients. Thirty-nine percent of patients aged 60 and under and 42 percent of patients 61 and over received prescriptions for 15 mg. doses. Forty-five patients accounted for the eighty-one flurazepam prescriptions for patients aged 61 and over. During the year covered by this study, one patient received ten small prescriptions for flurazepam, another six, and another five.

Discussion

As we reported previously,[4] the physicians monitored in this study are affiliated academically and tend to be judicious and careful in their prescribing. Their prescribing of hypnotics demonstrates these characteristics; they wrote less than half of the percentage of hypnotic prescriptions for all ages described in the Institute of Medicine Report and a much lower percentage of hypnotic drugs for elderly patients.[5] In fact, forty-five patients accounted for all prescriptions for hypnotics written for patients 61 years of age and over. Most of these prescriptions were for one month of treatment, with few or no refills, indicating short-term use and frequent reassessment of drug need—in short, excellent prescribing habits. (Of course, patients will pay for this careful supervision in somewhat higher prescription costs—at least in pharmacies that use the professional fee system of charging—as well as in increasing traveling and visits to the physician.)

The recommended decrease in flurazepam dose for patients over 60 years of age was not noted. At the time these prescriptions were being written, the report of increased adverse reactions from 30 mg. doses of flurazepam in older patients had not yet been published.[6] In any case, since that study was done in hospitalized patients, our prescribers might not have considered the findings applicable to their patients even if the information had been available. It is also possible that with the close supervision and the better health status of patients receiving flurazepam in this practice, the adverse effects that hospitalized elderly patients suffered would not occur.

Despite the conservatism of hypnotic prescribing by the monitored physicians, a few patients were given prescriptions for large numbers of flurazepam capsules, with many refills. We do not know the reasons for this apparently anomalous prescribing. All prescriptions directed continuous nightly administration. (At the time these prescriptions were written, the current recommendation for interrupted regimes was not being emphasized.) Flurazepam was the single most important drug prescribed, reflecting nationwide prescribing habits. Almost no barbiturates and very little glutethimide or chloral hydrate were prescribed despite the frequent use of these drugs in the past and the proved efficacy of barbiturates in elderly patients.[7] Some patients find that antihistamines provide effective hypnotic action for them. The prescribing of diphenhydramine thus may reflect the patient's perception of its hypnotic action or a belief on the part of some physicians that antihistamines are safer than hypnotic drugs for older patients. It has been shown that 50 mg. of diphenhydramine is significantly better than placebo and roughly equivalent to 60 mg. of pentobarbital as a hypnotic in at least one study of hypnotic efficacy.[8]

We did not include in our study the use of nighttime benzodiazepines other than flurazepam, tricyclic antidepressants, or OTC drugs because of the confusion of their category of use through diagnostic considerations other than insomnia. It is thus possible that the monitored physicians prescribed more hypnotics than our data show. We also have no data on the efficacy of the hypnotics or on whether patients had increased sleep problems after stopping the drugs.

Our data are at variance with the claims of casual or excessive prescribing of hypnotics for patients over the age of 60 years. Further study of the prescribing habits of other physicians is required to corroborate or refute the conclusions based on the findings in our sample. The presentation of these 1975 data thus seems appropriate particularly in the light of increasing recent criticism of the sort stated in the Institute of Medicine's 1979 report.

Notes

1. F. Solomon et al., "Sleeping Pills, Insomnia and Medical Practice," *New England Journal of Medicine* 300 (1979):803–808.
2. N.L. Trabert et al., "Physician Prescribing Patterns: Technical Aspects and Initial Analyses," *Drug Information Journal* 10 (1976):84–90.
3. M. Weintraub et al., "Digoxin Prescribing: Mostly Good News," *Journal of the American Medical Association* 242 (1979):445–448.
4. Ibid., p. 448.
5. Solomon et al., "Sleeping Pills," p. 806.
6. D.J. Greenblatt, M.D. Allen, and R.I. Shader, "Toxicity of High-Dose Flurazepam in the Elderly," *Clinical Pharmacology and Therapeutics* 21 (1977):355–361.
7. J.P. Morgan et al., "Mebutamate as a Hypnotic: Clinical Trial and Statistical Considerations," *Clinical Pharmacology and Therapeutics* 14 (1973):1001–1012.
8. G. Teutsch et al., "Hypnotic Efficacy of Diphenhydramine, Methapyriline and Pentobarbital," *Clinical Pharmacology and Therapeutics* 17 (1975):195–201.

16 Prescribing Psychoactive Drugs: A Question of Perspective

David E. Smith and
Richard B. Seymour

Physicians enter into the practice of medicine with limited training in the field of psychoactive substance abuse, but they are exposed to substance abusers, to the potential profits to be made in prescription-drug diversion, and to the temptation of personal abuse in a variety of medical settings. Although the situation may be improving, many practicing physicians, both consciously and unwittingly, are involved in the diversion of psychoactive drugs.

The Drug Enforcement Administration, which is charged with broad statutory responsibility for administering the laws that govern the distribution and use of legally manufactured drugs, cites the magnitude of its task. Presently, about one-half million registered private enterprises in this country supply drugs to those in need of medication. Through this drug-distribution system flow some 20,000 different brand-name products that are administered by law. The annual volume of these drugs includes approximately 185,000 pounds of opium derivatives, 45,000 pounds of synthetic opioids, 4,172 pounds of amphetamine, and more than a million pounds of barbiturates. Additionally, the law requires the monitoring of an estimated 2 billion dosage units of various tranquilizers, 60 million dosage units of stimulants, and more than 25 million four-ounce bottles of codeine cough syrup.[1] While most of these drugs are used legitimately, a significant amount arrives in the hands of this country's 2 million nonnarcotic drug abusers and 500,000 heroin addicts.

It is apparent from figure 16–1 that the physician is only one among many sources for the diversion of prescription psychoactive drugs.[2] In those instances where a physician deliberately or inadvertently is involved in drug diversion, however, there is a potential for contact and conflict with drug enforcement. For the sake of clarity, we have separated the physicians most likely to come into contact with drug enforcement into four categories.

Four Problem-Causing Physician Types

In the course of our clinic's related activities, we have studied nonnarcotic- as well as narcotic-drug-abuse epidemiology in the San Francisco Bay area.

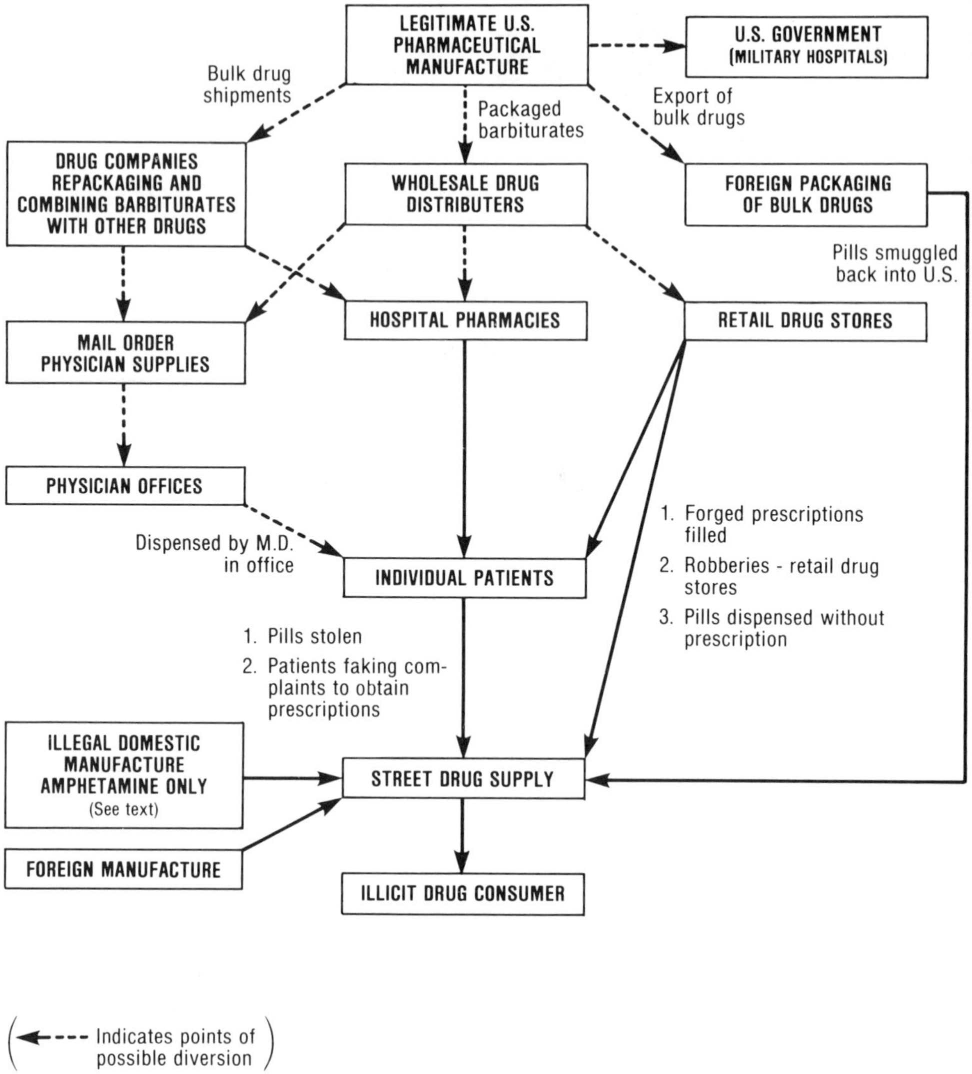

Source: *Journal of Psychedelic Drugs* (Winter 1972), p. 179.

Figure 16-1. Routes by which Amphetamine and Barbiturates Reach the Black Market

We found that a number of nonnarcotic drug abusers were not drug-culture oriented. We defined these individuals as nonstreetwise polydrug abusers.[3] Instead, they were obtaining their drugs from physicians. Since treatment programs should be designed to meet the needs of the client, we modified our polydrug research and treatment efforts in the early 1970s. In order to reach the physicians who were prescribing for the population, we joined forces with the San Francisco Medical Society, the California Medical Association, and the American Medical Association. To work for an improvement in the diagnostic and treatment skills of the practicing physician, we set up a phone-consultation service for physicians with substance-abusing patients. We provided emergency information for the surgeon who discovered his patient was drinking heavily when the patient went into post-operative delirium tremens and the obstetrician who realizes he is seeing a pregnant addict. At the same time, we started outreach training through the medical community, medical societies, and hospitals.

Through these activities, we found that a number of physicians had personal addiction problems. These comprised our first category, the addicted doctor—physicians who had drug or alcohol problems and who were concerned about their condition on the one hand and about losing their licenses on the other hand.

We also received inquiries from other types of physicians who were in potential or actual conflict with the law. These were dated doctors who, while attempting to practice good-faith medicine, had not maintained their expertise in psychoactive drugs and were writing inappropriate prescriptions out of ignorance about addicts and addictive behavior; script doctors who deliberately sell large numbers of prescriptions to patients for profit with no attempt to practice legitimate medicine; and drug-treatment doctors who chose to prescribe Schedule II psychoactive drugs at higher than usual doses in the course of their detoxification and maintenance work with addicts.

These categories of doctors, all of whom may come in contact with drug-enforcement or other regulatory agencies, are deserving of and require different approaches. In the following pages we have outlined these approaches and offered some possible solutions.

The Addicted Doctor

The addicted doctor needs treatment for his addictive disease. A collaborative effect by drug enforcement and medicine is essential to obtain such treatment.

In California, these physicians may come under the state's Diversion Program for Physicians. Legislation enacted in 1979 directed the Division of Medical Quality of the Board of Medical Quality Assurance to "seek ways to identify and rehabilitate physicians with impairment due to abuse of dangerous drugs or alcohol, or due to mental illness or physical illness affecting competency, so that physicians so afflicted may be treated and returned to the practice of medicine in a manner which will not endanger the public health and safety."[4] This legislation establishes the three major supports of physician diversion: (1) it allowed physicians on diversion to keep their licenses intact, even though the law may have been violated; (2) it established confidentiality for physicians in the program; and (3) it directed that appointments to the diversion-evaluation committees be made strictly on the basis of expertise.

The diversion-evaluation committee decides whether or not a physician is treatable on the basis of history and attitude. Once a candidate is accepted, treatment elements and a monitoring schedule based on the candidate's needs and circumstances are combined into an itemized treatment contract. The following are examples of items that may be included in these contracts:

Follow the directions of the assigned treating physician.

Abstain from alcohol or drug abuse.

Consent to body-fluid testing on a random schedule.

Participate in peer-support group meetings and/or Alcoholics Anonymous (AA) meetings with a specified frequency and with verified attendance.

Participate in individual psychotherapy.

Take Antabuse.

Practice in a supervised work setting, and get the approval of the committee before changing the work setting.

Voluntarily relinquish his or her Drug Enforcement Administration number.

Live in a specified treatment facility.

Participate in a certain number of hours (up to twenty-five) of continuing medical education related to appropriate prescribing practices. (These hours are in addition to those required for renewal of license in California.)

Cooperate with periodic exams by a psychiatrist who will report findings to the Diversion Evaluation Committee.

Encompassing the specifics, the contract is completed by a general statement: "I agree to adhere to the following terms and conditions of my treatment program and agree to accept supervision to assure my compliance with these terms and conditions. The Diversion Evaluation Committee will accommodate me with written verification of my participation in this treatment program if I so request."[5]

Since relapse into drug or alcohol abuse are strongly possible, each diverted physician is monitored by a case manager who helps the physician to understand and stay in compliance with his or her treatment contract and a compliance officer who directly monitors the physician's behavior.

At the end of a specified period of rehabilitation and monitoring, usually three to five years, the committee will interview the physician and determine if rehabilitation has been achieved and if the physician can return safely to unsupervised, unmonitored practice. If so, the diversion program is concluded, and the physician's file is purged. No records of participation in diversion remain.

The program has been in operation since 1980. It originally was estimated that about twenty people would be accepted the first year. As of October 1980, fifty-nine physicians were in various plans of diversion treatment.

Given an atmosphere of cooperation between regulatory agencies and the medical community, some form of the physician-diversion system, developed in California, is replicable in any state where the need for such a system is perceived. Costing approximately half of what eventual prosecution would, diversion is also effectively aiding public safety.

In addition, addicted physicians are treated in private voluntary treatment programs where a high degree of confidentiality is provided in order to intervene at an earlier stage in his addictive disease. The treatment principles remain the same although the interaction with the regulatory and enforcement agencies is quite different because of confidentiality issues.

The Dated Doctor

The dated doctor needs additional consultation and training in order to improve his prescribing practices. If educational attempts fail, then restrictions must be placed on the physician's license in order to protect the safety of patients. Probations, limitations on prescribing and practice, license removal, and mandatory diversion to education may be used in states like California (see appendix 16–A for a description of our prescribing-practice course).

The dated doctor often is caught up in the drug-enforcement net for prescribing psychoactive drugs, even if his intent is not criminal. He may not understand addictive behavior or recent information about the toxicity of a particular drug. As an example, the rapidly acting barbiturates were considered in the 1950s to be substances of relatively low abuse potential. They were prescribed widely by physicians all over the United States for sleep induction. Now there is growing awareness that these substances can be abused highly, and alternative sedative-hypnotic agents like benzodiazepines have largely replaced them. In addition, more emphasis is being placed now on nonpharmacological alternatives.[6] The situation with amphetamine is similar. In the early 1960s, amphetamine was prescribed for a wide variety of indications, and the awareness of its abuse potential was quite low. Now we appreciate that when the dose is increased to high levels, and when the route of administration is changed to an intravenous one, this drug can be extremely toxic.[7]

Another example is methaqualone (Quaalude) that initially was promoted as a safe alternative to barbiturates. In time, methaqualone displayed its high abuse potential equal to that of the rapidly acting barbiturates. However, many of the physicians did not learn the new information on abuse.

We believe that the approach to these physicians should not be prosecution by a criminal-justice system but training, continuing education, and consultation spurred by legal warnings and peer pressure from medical societies and hospitals. The vast majority of dated physicians will respond to this approach if it is presented through appropriate education and training techniques.

Since November 1979, the Haight Ashbury Training and Education Projects of the Haight Ashbury Free Medical Clinic have presented three two-day courses on the ethics and practice of prescribing psychoactive drugs. These courses were organized in cooperation with the California Medical Association and the Board of Medical Quality Assurance, with a focus on the misprescriber on probation. These courses were an extension of our ten-year training experience with continuing medical education programs for physicians in the alcohol- and drug-abuse areas. The reception of and obvious need for such training by physicians has led us to a policy decision of continuing development and ongoing presentation in the ethics and practice of prescribing psychoactive drugs.

Development of the courses occurred as a natural outgrowth of our physician-training activities in the treatment for addicted physicians. The California Board of Medical Quality Assurance, the California Medical Association, and the California Society for the Treatment of Alcoholism and Other Drug Dependencies were highly active in developing the disabled-physician program. In the process, they perceived a growing need for dealing with the misprescribing physician as well as the addicted physician. A series of conversations and meetings held in late summer 1979 resulted in the creation of a physician-training course that would help to educate the unintentional violator.

There is a level of physician hostility toward regulatory-agency representatives and vice versa that needs to be dealt with in such courses. There are conflicts in perception; an enforcement attitude exists that all misprescribing physicians should know better and are, therefore, script doctors; and many physicians see any interaction with enforcement a part of a possible entrapment. The panels provide an informed forum for these and many other concerns.

The ethics and practice of prescribing psychoactive drugs course has had the enthusiastic endorsement and support of both regulatory and medical agencies. We feel that it is replicable in any area where prescribing practices and misprescribing are a concern. The course has both symbolic and educational value that make it worth promoting and developing on a widespread basis. Then, too, there is the economic value of dollars saved in training a physician to be more aware of his prescribing ethics and practices rather than having to prosecute that same physician for making mistakes that make him a danger to society. As part of the overall regulatory approach to the control of prescription-drug abuse, we emphasize the need for an educational alternative and hope that other states will develop cooperative planning between enforcement and medicine in establishing annual prescribing-practice courses.

The Script Doctor

The script doctor should be prosecuted vigorously like any criminal who sells dangerous drugs for profit to the detriment of both the individual and society.

Let us stress at the outset our belief that a majority of the legitimately manufactured psychoactive drugs that are diverted into illicit channels by physicians come from script doctors. On the one hand, we believe that the vast majority of practicing physicians is well intentioned and not a major source of drug abuse. On the other hand, however, a few physicians are criminal. These doctors write quantities of prescriptions for profit.

The medical community has a responsibility to speak out against the script doctor and not to engage in some conspiracy of silence in order to protect the name of medicine. Properly approached, however, the problem of script doctors can be dealt with jointly by the interaction of drug enforcement and the medical community.

We have participated in reviews of prescribing patterns with law-enforcement officers of the California Diversion Investigation Unit. Of eleven

Bay-area physicians who prescribed 55 percent of Schedule II drugs in San Francisco, a decision to pursue nine of the eleven in criminal prosecution was approached jointly. Drug-abuse experts associated with the California Medical Society agreed to testify in court following this review.

This establishment of community standards and the development of prescribing-practice standards is desirable to counter the restrictive use of the *PDR* by the criminal-justice system as the only standard by which to define the practice of medicine. This is what happened in the Arnold Mandell case and other cases we have observed in which a one-dimensional approach to deviant prescribing is used rather than the multifactorial approach described in this chapter.[8]

It is our firm belief that the *PDR* is a guide and a contract between the drug manufacturer and the FDA. The practicing physician is not a party to that contract. The *PDR* gives the FDA-approved indications for drugs but does not define the standards of clinical medicine.

The Drug-Treatment Doctor

The drug-treatment doctor, if practicing responsible medicine, should be left alone to deal with the difficult problem of addictive behavior for the benefit of both the individual and society.

The drug-treatment physician may utilize unusual doses and unusual regimes of psychoactive drugs. He surely will use drugs outside the *PDR* listings like the well-documented use of phenobarbital in the treatment of sedative-hypnotic withdrawal.[9] We believe that many workers in drug enforcement do not understand this phenomenon and this legitimate interest of practitioners. The course described has the added advantage of exposing enforcement workers to this type of unusual and proper prescribing.

Conclusion

Deviant prescribing of psychoactive drugs has provoked much concern in an era in which prescription-drug abuse has become discussed widely. We described four types of unusual prescriber and the different approaches that could be taken toward the particular deviance. An educational alternative, a course on the ethics and practice of prescribing psychoactive drugs, is discussed and a course outline is provided in appendix 16–A.

Notes

1. K.A. Durrin, "Compliance, Who Is Responsible?" *Drug Enforcement* (Spring 1974).

2. D.E. Smith and D.R. Wesson, *Uppers and Downers* (Englewood Cliffs, N.J.: Prentice-Hall, 1974):3–6.

3. D.R. Wesson, D.E. Smith, and S.E. Lerner, "Streetwise vs. Nonstreetwise Polydrug Typology: Myth or Reality?" *Journal of Psychedelic Drugs* 7 (1975):121–134.

4. R. Shapiro, "California's Diversion Program for Physicians," *California Society for the Treatment of Alcoholism and Other Drug Dependencies Newsletter* 7 (1980):4–7.

5. Ibid.

6. D.E. Smith and M.E. Buxton, "An Alternative Approach to the Treatment of Drug Abuse" (Presented at the Women in Crisis Conference, Washington, D.C., 4 June 1980).

7. J.P. Morgan, "Amphetamine," in *Substance Abuse: Clinical Problems and Perspectives,* eds. J.H. Lowinson and P. Ruiz (Baltimore: Williams & Wilkins, 1981). p. 176.

8. J. Ketchum, *Fact and File of Opinion.* Distributed by the Arnold Mandell Defense Fund, 409 Clayton St., San Francisco, Ca. 1978.

9. D.R. Wesson, and D.E. Smith, *Barbiturates: Their Use, Misuse and Abuse.* New York: Human Sciences Press, 1977.

Appendix 16-A Prescribing Psychoactive Drugs: A Contemporary Focus on Clinical, Legal, and Ethical Issues

Day I

A.M.

8:15	Registration
9:00	Pretest
9:15	The Evolution of Prescribing Constraints
10:15	Break
10:30	Misused Prescription Drugs: An Overview of Pharmacology and Scheduling
11:15	Legal and Clinical Issues in Medical Practice A. Clinical Freedom and Deviant Prescribing B. Regulation of Physicians C. Enforcement and Discipline
12:15	Lunch
1:45	Case I: Physician in Difficulty (Small-group discussion)
3:00	Break
3:15	Case II: Unusual Request for Treatment (Small-group discussion)
4:00	Keeping It Legal (Professional Conduct Board Lawyer Defense Counselor)

Day II

A.M.

9:00	Guidelines for Prescribing and Not Prescribing A. Sedative-Hypnotics B. Benzodiazepines C. Psychostimulants
10:15	Break
10:30	D. Opioids E. Psychoactive Drugs and Special Patients: The Alcoholic and the Methadone Dependent
11:30	Panel discussion and review
12:10	Lunch
1:30	Patient Simulation
2:15	Small-group discussion
2:45	Response to Simulation and New Simulation
3:15	Break
3:30	Patients: Manipulated and Manipulating
4:15	Posttest and Evaluations
4:30	Adjourn

The following individuals made important contributions to this course-outline version: John N. Chappel, M.D.; Richard Corbett, M.D.; Jack Farrell; Gail Jara; Doreen Kagan; John P. Morgan, M.D.; Stephanie Ross; Richard B. Seymour; David E. Smith, M.D.; and Donald Wesson, M.D.

Educational Objectives, Day I

The Evolution of Prescribing Constraints

1. Outline the uses of opium before the Civil War.
2. Describe the changes in opioid occurring during and after the Civil War.
3. Relate the uses of morphine and heroin to the patent-medicine industry.
4. Describe the addict population in 1890; in 1910.
5. Define the interpretation of the Harrison Narcotics Act (1914) regarding use of opioids in addicted patients.
6. Describe amphetamine sources for illegal use in 1960.
7. Explain the failure of the government to remove the Benzedrine inhaler from the market.
8. List four important measures of the Controlled Substances Act that diminished amphetamine diversion.
9. Describe the impact of scheduling methaqualone; chlordiazepoxide.

Misused Prescription Drugs: An Overview of Pharmacology and Scheduling

1. Describe briefly the five schedules of the Controlled Substances Act.
2. Outline the relationship of the state schedules to the proposed federal schedules.
3. Place the following agents in the proper schedules:

Generic Name	*Trade Name*
Phenmetrazine	Dolophine
Heroin	Pre-Sate
Meperidine	Beta-chlor
Pentobarbital	Seconal
Fentanyl	Dalmane
Methyl-fentanyl	Biphetamine
Tetrahydrocannabinol	Desoxyn
Chlorazepate	Leritine
Methadone	Levodromoran
Oxazepam	Plegine
Ethchlorvynol	Ativan
Phentermine	
Glutethimide	

4. Discuss the relationships regarding scheduling, approved use, and pharmacological characteristics of Dalmane versus Valium, Mequin versus Doriden, Demerol versus Darvon.

Legal and Clinical Issues in Medical Practice

1. List four reasons, other than a desire for profit, that characterize deviant prescribing.
2. Describe the legal status of the approved indications in the package insert.
3. List some instances in which it is justified to prescribe narcotics to a known addict.
4. Outline some protective measures when you use amphetamine for an unapproved purpose.
5. Outline physician behaviors that show good faith in dealing with the problems of caring for a known misuser of a controlled substance.
6. Outline the steps for civil discipline (under the Professional Conduct Board) in your state.
7. Describe the circumstance under which a pharmacist may fill a phoned prescription for a controlled substance.
8. Justify the state's decision to curtail a physician's power to administer controlled drugs to a known addict.
9. Describe the likely behavior, regarding medical complaints, of an undercover investigator of a state or federal agency.
10. List some characteristics that are likely to describe the practice characteristics of a physician in trouble.
11. Describe the legal liabilities of dispensing or administering Schedule II controlled substances.
12. Discuss briefly the legality of prescribing controlled substances for yourself; your family.
13. Describe the success of rehabilitation of drug-dependent physicians.

Day II

Guidelines for Prescribing and Not Prescribing

Sedative-Hypnotics.

1. Compare the hypnotic dose to the intoxicating dose to the lethal dose in naive patients; tolerant patients.
2. Describe the current style of misuse of glutethimide.
3. List some drugs not usually classified that may be used for their sedative powers.
4. Discuss briefly the utility of the following agents to treat an agitated patient withdrawing from secobarbital dependence:

   chlorpromazine,
   diazepam,

pentobarbital,
oxazepam,
phenobarbital.

5. List the chief ingredients of OTC sleeping pills.
6. List the sleeping pills that are Schedule II controlled substances.

Benzodiazepines.

1. Compare the onset of action, the distribution in the body, and the time for excretion of diazepam to two of the following:
   chlorazepate,
   lorazepam,
   oxazepam.
2. Describe why REM rebound is less of a problem with flurazepam than oxazepam.
3. List some possibly predictive characteristics of an individual who will develop physical dependence to a benzodiazepine.
4. Criticize the belief in the 1960s that benzodiazepines were better sedative drugs than barbiturates because they had less likelihood to cause dependence and overdose death.
5. Draw a curve reflecting benzodiazepine prescribing relative to barbiturate prescribing from 1964–1974; 1974–1980.

Psychostimulants.

1. Which of the following psychostimulant agents are not Schedule II?
   Desoxyn,
   Biphetamine,
   Ionamin,
   Pre-Sate,
   Tenuate,
   Plegine,
   Ritalin.
2. List the usual ingredients found in preparations sold as street speed.
3. Outline a self-protective procedure to use when you have decided you must use amphetamine as an antidepressant.
4. Draw a graph depicting weight loss versus time in the successful dieter who loses twenty-six pounds.
5. List the approved indications for amphetamine use in your state. Discuss the special case of the use of amphetamine as an anorexiant.

Opioids

1. Discuss the issue of opioid potency.

2. Relate the effect oral dose to the effective parenteral dose of the following opioids:

   methadone,
   morphine,
   hydromorphone,
   meperidine.

3. List the ingredients of the following products:

   Darvocet-N,
   Percodan,
   Percoset,
   Tylox.

4. Outline the use and misuse of pentazocine (Talwin).
5. Outline a postoperative course of analgesia without using the letters *PRN*. Describe the rationale for doing so.

Psychoactive Drugs and Special Patients.

1. List five agents to which the alcohol-dependent patient is cross-tolerant.
2. List medications that may cause an Antabuse-type reaction.
3. Describe a circumstance in which an alcoholic patient may be oversensitive to sedation; resistant to sedation.
4. Describe benzodiazepine withdrawal imposed on alcohol withdrawal.
5. Outline a program of alcohol detoxification that does not use psychoactive drugs.
6. Describe the analgesic response of a methadone-maintenance patient given narcotic opioids.
7. Describe the analgesic needs of a methadone-maintenance patient who is severely injured.
8. Describe the clinical situation that may transpire when a methadone-maintenance patient is given pentazocine.
9. Describe the circumstances under which a practitioner may use methadone as an analgesic.
10. Pick out of the following list which agents may be analgesic in methadone-maintenance patients:

    acetaminophen,
    aspirin,
    methotrimeparazine (Levoprome),
    Darvon,
    Darvon Compound,
    Demerol.

Patients: Manipulated and Manipulating

1. List five to six physical problems that a deceptive patient may describe and imitate to obtain medication.
2. List five to six psychological problems that a deceptive patient may describe and imitate to obtain medication.
3. Describe three to four methods a patient may use to place pressure on a physician.
4. List five to six physician characteristics contributing to prescription-drug abuse.
5. Describe briefly some alternatives to psychoactive prescribing in the following conditions:

   Insomnia,
   Anxiety,
   Fatigue/depression.

Part V
Educating Consumers

17 Patient Package Inserts: A Review and a Perspective

Louis A. Morris

Any review of patient-package-insert studies must take into account that package-insert research is done in the arena of public-policy determination. Requirements for patient package inserts have been applied to only a few specific drugs. In 1970, the FDA required patient package inserts for oral contraceptives and, in 1977, for estrogenic drugs used during menopause. In the mid-1970s, however, the FDA began investigating the concept of requiring package inserts for a wide variety of drugs. This interest was announced in a 1975 *Federal Register* statement where the FDA solicited comment on the patient-package-insert concept and asked for advice on specific aspects of the program.[1]

At that time the FDA received about a thousand comments, mostly from individual consumers who stated that they favored receiving written information with prescription drugs. In addition to *Federal Register* notices, the FDA also held a number of meetings and symposiums where this issue was discussed more fully.[2] These discussions culminated in a proposed regulation that was published in 1979.[3] The proposed regulation also prompted a large response, but the response this time came from health professionals as well as consumers. On the one hand, health professionals stated that the FDA proposal, which if enacted, would have required patient package inserts for 375 drugs over a five-year period, was much too ambitious, that the inserts were too costly, and that they were unproven. On the other hand, about half of the responses came from individual consumers who stated, again almost unanimously, that they were in favor of patient package inserts and that their costs were dwarfed by their benefits.

After reviewing these comments, the FDA considerably scaled down the final regulation, which was published in September 1980.[4] Patient package inserts would be required for ten drugs or drug classes and would be evaluated over a three-year period to obtain data on their costs and benefits. The FDA also would evaluate plans for the inserts. Most of the costs attributable to patient package inserts are related to their delivery system. To reduce costs, the FDA allowed for a much greater flexibility for manufacturers in the method of delivery of the package insert to the pharmacy, permitted pharmacists to test other distribution mechanisms, and changed the regulation to require inserts for only new prescriptions, not refills. In April 1981, the FDA issued a stay on the effective date of the regulation, pending a review by the new commissioner. The patient-package-insert issue remains a highly controversial regulation for a number of reasons. For example, pharmacy groups are vocal in opposition to the requirement. Consumer organizations remain highly supportive of the concept and recently filed suit in federal court that seeks to declare the stay order unlawful and to allow the regulation to go into effect.

Research Questions

Given this delay and public debate, patient-package-insert research is refreshing because it permits decisions to be based on data rather than conjecture. At the time the FDA first decided to explore the possibility of requiring patient package inserts, we also initiated a research program. At that point we asked ourselves three conceptual questions: (1) What information do people need to know? (2) What is the effect of written drug information? (3) What is the best way to communicate this information?

Desire for Information

The issue of what information people need to know can be answered partially by asking people what they want to know. Over the years, a number of surveys have solicited people's viewpoints regarding the desirability of receiving written information with prescription drugs. Table 17–1 lists these studies, describes the sample surveyed, and lists the percentage of patients in that sample who said they would like to receive written information describing their therapy. In looking at the results listed in table 17–1, we can draw some tentative conclusions.

In 1973, when the Knapp study was done, only about 41 percent of the people surveyed said they wanted patient package inserts.[5] The people who said they wanted this information tended to be young and well educated.

Table 17–1
Patient Desire for Patient Package Inserts

Study	*Sample*	*Percent Desiring Inserts*
Knapp (1973)	1,321 (National)	41
Ryan and McMahon (1976)	83 (Oral contraceptive users, New Orleans)	94
Morris, Mazis, and Gordon (1977)	1,720 (Oral contraceptive users, national)	89–97

Table 17-1 continued

Study	*Sample*	*Percent Desiring Inserts*
Blackwell and Talarzyk (1977)	1,500 (Ohio)	77
Kanouse and Morris (1978)	145 (Hypertensive outpatients, Los Angeles)	97
Mellinger (1978)	172 (Oakland)	80
Roper Reports (1978)	2,002 (National)	64
Qube TV (1980)	394 (Columbus, Ohio)	62
DeKoek and Burnell (1980)	83 (Oral contraceptive, estrogen users, New Jersey)	77
Marshall, Hadsall, and Gourley (1981)	411 (Pharmacy patrons, Nebraska)	38
Harris Survey (1981)	1,500 (National)	92
Morris and Kanouse (1981)	438 (Washington, D.C.)	90

Sources: D.E. Knapp, "Consumers and Medication," *FDA Report no. FDA-D-ADNC-4* (Springfield, Va.: Technical Information Service, 1974).

J. Ryan, and F.G. McMahon, "Potential Effects on the Health Care System - 2." *Drug Information Journal* Supplement (1977):75-79.

L.A. Morris, M. Mazis, and E. Gordon, "A Survey of the Effects of Oral Contraceptive Patient Information," *Journal of the American Medical Association* 238 (1977):2504-2508.

R.D. Blackwell and D. Talarzyk, "Medical Attitudes and Behavior of Respondent Base" In *Consumer Attitudes Toward Health Care and Medical Malpractice* (Columbus: Grid, Inc., 1977), pp. 27-42.

D.E. Kanouse, and L.A. Morris, "Patient Package Inserts: Effect on Patient Knowledge, Attitudes, and Behavior" (Paper presented at the American Public Health Association Meeting, Los Angeles, Calif., October 15, 1978.)

G.D. Mellinger, *Public Judgements About Ethical Issues in Research* NIMH Grant 27337-03 (Oakland, Calif., 1978).

Roper Organization, Inc., *Roper Reports* 78-3 (New York, April 1978).

Qube TV (1980) as reported in *FDC Reports* (1980) S-5 (Washington, D.C., September 15).

L. DeKoek and S.K. Burnell, "Patient Attitudes to PPIs—A Pilot Survey of Three Demographically Distinct Areas," *Medical Marketing and Media* 5 (1980):36-44.

R.P. Marshall, R.S. Hadsall, and D.R. Gourley, "Nebraska Patients' Attitudes about Patient Package Inserts, *American Pharmacy* 21 (1981):57-59.

L. Harris, "Louis Harris and Associates Survey," reported in *Washington Drug Letter,* January 19, 1981.

L.A. Morris and D.E. Kanouse, "Consumer Reactions to Differing Formats of Drug Information" (Unpublished manuscript, Rockville, Md.: Federal Drug Administration, 1981).

More-recent national surveys like the Roper survey done in 1978 find that about two-thirds of people desire package inserts.[6] It is no longer just the young and well educated but also the elderly who state a desire for the inserts. Several of these studies solicited information from patients who received patient package inserts.[7] These patients were asked if they would like to receive written information for other drugs. The data suggest that people who have experience with patient package inserts are apt to endorse their availability for other drugs.

The only study done in recent years that indicates a lack of consumer support was that by Marshall, Hadsall, and Gourley.[8] Pharmacy students were stationed in thirteen Nebraska pharmacies. Eleven of these pharmacies were engaged actively in prescription-drug-counseling activities. Customers were asked if they felt the government should require that written information be given to all patients with each prescription medication dispensed. About 40 percent of patients felt that they wanted the written information, 55 percent were opposed, and 7 percent were undecided about such a program.

Effects of Patient Package Inserts

Measuring the impact of patient package inserts can be accomplished in two ways. First, the effects of already required inserts can be assessed in the general population, or second, the effect of either prototype or actual inserts in small patient populations can be measured.

To evaluate the oral-contraceptive patient package insert, a national survey was conducted in 1975.[9] Approximately 1,720 women currently using the pill and about 950 former users of the pill were interviewed in a door-to-door survey. The results indicate that 93 percent of the women currently using the pill said that they had received the patient package insert. The great majority of those who said they received it said they read it; however, only about half of these people remembered what was the most important warning information at that time (that oral contraceptives may cause blood clots). One of the questions asked solicited information on whether the patient package insert affected the frequency with which patients contacted their physician. Three-quarters of the respondents said that it did not. About two-thirds of the remaining subjects said there was a decrease in physician contact, and about one-third said that the package insert increased the frequency of physician contact.

The data relating to the rate of physican contact is interesting because patient package inserts have been criticized for changing this frequency in either direction.[10] If patient package inserts increase the frequency of physician contact, they are said to increase costs. If they decrease the frequency of physician contacts, they are said to interfere with the physician/patient relationship. These criticisms suggest the need for careful analyses of package-insert effects. On the one hand, it is hoped that package inserts would decrease the nuisance calls of which physicians complain regularly. On the other hand, it is hoped that the inserts would increase patient sensitivity to what constitutes a warning signal of a serious adverse drug effect. This would allow people to call their physician when there might be a preventable problem that can be corrected by early physician intervention.

The data from the oral-contraceptive study also indicated that the major reason for contacting the physician was the experience of a reaction not mentioned in the insert. At the time the oral-contraceptive survey was completed, there was a two-tier delivery system for the patient package insert. First, a small insert was prepackaged by the manufacturer and delivered with the dispensed medicine. Second, if the patient wanted more information, she was advised to ask her physician for a copy of a brochure that more fully described the risks and proper use of oral contraceptives. Whereas most women said they received the insert, only about a third said they received the brochure. If it was received, the great majority said that they read the brochure. There were two types of brochures. One type was printed by individual manufacturers, and the second was much shorter, printed by the American Medical Association. Women were more apt to say they saved the manufacturer brochure for future use rather than the American Medical Association brochure. The results of the oral-contraceptive survey were utilized in 1977 when the FDA issued a revision of the oral-contraceptive patient package insert. The revised insert contained greater detail about some of the more recently discovered risks of the pill. In addition, the delivery system was changed so that both the brochure and the insert were delivered directly with the dispensed medication.

In addition to the oral-contraceptive PPI, it is possible to evaluate the effects of the patient package insert for estrogens used primarily for menopausal symptoms. Figure 17–1 displays sales results for oral Premarin, which holds a high percentage of the estrogen market. Sales for the most popular dosage form of the drug, 1.25 mg. tablets, are displayed with several events noted that might be expected to influence sales. As evidenced in the figure, this downward sales trend was initiated in 1976, following publication of studies that first linked the use of estrogens with increased rates of endometrial cancer. Events such as senate hearings, an *FDA Drug Bulletin*[11] article, and a revision of the physician labeling of 1976 appear to have contributed to this downward sales trend. In 1977, a patient package insert was required for estrogen. It appears that in 1978 there was another dip in the curve; however, it is impossible to be fully certain of the contribution of the patient package insert independently of the other influences.

In addition to large-scale studies, patient package inserts have been assessed in smaller scale studies of patients. The effect of patient package inserts have been measured on at least four different parameters: knowledge

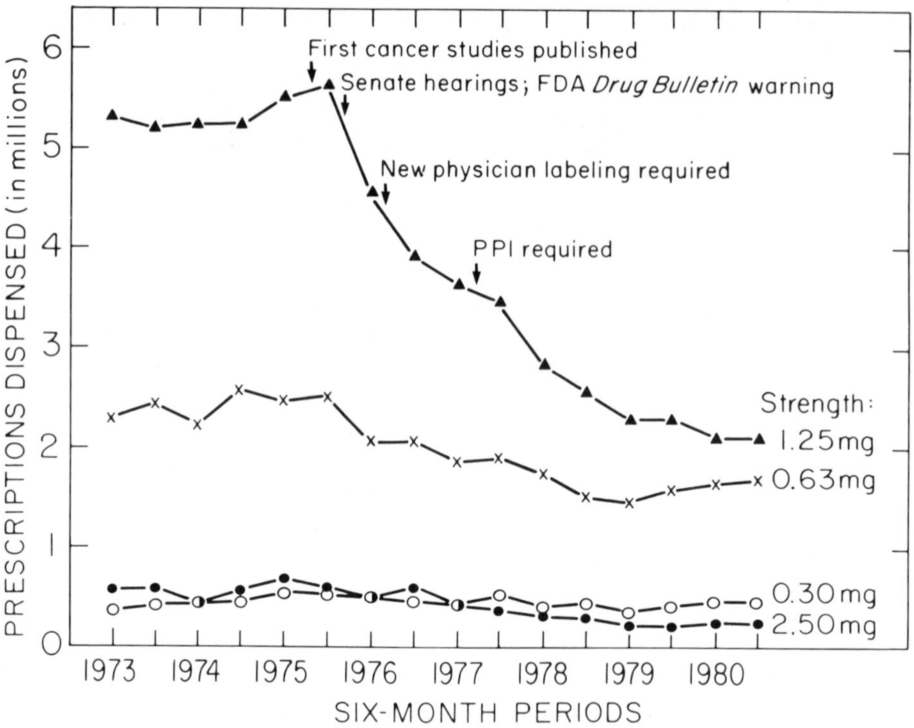

Source: Data from National Prescription Audit of IMS America, Ambler, Pa.

Figure 17-1. Total Prescriptions of Oral Premarin Dispensed, by Strength, Semiannually, 1973 through 1980

gained from reading PPIs, compliance with the therapeutic regimen, the effects of written information on therapeutic outcomes, and a determination on how the patient package insert influences the frequency of side effects (that is, does the listing of side effects in a patient package insert increase the incidence of suggestion-induced side effects?).

The following tables display the results of these studies: Table 17-2 for antibiotic drugs, table 17-3 for drugs used on a long-term basis, and table 17-4 for miscellaneous mixtures of drugs. In examining the results for antibiotic drugs, it is clear that patient package inserts consistently increase knowledge. In the majority of these studies, there is an increased rate of compliance with the therapeutic regimen. The two studies that have looked at therapeutic outcomes do find some improved effects; however, none of the studies have found an increase in the incidence of side effects related to patient package inserts.

Table 17-2
Studies Assessing Written Information for Antibiotic Drugs in Patient Populations

	Effects			
Study	*Knowledge*	*Compliance*	*Therapeutic Outcomes*	*Side Effects*
Sharpe and Mikeal (1974)		I[a]		
Madden (1973)	I	I		
Mattar, Markello, and Yaffee (1975)	I	I		ND[b]
Linkewich, Catalano, and Flack (1974)		I		
Lima et al. (1976)		I		
Eklund and Wessling (1974)	I	ND		
Colcher and Bass (1972)		I	I	
Leistyna and Macaulay (1966)			I	
Suveges (1977)	I	ND		ND
Crichton (1977)	I			

Sources: T.R. Sharpe and K.L. Mikeal, "Patient Compliance with Antibiotic Regimens," *American Journal of Hospital Pharmacy* 31 (1974):479–484.

E.E. Madden, "Evaluation of Outpatient Pharmacy Patient Counseling," *Journal of American Pharmaceutical Association* 13 (1973):437–443.

M.E. Mattar, J. Markello, and S.J. Yaffee, "Pharmaceutic Factors Affecting Patient Compliance," *Pediatrics* 54 (1974):101–108.

J.A. Linkewich, R.B. Catalano, and H.L. Flack, "The Effect of Packaging and Instruction on Outpatient Compliance with Medication Regimens," *Drug Intelligence and Clinical Pharmacology* 8 (1974)10–15.

J. Lima et al., "Compliance with Short-term Antimicrobial Therapy," *Pediatrics* 57 (1976): 383–386.

L.H. Eklund and A. Wessling, "Evaluation of Package Enclosures for Drug Package," *Lakartidningen* 73 (1976):2319–2320.

I.S. Colcher, and J.W. Bass, "Penicillin Treatment of Streptococcal Pharyngitis," *Journal of American Medical Association* 222 (1972):657–659.

J.A. Leistyna and J.C. Macaulay, "Therapy of Streptococcal Infections," *American Journal of Diseases of Children* 111 (1966):22–26.

L. Suveges, "The Impact of Counseling by the Pharmacist on Patient Knowledge and Compliance" (abstract) (Paper presented at the McMaster Symposium on Compliance with Therapeutic Regimens: Hamilton, Ontario, Canada: May 28, 1977).

E.F. Crichton, "Patient Recall of Medication Information" (abstract) (Paper presented at the McMaster Symposium on Compliance with Therapeutic Regimens: Hamilton, Ontario, Canada: May 28, 1977.

[a]I denotes an increase by information.

[b]ND denotes no difference caused by information. ND under side effects refers to the finding that written information did not increase the occurrence of side effects.

Table 17-3
Studies Assessing Written Information for Drugs Used on a Long-Term Basis in Patient Populations

	Effects			
Study	*Knowledge*	*Compliance*	*Therapeutic Outcomes*	*Side Effects*
Hecht (1974)		ND[b]		
Clark and Bayley (1972)	I[a]			
Sackett, Haynes, and Gibson (1975)	I	ND		
McKenney, Slining, and Henderson (1973)	I	I	I	
Bentz and Deliganis (1974)	I			
Rosenberg (1971)	I		I	
Hladik and White (1976)	I			
Fleckenstein, Joubert, and Lawrence (1976)	I			
Maiman, Green, and Gibson (1977)			ND	
Ley, Jain, and Skilbeck (1976)		I		
Deberry, Jefferies, and Light (1975)	I			
Dwyer (1977)	ND	ND		
Kanouse, Morris, and Kent (1980)	I	ND	ND	ND
Myers and Calvert (1978)		I		ND
Ferencz (1981)	I	I		
Udkow et al. (1979)	I			
Laher et al. (1981)	I			

Sources: A.B. Hecht, "Improving Patient Compliance by Teaching Outpatients," *Nursing Forum* 8 (1974):112–129.

C.M. Clark and E.W. Bayley, "Evaluation of the Use of Programmed Instruction for Patients Maintained on Warfarin Therapy," *American Journal of Public Health* 62 (1972):1135–1139.

D.L. Sackett, R.B. Haynes, and E.S. Gibson, "Randomized Clinical Trail of Strategies for Improving Medication Compliance in Primary Hypertension," *Lancet* 1 (1975):1205–1207.

J.M. McKenney, J.M. Slining, and H.R. Henderson, "The Effect of Clinical Pharmacy Services on Patients with Essential Hypertension," *Circulation* 48 (1973):1104–1111.

P.M. Bentz and S.G. Deliganis, "Protocol: Patient Medication Education," *Northwest Medical Journal* 3 (1974):33–40.

S.G. Rosenberg, "Patient Education Leads to Better Care for Heart Patients," *Nursing Forum* 8 (1971):112–129.

W.B. Hladik and S.J. White, "Evaluation of Written Reinforcements Used in Counseling Cardiovascular Patients," *American Journal of Hospital Pharmacy* 33 (1976):1277–1280.

L. Fleckenstein, P. Joubert, and R. Lawrence, "Oral Contraceptive Patient Information: A

Questionnaire Study of Attitudes, Knowledge, and Preferred Information Sources," *Journal of the American Medical Association* 235 (1976):1331.

L.A. Maiman, L.W. Green, and G. Gibson, "Randomized Clinical Trails to Evaluate Patient Education for Self Management by Adult Asthmatics" (Paper presented at the American Public Health Association, Washington, D.C., November 1977).

P. Ley, V.K. Jain, and C.E. Skilbeck, "A Method for Decreasing Patients' Medication Errors," *Psychological Medicine* 6 (1976):599–601.

P. Deberry, L.P. Jefferies, and M.R. Light, "Teaching Cardiac Patients to Manage Medications," *American Journal of Nursing* 75 (1975):2191–2193.

F.R. Dwyer, "An Experimental Study of Consumer Use of Supplemental Drug Information," (Ph.D. Thesis, University of Minnesota, Minneapolis, Minn., 1978).

D.E. Kanouse, L.A. Morris, and J.T. Kent, "Effects of a Prototype PPI for Thiazide Drugs" (Unpublished manuscript, 1982).

E.D. Myers, and E.J. Calvert, "Knowledge of Side Effects and Perserverance with Medication," *British Journal of Psychiatry* 132 (1978):526–527.

N. Ferencz, "The Effect of the Estrogen Patient Package Inserts on Patient Compliance With Physician's Instructions," *Contemporary Pharmacy Practice* 4 (1981):45–48.

G. Udkow et al., "The Safety and Efficacy of the Estrogen Patient Package Insert: A Questionnaire Study," *Journal of the American Medical Association* 242 (1979):536–539.

M. Laher et al., "Educational Value of Printed Information for Patients with Hypertension," *British Medical Journal* 282 (1981):1360–1361.

[a]I denotes an increase by information.

[b]ND denotes no difference caused by information. ND under side effects refers to the finding that written information did not increase the occurrence of side effects.

Table 17–4
Studies Assessing Written Information for a Miscellaneous Mixture of Drugs in Patient Populations

	Effects			
Study	*Knowledge*	*Compliance*	*Therapeutic Outcomes*	*Side Effects*
Clinite and Kabat (1976)	I[a]	ND[b]		
Beardsley, Johnson, and Wise (1977)	I	I		
Weibert (1977)	I			ND
Greiner (1972)			ND	
Wandless and Davie (1977)	I			
MacDonald, MacDonald, and Phoenix (1977)	I	I		
Boyd et al. (1974)	I	I		
Newcomer and Anderson (1974)	I	ND		I
Fox (1969)	I			
Paulson et al. (1976)	I			

Table 17-4 continued

	Effects			
Study	*Knowledge*	*Compliance*	*Therapeutic Outcomes*	*Side Effects*
Rosser and Fleet (1971)		I		
Doyle (1977)	I			
Ellis et al. (1979)	I			
Benson et al. (1977)	I			
Noyes and Gordon (1975)	I			

Sources:J.C. Clinite and H.F. Kabat, "Improving Patient Compliance," *Journal of the American Pharmaceutical Association* 16 (1976):74–76.

R.S. Beardsley, C.A. Johnson, and G. Wise, "Privacy as a Factor in Patient Counseling," *Journal of the American Pharmaceutical Association* 17 (1977):366–368.

R.T. Weibert, "Patient Package Inserts: Potential Distribution Problems," *Drug Information Journal* 11 (1977):45–49.

G.E. Greiner, "The Pharmacist's Role in Patient Discharge Planning," *American Journal of Hospital Pharmacy* 21 (1972):72–76.

I. Wandless and J.W. Davie, "Can Drug Compliance in the Elderly be Improved? *British Medical Journal* 1 (1977):359–361.

E.T. MacDonald, J.B. MacDonald, and M. Phoenix, "Improving Drug Compliance After Hospital Discharge," *British Medical Journal* 2 (1977):618–621.

J.R. Boyd et al., "Drug Defaulting Part II: Analysis of Noncompliance Patterns," *American Journal of Hospital Pharmacy* 31 (1974):485–491.

D.R. Newcomer and R.W. Anderson, "Effectiveness of a Combined Drug and Patient Teaching Program," *Drug Intelligence and Clinical Pharmacy* 8 (1974):374–381.

L.A. Fox, "Written Reinforcement of Auxiliary Directions for Prescription Medications," *American Journal of Hospital Pharmacy* 26 (1969):334–341.

P.T. Paulson et al., "Medication Data Sheets—An Aid to Patient Education," *Drug Intelligence and Clinical Pharmacy* 10 (1976):448–453.

W.W. Rosser and D.C. Fleet, "How Patients Follow Hospital Discharge Instructions in an Urban Family Practice," *Canadian Family Physician* 20 (1971):57–59.

C. Doyle, "Factors Influencing the Misuse of Medication by the Older Person," (Social Planning and Review Council of British Columbia, Vancouver, B.C., 1977).

D.C. Ellis et al., "Doctor's Orders: Controlled Trial of Supplementary Written Information for Patients," *British Medical Journal* 278 (1979):1285–1286.

H. Benson et al., "Patient Education and Intrauterine Contraception: A Study of Two Package Inserts," *American Journal of Public Health* 67 (1977):446–449.

R.W. Noyes and W.H. Gordon, "Patient Information Drug Package Leaflet," Exhibit #1304, American Medical Association Meeting, Atlantic City, N.J., 1975

[a]I denotes an increase by information.

[b]ND denotes no difference caused by information. ND under side effects refers to the finding that written information did not increase the occurrence of side effects.

In studies that have looked at the effects of patient package inserts for drugs used on a longer-term basis, again relatively consistent knowledge differences are shown. For compliance data, however, results are more mixed. Some studies show an increase while others do not. No increase in side effects is found. For studies that examined a miscellaneous mixture of drugs, the results again are consistent with the long-term drug studies—clear increases in knowledge and some mixture of results related to whether or not patient package inserts increase compliance. The Newcomer and Anderson study has found an increase of reporting side effects associated with patient package inserts.[12]

In reviewing these studies, one must totally realize that many of the studies concurrently examined a number of educational interventions in addition to written information. For example, pharmacist counseling was utilized frequently in addition to package inserts.

Overall, the studies find that written information clearly increases patient knowledge about drugs. However, this knowledge is not necessarily translated into behavioral changes. Where the behaviors requested in the insert are relatively simple ones, such as finishing a full course of therapy for antibiotics, there is a greater probability of success. Suggestion-induced side effects are not normally seen in these studies.

How To Communicate Patient-Package-Insert Information

The communication issue covers two different issues: (1) What is the appropriate content for patient package inserts, and (2) what is the most cost-effective means of delivering this information to the patient? Although these issues are interdependent (as certain distribution means would necessitate certain styles of information presentation), for the most part they can be examined separately. However, the criteria for evaluating successful communication changes depending upon the issue examined. On the one hand, package-insert content is evaluated by clinical or experimental means (that is, which of several alternative contents works best?). On the other hand, an economic basis is used to evaluate the package-insert delivery system (that is, which of several alternative distribution methods costs least for equal benefits?).

The FDA has examined the content of patient-package inserts in a number of different studies. Our first effort at examining their content was to utilize small focused group interviews.[13] Eight to ten consumers drawn from the population were asked to discuss their reactions to different examples of package inserts. Several styles of presentation were shown to the groups. In addition, inserts have been studied using different styles of presentations in analog studies where college students or more-representative groups of consumers are asked their reactions to different styles of presentations.[14] The most representative study in this vein is one being conducted by the Rand Corporation.[15] Again different styles of package-insert presentations were tested in an outpatient population. The subjects were patients obtaining prescriptions for study drugs from a random sample of pharmacies in the Los Angeles area.

Some of the content features we have examined include the amount of information presented, tone, and language complexity (readability level). Package-insert influences are assessed on variables indicating changes in knowledge, attitude, compliance, side effects, and clinical course.

Thus far, our initial conclusions from the content studies are that writing a patient package insert is more similar to painting a picture with words than to drafting a novel. Documents need to be designed to meet specific knowledge objectives. Patient memory appears to be the bottleneck for the communication effectiveness. People have finite capacities for remembering details, and they appear to remember best what they consider the most important information. Therefore, the relative emphasis of information in the insert helps to determine what information in an insert will be best remembered. The data obtained thus far may be explained by what is already known from research literature about how people process information. As we move to larger population studies, one question that needs to be answered is whether or not memory will remain a major problem in patient-package-insert communication or whether or not exposure and attention factors will determine the effectiveness.

The issue of how to distribute patient package inserts is phrased in terms of cost-effectiveness and is a major focus of current debate. Many pharmacy groups have suggested that mandatory regulations are not needed because voluntary systems are adequate. In addition, several people have suggested that rather than the FDA-mandated system (distributing a separate leaflet with each new prescription), other alternatives would work equally well at less cost. Some suggested alternatives include placing a looseleaf book in the pharmacy that the patient could consult while the prescription is being filled, having the information in an open rack where the customer could pick out the one he or she needs or having the patient request the document from the pharmacist.

There has been some evaluation of these issues. A pair of unpublished market-research reports has examined the distribution of patient package inserts under mandatory and voluntary systems. Recently, Eli Lilly voluntarily decided to institute an insert for their Darvon products. They sent inserts to 50,000 pharmacies throughout the United States. Lilly conducted a telephone survey of 200 pharmacists to determine if the insert was received and if it was being dispensed. About 85 percent of the pharmacists said that they had received and were dispensing the inserts.

To obtain converging data on patient-package-insert dispensing, observers in an FDA evaluation visited 103 pharmacies chosen at random in seven cities to obtain prescriptions for Darvon products. Only 7 percent of the people filling prescriptions received a copy of the package insert. If they then requested a copy of the insert, an additional 34 percent received one. Overall, the majority of the people (59 percent filling prescriptions did not receive an insert even when they requested it. In comparing those data to mandatory patient package inserts (from a similar study of estrogens), 39 percent of the patients received one spontaneously, 55 percent received one if it was requested, and 6 percent did not receive one.[16]

One of the market-research studies has compared two different voluntary systems for dispensing a patient package insert for diazepam (Valium). The Hoffman-La Roche Company field tested a book placed at the pharmacy counter compared to a patient package insert distributed spontaneously by the pharmacist. The test was conducted in three cities: Boston, Atlanta, and Dallas/Fort Worth. Over 42,000 interviews were conducted to find about 800 people who had received a prescription for diazepam during the test period. Only 7 percent of the subjects said that they saw the insert. This low percentage of distribution was attributed by Hoffman-La Roche to low cooperation rates by pharmacists. When pharmacists were asked to compare the booklet in the pharmacy to the insert spontaneous-dispensing system, the spontaneous-dispensing system was preferred. However, with only a single insert to be dispensed, this comparison is of questionable value.

After an extensive review, including new hearings in September and October 1981, the FDA decided to propose a revocation of the patient-package-insert rule. The rationale for the proposed revocation was that the private sector had initiated steps to improve patients' knowledge of prescription drugs and that these privately initiated systems may prove to be more effective than a mandated program.

The basic goal of the patient-package-insert program—to educate patients more fully about prescription drugs—remains an FDA objective. A multifaceted, private-sector approach is now the primary means of achieving this goal. To encourage private-sector action, the FDA has established a committee on patient education. Some recent private-sector programs include the following:

The American Medical Association is preparing patient leaflets to be distributed by physicians.

The Retired Persons Pharmacy Service, a mail-order pharmacy serving about 3 million people and affiliated with the American Association of Retired Persons, is distributing leaflets written especially for the elderly.

Biomedical Information Corporation is distributing to physicians, at no cost, patient-information sheets that describe various indications and their treatments.

The Ciba-Geigy Corporation has provided initial funding for a consortium of consumer and professional groups. The consortium will coordinate programs seeking to improve patient knowledge about prescription drugs.

Conclusion

An increase in patient responsibility for, and control of, health care is a desirable goal. Such an increase surely depends upon increased knowledge about drugs (among other interventions). Despite some obvious problems, the program in patient package insert's is a workable, potentially useful step toward this goal.

Notes

1. *Federal Register* 40, no. 216 (November 7, 1975):52075–52076.
2. A.D. Berton, "Drug Information for Patients: The Patient Package Insert." *Drug Information Journal* (1977):1155; and A.M. Meyers, "Patient Package Inserts. Content and Format," Proceedings of FDA-Sponsored Conference December 11–12, 1978. (Springfield, Va.: National Technical Information Service, Publication no. 298184).
3. *Federal Register* 44, no. 131 (July 6, 1979):40016–40041.
4. *Federal Register* 45, no. 179 (September 12, 1980):60754–60817.
5. D.E. Knapp, "Consumers and Medication," FDA Report, no. FDA-D-ADMC-4 (Springfield, Va.: Technical Information Service, 1974).
6. Roper Organization, Inc., *Roper Reports* 78-3 (New York: April 1978).
7. L.A. Morris, M. Mazis, and E. Gordon, "A Survey of the Effects of Oral Contraceptive Patient Information," *Journal of the American Medical Association* 238 (1977):2504–2508; D.E. Kanouse and L.A. Morris, "Patient Package Inserts: Effect on Patient Knowledge, Attitudes, and Behavior." Paper presented October 15, 1978, at the American Public Health Association Meeting, Los Angeles, California; and L. De Koek and S.K. Burnell, "Patient Attitudes to PPI's—A Pilot Survey of Three Demographically Distinct Areas," *Medical Marketing and Media* 5 (1980):36–44.
8. R.P. Marshall, R.S. Hadsall, and D.R. Gourley, "Nebraska Patients' Attitudes about Patient Package Inserts," *American Pharmacy* 21 (1981):57–59.

9. L.A. Morris, M. Mazis, and E. Gordon, "A Survey of the Effects of Oral Contraceptive Patient Information," *Journal of the American Medical Association* 238 (1977):2504–2508; and M. Mazis, L.A. Morris, and E. Gordon, "Patient Attitudes about Two Forms of Printed Oral Contraceptive Information," *Medical Care* 16 (1978):1045–1054.

10. A. Gross, "Assessment of Value of Information for Patients," *Journal of the American Medical Association* 240 (1978):1240; and R. Lanzillotti and R. Blair, "An Economic Analysis of the Food and Drug Administration's Proposed Patient Package Insert Program." Unpublished manuscript submitted to the Food and Drug Administration, Rockville, Md., November 1977).

11. *FDA Drug Bulletin* (February–March 1976):18–20.

12. D.R. Newcomer and R.W. Anderson, "Effectiveness of a Combined Drug and Patient Teaching Program," *Drug Intelligence and Clinical Pharmacy* 8 (1974):374–381.

13. A. Myers et al., "Consumer Reactions to Prototype PPIs for Prescription Drugs" *A Focus Group Analysis* (Springfield, Va.: National Technical Information Service, 1980).

14. L.A. Morris and D.E. Kanouse, "Consumer Reactions to Differing Formats of Drug Information." Unpublished manuscript submitted to the Food and Drug Administration (Rockville, Md., 1981); L.A. Morris, A. Myers, and D.G. Thilman, "Application of Readability Concepts to Patient-Oriented Drug Information," *American Journal of Hospital Pharmacy* 37 (1980):1504–1508; and L.A. Morris and D.E. Kanouse, "Consumers' Reactions to Differing Amounts of Written Drug Information," *Drug Intelligence and Clinical Pharmacy* 14 (1980):531–536.

15. Rand Corporation, "Effects of Patient Package Inserts as a Function of Critical Variations:" FDA Contract, no. 5 223-78-3009 (Santa Monica, Calif., 1978).

16. L.A. Morris et al., "Estrogen PPI's—An FDA Survey," *American Pharmacy* NS 20 (1980):318–322.

18 Reporting Drug Truth in the Media

Charles Winick

What have the mass media been saying about prescription drugs? The answers to this question are important because the media can represent a significant service of role validation for professional participants such as physicians, nurses, and pharmacists in this country's system of delivering medical services, as well as provide information and raise questions for legislators and administrators and, especially, for the patients who take the drugs.

A patient taking prescription drugs may receive some information about them from the prescriber, in terms of the nature, specific context, and expected effects of the prescription. Such information could, however, be interpreted by patients in the light of their knowledge of the product as obtained from sources such as friends and observations of media content. The latter may be so important that the well-known and widely distributed journal *Drug Therapy: The Journal of Clinical Therapeutics* carries, in every issue, a feature called "What Your Patients Are Reading." This feature summarizes and critiques five or six articles on medication and treatment that currently are appearing in popular magazines.

Several physicians on the staff of a major medical center that services chronically ill children encountered significant problems because of the increase in media reporting of developments in health research.[1] Patients and their families may be vulnerable to mass-media reports because their hopes for therapeutic benefit are usually intense. Patients with nonchronic ailments may encounter news or information in the media that affect the expectations the patients bring to the treatment situation.

Legislators and regulatory agencies may be responsive to media content. Pharmaceutical manufacturers not only are subjects of media attention but also could be obtaining impressions of public perceptions of their products from media representations. An article in *The New York Times* on the prescription-writing activities of a physician on the staff of a major drug manufacturer led to the physician's resignation on the very next day.[2]

In order to obtain information on the parameters of media reporting on prescription drugs, a content analysis was conducted of mass-media content concerned with prescription medications for the calendar years 1979 and 1980. The media covered were popular magazines as measured by the over 300 publications cited in the *Magazine Index;* television, as measured by the news and talk programs presented on the three commercial networks, one public television station, and three independent commercial stations in New York City; and newspapers, as measured by news stories in *The New York Times* and the *New York Daily News.*

The television-network flagship stations in New York City (WABC, WCBS, WNBC) are typical of network-owned or -affiliated stations nationally. The three independent stations (WOR, WPIX, and WNEW) are reasonably representative of other independents, and the public channel (WNET) is typical of other public stations. *The New York Times* is a so-called newspaper of record, and the *New York Daily News* is a morning tabloid with the second-largest circulation of any daily newspaper in the United States.

Methodology

There were 482 magazine articles, 189 television programs, and 291 newspaper reports, for a total of 962 communications. The magazine articles and newspaper reports were concerned entirely with subjects related to prescription drugs. Thus, all the tabulated content in these two media was devoted to prescription drugs. The television material, however, usually was part of a news program or a talk show or part or all of a public-service show, documentary program, or special.

During the two years studied, another 81 magazine articles, 11 television programs, and 13 newspaper communications appeared that had relevant content, judging from various indexes, but the original or a summary of which could not be obtained. There is no way of knowing how these 105 unavailable items might have affected the overall results of the current study, but it would seem unlikely that they could have added new content dimensions.

Although the communications were of varying lengths and degrees of importance in the magazine, television program, or newspaper, they were not weighted. Because several different media were involved, there was no systematic way to weight them quantitatively for factors such as length, size of audience, degree of prominence within the medium, day of the week of appearance, anticipated pass-along audience, multisensory impact of television, and editorial environment of the item. Thus, all items are given the same weight.

Categories of Content

The title of every story or relevant feature was listed, and either the original or a summary was viewed/read. A series of content categories were estab-

Table 18–1
Media Content Related to Prescription Drugs, by Category

Category	*Percent of Total*
Effects of prescription drugs	34
New drugs and uses	24
Consumer considerations and economics of prescribing	20
Role of physicians, nurses, and pharmacists	14
Regulation of prescription drugs	8

lished on a tentative basis and employed on a sample of content in order to see how adequate the categories were for the materials. A total of thirty-five categories were finally established. For ease of discussion, the thirty-five categories were grouped into five larger categories, set forth in table 18–1 along with the percentage of the total number of communications represented by each one. Each story, article, or broadcast was counted only once; if it straddled two or more content categories, it was assigned to the one to which it was most centrally related.

Effects. The largest single category, accounting for 34 percent of the total, dealt with the effects of the drugs, as set forth in table 18–2. The tranquilizing drugs, especially Valium, represented the largest single category by an overwhelming margin (8 percent). The addiction/abuse potential of tranquilizers was the theme of 7 percent of the stories, with side effects and toxicity close behind (6 percent). Celebrities' drug habits and experiences accounted for 4 percent.

Populations on which drugs are tested (3 percent) and drug interactions with alcohol and other drugs (2 percent) were responsible for a number of stories. Estrogens, overmedication, and various public-health-related stories each accounted for 1 percent.

A previous content analysis of a sample of 108 articles on diazepam, appearing in general-circulation magazines between 1974 and 1977, concluded that 75 were negative, 18 were positive, and 15 were neutral.[3] The negative tone of so many of the discussions of Valium in the latter study, in the current content analysis, and in widely read books (see, for example, Gordon[4]) is noteworthy in view of the recurring finding that approximately one-fifth of all prescriptions involve tranquilizers.[5] It is possible that tranquilizer use might be greater if it received more media support, or perhaps media support only recently has declined.

Overall, over three-fourths (77 percent) of these communications in the current study present a questioning or negative view of the effects of prescription medications. Presumably, horror stories and difficulties are more

Table 18-2
Effects of Prescription Drugs

Subject of Communication	*Percent of Total*
Valium and other tranquilizers	8
Addiction and abuse potential (athletes, drivers, other special groups, parents/children, and so forth)	7
Side effects, long-term effects, and toxicity (for example, diethylstilbestrol)	6
Experiences of celebrities with prescription drugs	4
Testing drugs (for example, prisoners, Central Intelligence Agency, military, animal studies, etc.)	3
Drug interactions with alcohol and other drugs	2
Estrogen hazards	1
Overmedication	1
Swine-flu innoculation, influenza shots, other public-health matters	1
Other	1
Total for category	34

newsworthy than positive reports or experiences. Publications and television stations may feel they are serving their audiences best by informing them about possible hazards and problems relating to prescription medications rather than by conveying positive achievements.

A study of the relationship between media coverage and public opinion on scientific issues suggests that the public is usually conservative and would rather be safe than sorry, so that the media presentation of problems works to the detriment of acceptance of new technology.[6] This attitude may be related to the conservative attitudes of Americans toward mood-modifying drugs, documented by Manheimer and his associates.[7] There has also been considerable scholarly denunciation of Americans' allegedly uncritical use of drugs—notably, mood-modifying substances.[8]

New Drugs and New Uses

Table 18-3 gives the details of the 24 percent of the publications and broadcasts that were concerned either with new drugs or new uses of existing drugs. The disease that drew the largest single number of communications was cancer (7 percent), with drugs for cardiovascular conditions frequently cited (4 percent). Psychoactive drugs—notably, lithium—were discussed often (4 percent). A variety of new so-called miracle drugs (4 percent) and

Table 18–3
New Drugs and New Uses

Subject of Communication	*Percent of Total*
Cancer-treatment drugs	7
Cardiovascular drugs	4
Lithium and other psychoactive drugs	4
Prostaglandins, beta-blockers, dynorphins, other miracle drugs	4
Procedures for testing new drugs	1
Ritalin, new uses	1
Recall of new drugs	1
Marijuana as a therapeutic drug for cancer, glaucoma, and so on	1
Other	1
Total for category	24

testing procedures (1 percent) also figured as subjects. Problems leading to recall of new drugs (1 percent) and marijuana as a therapeutic drug (1 percent) accounted for other content.

Since magazines, television, and newspapers are event oriented, it is not surprising that the subject of new drugs and new uses of existing medications represent important content. The public has been so sensitized to cancer and cardiovascular conditions that there is a built-in audience for stories on chemotherapy developments in treating these conditions. The methodology for testing drug efficacy and safety, and reports of field and other trials, are of continuing interest. Usually, reports of new medications or new uses of extant medications derive from studies in scholarly journals or presentations by scientists to professional groups. In the case of cancer chemotherapy, popular-science writers regularly are invited to attend seminars specifically designed to provide valid current information for mass media.

Sensational large-circulation tabloid weekly newspapers like the *Enquirer* and *Star,* not included in this study, carry articles on new drugs in almost every issue. The media analyzed in the current survey are relatively conservative in their coverage of new medications compared to the large-circulation tabloid weeklies.

Many physicians and clinics have had the experience of patients arriving for treatment with a newspaper or magazine clipping describing a new drug the patient felt was relevant to his condition. If the clipping or television report was exaggerated or if the drug was inappropriate for the patient's condition, the patient might feel let down or have less confidence in the physician. The volume and quality of media communications on new drugs or new uses of old drugs thus could interact directly with patients' expectations of treatment.

Consumer Considerations

One-fifth of the materials were concerned with consumer considerations and the economics of prescribing, as summarized in table 18–4. The most frequently discussed subject was generic drugs, especially their price, quality, and availability (6 percent). Medicaid and Medicare policies on prescriptions were fairly frequent (3 percent) themes, as were reports on pharmaceutical manufacturers (3 percent), advertising (2 percent), and medicine-chest contents (2 percent). Foreign products, quality control, and the growing number of prescription products each accounted for 1 percent.

Consumerism has been of growing importance in the health field in recent years, and the issue of generic drugs has represented a significant focus of consumer concern. In the current study, television and magazines were particularly likely to deal with generics and Medicaid/Medicare practices. Exposés and discussions of pharmaceutical companies and their profits tended to appear in newspapers and magazines, which also often carried information on the contents of medicine chests.

A few consumer-advocate groups receive a large proportion of the media attention. It is possible that these high-visibility groups have learned how to present their press releases and conferences in a manner that facilitates their media access. Someone like Dr. Sidney Wolfe of the Center for

Table 18–4
Consumer Considerations and Economics of Prescribing

Subject of Communication	*Percent of Total*
Generic drugs—price, quality, availability	6
Medicaid and Medicare policies and practices on prescriptions	3
Practices and profits of pharmaceutical manufacturers	3
Content and effects of advertising	2
Medicine-chest contents	2
Foreign pharmaceutical manufacturers and products	1
Quality control	1
Proliferation of prescription drugs	1
Other	1
Total for category	20

Science in the Public Interest is a kind of brand name that is easily recognizable. In contrast, industry representatives tend to be less well known and seldom give rejoinders to the many charges directed against the industry. It is possible, of course, that they attempt rejoinders that are not conveyed by the media because an attack may be more newsworthy than an answer to it.

The U.S. health industry currently accounts for approximately $130 billion in expenditures per year. The size of this outlay and the increasing number of Americans who are living longer and who are subject to various maladies of old age for which they will be taking medications make it likely that the consumer dimension will remain an important part of media treatments of prescription drugs. As Medicaid and Medicare remain features of the health landscape, their policies with respect to matters like generics, fraud, or drug efficacy will continue to attract media concern.

Pharmaceutical manufacturers represent popular subjects for articles and media reports because the industry, in the eyes of its critics, earns so much money on its capital investment, while to its proponents, it takes immense financial risks in the attempt to develop new medications. There is spirited debate over the amount and quality of ethical-drug advertising, foreign firms, and trends in Medicaid and Medicare.

Role of Physicians, Nurses, and Pharmacists

The role of physicians, nurses, and pharmacists was the theme of approximately one-seventh (14 percent) of the materials, as summarized in table 18–5. Two related subjects tied for first place (3 percent) in this category:

Table 18–5
Role of Physicians, Nurses, and Pharmacists

Subject of Communication	*Percent of Total*
Ease and lack of controls of physician prescription writing	3
Dr. Feelgood approach	3
Ethics of some prescription writing (especially executions, nursing homes)	2
Patients' pressures on prescribers	2
Nurses and pharmacists as prescribers	1
Physicians and appetite suppressants	1
Over- and underprescribing	1
Other	1
Total for category	14

the lack of supervision of doctors' prescription writing and the activities of so-called Dr. Feelgood script doctors. Ethical problems related to writing prescriptions in special situations like nursing homes or participation in executions by drugs in various states represented 2 percent, as did patients' pressures on prescribers. The role of prescription medications in treatment of overweight and over- and underprescribing practices each accounted for some (1 percent) items.

Almost all of the communications concerned with physicians' prescription practices raise questions about their motivations, skill, wisdom, morality, and yielding to patients' requests. Materials dealing with the new role of nurses and pharmacist prescribers typically praise this development. A number of the reports and stories were based on case histories of specific physicians or other prescribers who represented some extreme variety of activity.

Regulation of Prescription Drugs

Government and other official regulation of prescription drugs accounted for approximately one-twelfth (8 percent) of the items published or broadcast. The FDA figured in analyses of its procedures (3 percent) and critiques of its being too rigorous or not rigorous enough (2 percent). Information about the drugs on labels, package inserts, and other places (1 percent) and the issue of regulating advertising to physicians (1 percent) also figured in these materials, which are summarized in table 18-6.

Reports on the FDA usually find the agency wanting in some respect—for example, it exercises too much diligence or not enough diligence, provides too much or not enough control or direction, and so on. Media comments on information to be contained on labels and packages recommend such information's use, while comments on advertising addressed to physicians usually call for its regulation or minimization.

Table 18-6
Regulation of Prescription Drugs

Subject of Communication	*Percent of Total*
Description, length, and uncertainty of FDA procedures	3
FDA procedures too rigorous or not rigorous enough	2
Information on labels, safety inserts, and so on	1
Regulation of advertising to physicians	1
Other	1
Total for category	8

Of the five categories of communications, this regulation category had the largest proportion (74 percent) of negative or critical content. All government agencies that engage in regulatory activities are likely targets for criticism; however, there is no way of knowing whether or not prescription-drug-regulation activities are criticized proportionately more than other regulators.

Discussion

In other subjects related to science and medicine that are discussed by mass media, certain prominent personalities such as Dr. Linus Pauling or Dr. Michael DeBakey are sufficiently famous so that their views on a particular controversy may be sought and presented by interviewers. Although a number of distinguished scientists work in the field of prescription drugs, none has become enough of a national media celebrity to be sought out regularly in order to give an opinion. However, authorities are referred to and quoted by the media more often than specific studies or findings are cited. Especially in the case of television, it is easier to get a statement from an authority than to give the results of an investigation or study in the third person. Even when a study is being reported, it tends to be presented through a personality.

The media probably are interested in scientist-spokespersons who will speak unequivocally and clearly about a drug or its effects rather than the kind of cautious scientist who is likely to make an equivocal statement. The scientists who are interviewed and quoted thus often tend to be relatively committed to a particular viewpoint rather than to be disinterested contributors to knowledge.

Most of the communications presented in the three media studied are separate and discrete, with minimal reference to work that had taken place earlier. Typically, the so-called news hook of the report is presented as hard news of some recent specific development rather than as a report of a trend.

Approximately 32 percent of all the communications linked the hard news to some significant underlying issue, which might be ethical, economic, training, or consumer in nature. This is a relatively high proportion considering the immediate deadline orientation of newspapers and television. In terms of issues, television was much more likely than magazines or newspapers to present a balanced overview. Television traditionally tries to present all sides of a controversial issue, in accordance with Federal Communications Commission guidelines. A sharp disagreement between spokespersons for different viewpoints also can make for the kind of conflict that is exciting for the audience. Such disagreements are less likely to be found in a newspaper or magazine article, which can be more one-sided because it is signed by the reporter or writer.

An effort was made to determine the extent to which the communications represented media events or activities that were generated for the primary purpose of reaching the media. For 53 percent of the communications, no determination of this matter could be made. Where an estimate could be made on whether or not the immediate stimulus for the coverage was a desire for access to media, about half of the 47 percent remaining communications appeared to be media events. Thus, slightly less than a fourth of all the communications, using this admittedly crude measure, seemed to result from a press conference or a similar effort to contribute to public opinion. It is possible that the subject of prescription drugs is sufficiently salient to editors and other media gatekeepers so that it is not very difficult to get such materials in print or on the air. Prescription drugs presumably are used in conditions that are serious enough to make people concerned. A number of the conditions treated by drugs, such as cancer, cardiovascular conditions, and mental illness, have connotations that resonate for large numbers of people.

The same conditions or illnesses, like the aforementioned three, occur over and over again in media discussions of prescription drugs. Although literally thousands of prescription drugs are sold in the United States, relatively few are the subjects of media interest. In this, the media practice is analogous to that of typical physicians, who tend to prescribe a limited number of drugs on a regular basis (see chapter 21). Only 182 named products could be identified in the current study.

Radio was not included in the current study because of difficulties in obtaining station program logs. Since over 8,000 radio stations exist in the United States, the problems of getting an adequate sample are substantial. Radio is such a ubiquitous medium—the average home has four radios—that its content related to prescription drugs could be substantial in terms of volume and impact.

Future studies should include radio as well as entertainment programs on television and movies. There can be little doubt that television dramas, soap operas, situation comedies, and movies on television and in a theater communicate content dealing with prescription drugs, which may have considerable impact on their audiences.

In the case of evening network television, thirty different series were built around physicians between 1954 and 1977.[9] Seven of these series ran for five or more years (for example, "Marcus Welby, M.D."; "Medical Center"). In many episodes of these series, the physician writes a prescription for his or her patient. Prescription-drug practices in such television series may have enormous impact on their regular viewers.

Daytime daily television dramas, or soap operas, have a significant medical plot and character component (for example, "General Hospital," "The Doctors," "All My Children"). They have considerable plot and character activity relating to prescriptions—the setting in which they are written, filled, and taken and their consequences.

The same kinds of considerations apply to entertainment movies. A complete study of mass-media content relating to prescription drugs would include movies, the electronic media, and popular books. The impact of the mass media on the different groups concerned with prescription drugs is potentially so significant that a full analysis of their content could be very instructive.

Notes

1. M.H. Rourk et al., "The News Media and the Doctor-Patient Relationship," *New England Journal of Medicine* (19 November 1981):1278–1280.
2. M. Orestres, "Drug Executive Resigns over Insomnia Program," *The New York Times,* 1 December 1981, p. B3.
3. D.E. Smith, project director, Benzodiazepine Research and Physician Training Project, San Francisco, personal communication, May 1981.
4. B. Gordon, *I'm Dancing as Fast as I Can* (New York: Harper & Row, 1979).
5. R. Cooperstock and H.L. Lennard, "Some Social Meanings of Tranquilizer Use," *Sociology of Health and Illness* 1 (1979):331–347.
6. A. Mazur, "Media Coverage and Public Opinion on Scientific Discoveries," *Journal of Communication* 31 (1981):106–115.
7. D.I. Manheimer et al., "Use of Mood-Changing Drugs among American Adults," in *Sociological Aspects of Drug Dependence,* ed. C. Winick (Cleveland: CRC Press, 1974), pp. 103–111.
8. H.L. Lennard et al., *Mystification and Drug Misuse* (San Francisco: Jossey-Bass, 1971).
9. J. Liebmann-Smith and S.L. Rosen, "The Presentation of Illness on Television," in *Deviance and Mass Media,* ed. C. Winick (Beverly Hills: Sage, 1978), pp. 79–94.

Part VI
Educating Prescribers and Future Prescribers

19 Clinical Education Is Scarcely Enough: A Seminar Course in Social Issues in Prescribing

John P. Morgan, Michael Weintraub, and *Doreen V. Kagan*

This chapter reports an updated expanded version of a seminar course for medical students that focused on the social determinants of prescription-drug use. Students and instructors discussed social, economic, and philosophical determinants of physician, patient, and third-party behavior pertinent to drug giving and taking. The course format incorporates a series of packets including a brief essay relevant to the discussion, a series of questions to stimulate discussion, and selected references, all of which are available for students prior to the seminar. The positive response to an earlier version of this course and the discovery of new material and new sources of material applicable to patterns of drug utilization have encouraged us to produce this version. We hope that other medical educators may find the material useful to teach important concepts that receive too little attention in medical instruction.

Ten years ago, we published a course outline on this topic.[1] We recently have had the opportunity and support to revise and update the course. Our rationale for carrying out the course is unchanged. Students of medicine are little exposed to a comprehensive view of drug use in our society. Their education in pharmacology and therapeutics focuses necessarily on the issues of drug efficacy and toxicity. A wider view entails the recognition of nonpharmacologic or social uses of drugs and economic and legislative interventions into those uses. Drugs are used not only to treat disease but also to serve psychological, ideological, aesthetic, religious, and economic functions. Our culture is ambiguous about the use of medications, and daily we are exposed to articles and opinion about overmedication, too rigid (or too lax) controls on the channels of drug delivery, and a constant ambivalence about the fruit of pharmaceutical technology.

We initially presented this course for a few students as a seminar series

The preparation of this work was supported in part by Roche Laboratories. The help of Mr. Steven Janofsky, medical librarian at the School of Biomedical Education, City College of New York, was essential to the project.

incorporated into a second-year pharmacology course, and it has been utilized in that setting and others. One of us now directs such a course and has incorporated it for the entire enrollment. Our students reviews, although occasionally mixed, have been positive.

The format of presentation is unchanged. Students receive a packet of materials prior to the class session. The packet includes a brief statement outlining the topic, a few references, and a series of pertinent questions to guide and provoke discussion. Student discussion is always enthusiastic, often heated, and nearly always appropriate. They quickly decide that these issues will affect their future lives (and livelihoods) and welcome the opportunity to learn about them.

The understructured no-lecture format seems essential. There are few right answers and attitudes, and the didactic goal is to provide a framework within which the student can decide a personal course of action. The instructors scarcely could maintain an objective stance. The outlines, questions, and articles chosen reflect a point of view, but we have attempted a balanced presentation and have identified our own biases.

The preparation of the earlier outlines was difficult because we found it hard to locate appropriate articles. That difficulty is largely gone now. The continued importance and visibility of these questions generated two tools for locating articles. The Addiction Research Foundation of Ontario published, in 1977, "The Ethical Pharmaceutical Industry and Some of Its Economic Aspects: An Annotated Bibliography."[2] The American Medical Association now publishes *Medical Socioeconomic Research Sources,* an indexing service with many headings keyed to the social and economic aspects of pharmacology (now, unfortunately, discontinued since 1980). This volume contains chapters nearly always appropriate to our topics, and we have taken this opportunity to phrase questions and topics so as to refer to many of them.

In earlier versions of this course, the questions have been focused committedly and narrowly on the reprints. In this version we have moved away from this focus and our questions are general. This shift in focus modifies the need to use these identical articles and the need to replace missing articles in every instance.[3]

Some qualified and constructive critics of this work have felt that the publication of a series of questions without sharing our opinions of the answers is wrong. We have been working on a series of answer essays and other teaching packets. If those who are interested write and ask for them, we will be happy to send them. The course always has been called the *Patterns of Drug Utilization,* and that heading has been retained for the packets.

Patterns of Drug Utilization I: The Big Picture—Patterns of Ethical Drug Utilization

In this first session of a series of seminars on the patterns of drug utilization, we have presented an overview of prescription-drug usage in the United States. This and subsequent sessions will include a brief introduction, some questions to discuss, and a few references you must read prior to the class if the course is to be successful.

This packet should give you a view of the magnitude of prescription-drug use in the United States, some idea of the cost, and some idea of popular categories and popular drugs.

Some of the critical articles document a high rate of psychotropic and antibiotic prescribing and lament that generic prescriptions are still written much less often than brand-name prescriptions.

The total retail cost estimated may approximate 9 billion now, although precise figures are hard to obtain. If prescription-drug costs are calculated on a per capita rate, Americans spend approximately $50 per year. (Those who actually purchase prescriptions obviously spend more.)

A variety of pharmacy-based surveys yield data based on drugs prescribed, new prescriptions versus refills, branded prescriptions versus nonbranded, and so forth. We often have utilized the information provided by a commercial firm, IMS America, that sells such data to drug companies and others and publishes an annual summary. We have enclosed material from the 1980 IMS National Prescription Audit. (An alternative source is the annual New York State survey published by the Albany College of Pharmacy. The 1980 survey was published in *Medical Marketing and Media* in April 1981).

Questions

1. Does the $50 per capita figure surprise you? Did you think the total was much higher? Do Americans spend more for alcohol, cigarettes, shoes?
2. Why has the prescribing of nonbranded drugs increased proportionately in recent years?
3. How does the prescription volume of vitamins relate to the incidence of vitamin deficiency in the United States?

4. Why are hormones so high in terms of refill-to-new ratio and antibiotics relatively lower?
5. Eleven brand new chemical entities entered the market in 1980. If an average new prescription cost was $7, what might the cost be for a new chemical entity?
6. What are some factors that cause an enormous elasticity of this market? For example, at least 8,000 drug products are listed in the *PDR,* and all must sell something to be there, yet the most popular 200 drugs represent 70 percent of the market.
7. Why has prepaid drug insurance coverage grown rapidly in the United States?
8. What percentage of visits to a primary-care physician leads to a prescription?
9. Why are DOs (Doctor of Osteopathy) more likely to dispense drugs than GPs of the MD persuasion?
10. Why has dexedrine fallen from the list of the most popular 200 drugs?

References

1. Anon. National Prescription Audit General Information Reports, 19th ed. (Ambler, Pa. International Marketing Systems), pp. 1–18, 33–34, 39–42, 47.

2. "A Profile of Primary Care Physicians." *National Disease and Therapeutics Index Review* 6 (June 1975):1–12.

3. Wertheimer, A.I., "An Empirical Overview," this volume.

Patterns of Drug Utilization II: The Age of Valium

Most discussions in the patterns-of-drug-utilization seminars tend to slide toward benzodiazepines sooner or later. We have decided, therefore, to approach this topic in our second unit.

Valium has been the most commonly prescribed drug in the world. The worldwide market for benzodiazepines went over $1 billion around 1975. An intense argument is being carried out about the insouciance with which the drug is prescribed and taken. Many critics feel that the drug has physical dangers including a dependence potential, but more often their criticisms relate to a feeling that the drug is used inappropriately to combat problems that people should be able to deal with themselves. There is a continued call that counseling and attention to patients' needs by the physician will decrease the use of the agents.

Questions

1. What is the physical-dependence liability of Valium?
2. To what extent does Valium prescribing depend upon psychiatric diagnosis?
3. Discuss this statement: Patient receptivity of a drug converts the prescribing act into market demand.
4. Under what circumstances would you prescribe Valium or Librium for an alcoholic patient?
5. Discuss future benzodiazepine use in light of the fact that some researchers recently have reported that a central nervous system protein analogous to the opiate receptor seems specifically to bind benzodiazepines.
6. Why are women and elderly people more likely to receive benzodiazepines than youthful men?
7. Why not make Valium an OTC drug?
8. Speculate on the potential difference in benzodiazepine in-hospital consumption if it is made available on demand rather than on physician order.
9. Preliminary data indicate that many individuals who are physically dependent on benzodiazepines were once or are concurrently physically

dependent upon alcohol. What relationships between these agents might exist?

10. Some references indicate a downtrend in benzodiazepine use (particularly Valium) since 1974. Why might this have occurred?

References

1. Carpenter, T. I'm Writing as Fast as I Can. Two Cheers for Valium.'' *Village Voice,* 7 January 1980, pp. 1, 17, 18, 19.

2. Cooperstock, R. ''Some Comments on the Clinical Appropriateness of Prescribing, this volume.

3. Hollister, L. ''Valium: A Discussion of Current Issues.'' *Psychosomatics* 18 (January 1977):1-15.

4. Uhlenhuth, E.H.; M.B. Balter; and R.S. Lipman. ''Minor Tranquilizers: Clinical Correlates of Use in an Urban Population.'' *Archives of General Psychiatry* 35 (1978):650-655.

Patterns of Drug Utilization III: Noncompliance

Our society is referred to as overmedicated, yet overprescribed but not medicated may be more accurate. Evidence indicates that about one-third of patients never take prescribed medication (10 percent may not even fill the prescription), that one-third take some of the medication, and that only one-third take nearly all the medication. Underadherence to the therapeutic regimen is now discussed commonly, and many physicians attempt to assess the compliance of their patients. Some simply ask; others use pill counts or carry out serum drug measurements where applicable. We have learned a few things about the determinants of compliance—why people take or do not take their drugs. Some factors that decrease compliance, like complex regimens, are under physician control. Characteristics of patients such as age, educational level, and even their understanding of disease and medication do not adequately predict compliance. Now that physicians are aware of noncompliance and how it can thwart achieving the therapeutic goal, the next step has become compliance-insuring strategies (patient education, special medication dispensers, depot formulation medication). Some writers believe that noncompliance is a manifestation of the patient's right to decide (for example, Slack). The need for rigid adherence to the regimen implies that the doctor knows best. However, physician omniscience is being challenged by patient package inserts and consumerist approaches to health care. Other health professions (pharmacy, nursing) see compliance assurance as their valid role. The issue of patient adherence to medication has moved from a rarely considered aspect of therapeutics to another potent example of the impact of social forces on prescribing.

Questions

1. What is society's stake in compliance with antituberculosis therapy? with antihypertensive therapy? with anti-anxiety therapy?
2. What are the potential medical benefits of noncompliance?
3. Older patients have been described as either less compliant or more compliant with medical treatment. Which is it and why the confusion?
4. A patient tells you that he stopped taking the digoxin you prescribed about two months ago. What should you do?
5. What are the potential benefits to the physician of assessing compliance?

6. A physician's office can be compared to a restaurant; for the practice's survival the tables must be filled and emptied many times. How may compliance assessment effect this concept?
7. Can a pharmacist afford the time to discuss compliance with patients?
8. What are the patient's options if he becomes confused about his medications?
9. Is it appropriate just to offer comments about compliance and have patients decide what to do for themselves?
10. In a drug-failure clinic what percentage of patients is noncompliant? What explanation do you have for the others?

References

1. Haynes, R.B.; D.C. Sackett; and W.T. Taylor. "Manipulation of the Therapeutic Regimen to Improve Compliance: Conceptions and Misconceptions." *Clinical Pharmacology and Therapeutics* 22 (August 1977): 125–130.

2. Slack, W.V. "The Patient's Right to Decide." *Lancet* 2 (1977):240.

3. Stimson, G.V. "Obeying Doctor's Orders: A View from the Other Side." *Social Science and Medicine* 8 (1974):97–104.

4. Weintraub, M. "Capricious Compliance and Intelligent Noncompliance." In *Patient Compliance,* ed. by L. Lasagna (Mt. Kisco, N.Y.: Futura Pub. Co., 1976), pp. 39–47.

Patterns of Drug Utilization IV: Controls on Physicians. Part I—Friendly Persuasion

A variety of controlling factors influence physician prescribing. One group of factors might be labeled friendly persuasion. These interventions, usually with an eye to cost control, include third-party (governmental or private) limitations of payments for certain drugs or certain types of prescribing, county and state medical societies taking the pledge to not prescribe amphetamine for obesity, and the hospital formulary with its various levels of control. None of these subjects the physician to overt penalties or even always to direct criticism. However, because they may increase patients' out-of-pocket cost or cause inconvenience, the physician will hear about them, often with passion. The formulary or other official drug lists also carry the message of peer approval. Many physician prescribers will follow these directives simply because of that.

Questions

1. Why is it true that the wider the formulary jurisdiction (for example, more than a single hospital) the less effective it is in controlling costs?
2. What are the options open to a physician whose favorite tetracycline has been removed from the formulary at the hospital where he practices?
3. Some hospitals require consultation with an infectious-disease expert before using a new aminoglycoside antibiotic. Why is this done? Does this maneuver have different goals than merely helping the doctor to use a new drug intelligently?
4. How may formularies stifle innovative prescribing? How may they promote innovative prescribing?
5. Your patient requests a prescription for a decongestant-antihistamine because her prescription plan will not pay for an OTC preparation. What will you do?
6. What actions do third-party payers take to save money? In which instances does this not represent encouragement of good prescribing?
7. Why have third-party-payment plans for outpatient prescriptions grown so rapidly in the past few years?

8. There are few instances of restriction of physician rights to prescribe available drugs. Drugs released to the market are normally available for all prescribers in the United States. Can you think of some ways that prescribing might be restricted on certain available drugs?
9. Does the requirement of a small co-payment fee (50¢ to $1) on prescriptions limit the number of prescriptions under prepayment plans?
10. Describe what might happen when a state Medicaid program declines to pay for benzodiazepine use.

References

1. Berti, T.; L. Bozzini; and N. Martin. "Therapeutic Hospital Formulary for a Better Use of Drugs." *Pharmacological Research Communications* 11 (1979):379–387.

2. Morgan, J.P. "Watching the Monitors: 'Paid' Prescriptions, Fiscal Intermediaries and Drug Utilization Review." *New England Journal of Medicine* 296 (1977):251–256.

3. "Telltale Trails Left by Overprescribers Lead to Peer Pressure." *Legal Aspects of Medical Practice* 7 (1979):36–37.

4. Weintraub, M. "What's in the Hospital Formulary?" *Drug Therapy,* Hospital ed. (February 1976):45–48.

5. ———. "Effective Functioning of the P&T Committee: One Chairperson's View." *Hospital Formulary* 12 (1977):260–263.

Patterns of Drug Utilization V: Controls on Physicians. Part II—Pointed Constraints

In this packet on physician control, we examine some more-pointed constraints that affect physician prescribing. These constraints may lead to penalties including loss of license or even criminal prosecution. Two issues are considered, and in at least one instance, the two are closely related.

First, there is a long history of societal attempts to control physician prescribing of psychoactive drugs that may be abused. Second, there are increasing attempts to curtail physician prescribing of drugs for indications that are not listed in the official packet insert (collected in the *PDR*).

One constant theme in dangerous-drug legislation is the distrust (earned and unearned) of physicians by legislators. This distrust has culminated in the 1970 federal Controlled Substances Act. This act and state adaptations of it often make it illegal for a physician to prescribe any controlled substance for a "known addict or habitual abuser" of drugs. Physicians who greedily sell narcotics and psychostimulants (directly or by prescription) have been caught because they operate outside these guidelines. The issue under debate is that legitimate physicians also occasionally are caught up in the wide net of the law.

The package insert constitutes a legal document agreed upon by the FDA and the manufacturer of the drug to which practicing physicians have no input. It contains guidelines that allow the manufacturers to advertise for certain indications. Historically, it was not designed to limit physician usage of a drug. The anti-arrythmic effect of lidocaine was not stated in the package insert for a full five years after its usage for that purpose clearly was established. The FDA consistently has denied that it wishes the insert to serve as a guide for practice. However, it has been used in prosecution of physicians by some state jurisdictions and in malpractice cases where a plaintiff's attorney will try to use the insert as a substitute expert witness.

Questions

1. Can you list and describe the five schedules of drugs subject to abuse under the Controlled Substances Act?
2. Place acetyl methadol, pentazocine, LSD, cannabis, and codeine with aspirin into their proper schedules.

3. You wish to treat severe anxiety in a young man who had once been on methadone maintenance. Can you use a benzodiazepine without getting into trouble?
4. Can you describe a situation where not exceeding the guidelines in the package insert constitutes bad practice?
5. A physician treats a patient who has severe chronic pain with a combination of amphetamine and morphine. What is the rationale? Is this legal?
6. Why is the package insert a particularly fearsome issue for pediatricians?
7. Which anorexiants are in Schedule II? Which are in Schedule III?
8. Why does Ralph Nader's Health Research Group wish there to be s specific list of indications for prescription drugs to be incorporated into law?
9. Describe some situations in which physicians (who are not script doctors) exceed usual amounts of dangerous drugs prescribed.
10. Outline a situation in which a drug is used for a nonapproved indication. How often does this happen?

References

1. Calesnick, B. "Controlled Substances." *American Family Physician* 16 (1977):180–181.

2. Committee on Drugs. "Unapproved Uses of Approved Drugs: The Physician, the Package Insert and the FDA." *Pediatrics* 62 (1978):262–264.

3. Cohen, S. "The Prescription of Controlled Substances: What's Right and What's Wrong?" National Institute of Drug Abuse Monograph Series #27. (Washington, D.C., 1979), pp. 1–16.

4. Mundy, G.R.; L. Fleckenstein, and J.M. Mazzullo. "Current Medical Practice and the Food and Drug Administration." *Journal of the American Medical Association* 229 (1974):1744–1748.

5. Sadowsky, D. "Narcotic Legislation in New York State." *NY State Journal of Medicine* 75 (1975):2258–2261.

6. Tennant, F.S. and G.F. Uelmen. "Prescribing Narcotics to Habitual and Addicted Narcotics Users." *Western Journal of Medicine* 133 (1980):539–545.

Patterns of Drug Utilization VI: The FDA

The FDA appears to have no friends, only critics. The FDA's scientific and administrative staff must supervise the Pure Foods Act, the Hazardous Substances Act, toy safety and product safety, in addition to drug (prescription and OTC) and cosmetic safety.

In the past (particularly prior to 1962) the agency was thought to be entirely too soft and friendly toward its so-called enemy—the pharmaceutical industry. Following thalidomide and the 1962 Kefauver-Harris Drug Act, it has become increasingly difficult for the industry to get drugs on the market. Recently, therefore, many critics have complained that a host of valuable drugs is available abroad but that the FDA, acting primarily out of fear, has prevented their release here, causing the drug lag.

The FDA is still beset by consumerist criticism. The FDA, to consumers, moves too slowly to remove or curtail use of hazardous items. Critics also dispute the existence of a drug lag.

In terms of power, recall that the FDA receives its right to be involved in drug regulation because of the federal government responsibility to regulate interstate commerce. The agency neither regulates the practice of medicine—a responsibility of the individual state—nor controls how a state may decide on the intrastate manufacture, distribution, and use of certain therapeutic agents such as laetrile.

Questions

1. If the FDA protects consumers from bad drugs, who insures the consumer of needed drugs?
2. Explain the drug lag.
3. Why are new chemical entities usually tested first abroad?
4. Imagine testing a drug for safety but not efficacy as the FDA once did. Explain this in the light of what you have learned about the therapeutic index.
5. What are some social forces that led to the approval of twenty new major tranquilizers by the FDA's psychopharmacology division while the cardiovascular group approved no cardiovascular drugs?

6. A new drug is very good for a disease. However, it is invariably toxic for 10 percent of takers, and half of that 10 percent die because of drug toxicity. What else do you need to know (as an FDA monitor) to decide about approval?
7. A drug is good for disease X; reports filter in that it is good for disease Y as well. What else would you like to know to decide about approval of that indication?
8. Can you briefly describe the differences in the FDA's powers after important legislation in 1906, 1938, 1962?
9. Why is the agency more often criticized for releasing dangerous drugs than for delaying needed drugs?
10. Will the agency be responsive to the political pressure of an antiregulatory administration and increase new drug approvals in the 1980s?

References

1. Herzog, J. "Recurrent Criticisms: A History of Investigations of the FDA." *Medical Marketing and Media* 13 (1978):41–45.

2. Hollister, L.E. "The FDA Ten Years after the Kefauver-Harris Amendments." *Perspectives in Biology and Medicine* 17 (1974):242–249.

3. Morgan, J.P. "The Drug Lag: Good or Bad?" *Journal of the American Pharmaceutical Association* NS17 (September 1977):553.

4. Nightingale, S. "The FDA's Role in Appropriate Drug Use," this volume.

Patterns of Drug Utilization VII: Generic Prescribing and Drug-Product Selection

A majority of states have now enacted laws affecting retail pharmacies by repealing previous antisubstitution laws. The new regulations allow or even mandate pharmacist substitution of generic drugs for brand names written by the physician. In addition, there is renewed pressure on physicians to increase generic-drug prescribing. Generic drugs and alleged savings from their use have been a source of discussion for many years.

There are at least two important questions concerning generic prescribing: (1) Are generic versions comparable to their chemical equivalents in quality and bioavailability and therapy? (2) What is the savings to the consumer when a generic prescription is presented or when a pharmacist selects a generic product?

The professional role of pharmacists, the societal cost of decreased innovation by pharmaceutical manufacturers, the benefits of increased competition, and other serious problems are also numbered in the generic-drug controversy. As in every step of the process of prescribing drugs, major social forces—consumerism, capitalism, legal constraints, and the role of other professionals—impinge on the therapeutic process implied in writing a prescription. On which side of the controversy do the angels line up? What stance should you take as a prescribing physician?

Questions

1. Can physicians lower costs by learning about and prescribing less costly alternative drugs?
2. In 1974–1975, consumers decreased their beef purchases in protest against high costs. The price of beef did decrease. Could a similar action have an influence on the price of cephalexin, amoxicillin, or tetracycline?
3. Are prices within a pharmacy relatively stable? If not, why not?
4. Although laws now exist allowing prescription-drug price advertising, barriers still exist that prevent patients from obtaining savings. What are some of these barriers and how can they be overcome?
5. Pharmacists often do not fill generically written prescriptions with non-brand-name drugs. Can you describe some reasons for this?

6. What are the economic advantages to a pharmacist to substitute? Why might he not take advantage of them?
7. Who manufactures generic products?
8. Some consumer groups propose another way of decreasing drug costs. They want to decrease the patent period on drugs to less than the current seventeen years. What are the implications of this proposal?
9. What is the structure and impact of a state formulary?
10. Can you list factors of various state drug-product selection laws that are associated with increased dispensing of generic drugs?

References

1. Berki, S.E.; M.B.A. Richards; and H.A. Weicks. "The Mysteries of Prescription Pricing in Retail Pharmacies." *Medical Care* 15 (1977):241–250.

2. Francetic, I.; L. Lasagna; M. Weintraub; and F.E. Karch. "Prescription Prices under the New York Generic Substitution Law." *Annals of Internal Medicine* 92 (1980):419–423.

3. T. Goldberg, and C. DeVito. "The Impact of State Generic-Substitution Laws," this volume.

4. Hecht, A. "Generic Drugs: How Good Are They?" DHEW Publication no. 78-3068. Washington, D.C.: FDA, 1977.

5. Sharpe, T.R. "Economic Issues in Antisubstitution Controversy." *American Journal of Pharmacy* (March–April 1977), pp. 53–59.

Patterns of Drug Utilization VIII: The Drug Industry

Taking a middle road in writing about the U.S. (or multinational) pharmaceutical industry guarantees a lonely journey. Writers either extol the virtues or excoriate the excesses of the industry. In the past, academic writers provided much criticism of the actions of drug sellers (particularly promotional policies), but today, some academics are angered by the restrictive policies of the FDA and defend the industry.

In fact, perhaps too much of the cited references defend the industry. This is partially in reaction to the popular media's tendency to criticize pharmaceutical firms for actions that are tolerated easily in sellers of soaps and automobile tires.

Some economists argue that the United States is served best by a relatively unfettered industry and even call for repeal of the 1962 FDA amendments. Others still wish to restrain (appropriately) mercantile freedom because the public needs protection.

Many writers are pessimistic about the future of the industry for reasons even other than the complaints of economic restraint.

Questions

1. Comment on molecular manipulation as:
   A means to profit,
   An important mechanism to discover new drugs.
2. What is the current cost of bringing a new drug to the market?
3. What are the chief reasons for tightly regulating new drug marketing and human testing?
4. What is the drug industry's profit margin and how does it compare to other manufacturing concerns?
5. What is the usual length of patent protection afforded to a new chemical entity? When is the patent declared in the economic life of the drug?
6. Why do the twenty large innovative firms claim that a program to reduce drug costs to consumers (for example, decreased patent protection, drug-substitution laws) will adversely affect research?
7. Can you describe what happens when a popular drug (for example, Librium, Thorazine) goes off patent exclusivity?

8. How many patients will benefit from a new antihypertensive? a new antimetabolite? a new antibiotic? a new benzodiazepine?
9. Cimetidine has become the greatest dollar-volume drug in the United States. Can you discuss some reasons why?
10. The preparation of this course outline was supported by Roche. How do you feel about that?

References

1. Arcieri, G. "Process of Developing a New Antimicrobial Drug." *Annals of Internal Medicine* 89 (1978):838–841.

2. Brozen, Y. "The American Drug Industry: Private Enterprise or Public Utility?" Reprint no. 79. (Washington, D.C.: American Enterprise Institute, Center for Health Policy Research, November 1977. (Available from AEI, 1150 17th N.W., Washington, D.C. 20036. Cost = $.35.)

3. Lasagna, L. "Drug Discovery and Introduction: Regulation and Overregulation." *Clinical Pharmacology and Therapeutics* 20 (1977):507–511.

4. "MD's in the Drug Industry's Pocket." *Science for the People* 8 (1976):6–9, 20–21.

Patterns of Drug Utilization IX: Social and Cultural Determinants of Drug Use

It is extremely difficult to separate cultural components from more-personal (psychological) components that contribute to a pattern of drug use. Included in the latter are issues of compliance and placebo response. We have generated a unit on the larger cultural determinants of drug use because such factors are probably important, although we understand them very little. Volumes have been written on social and cultural determinants of health care, health expectations, and health seeking. Clearly, these issues also may determine how a defined community or individual representative of that community might approach medication and its use. There is, however, little systematic study of patterns of drug use (and drug seeking) of ethnic, social, or cultural groups.

We have identified a few papers that can serve as an introduction to this topic. We are well aware that our definitions are unclear. We have even included here the refusal of certain creative people to utilize prophylactic lithium as representing a cultural determinant of drug nonuse. Probably the most we can say is that certain norms of behavior in any social grouping modify the use of prescription drugs. In the future, we may even understand a few of them.

Questions

1. Are there cultural variants in the response to pain? Do pain thresholds vary in this fashion?
2. Why are patients loath to discuss home remedies with their physicians?
3. Do physicians believe in a wisdom of the body?
4. Why are unproved remedies (vitamin E, ginseng root) now discussed almost entirely in language that utilizes apparently scientific terms?
5. Compare a hypomanic patient who refuses Lithium to a recovered psychotic who refuses Thorazine because it makes him jittery.
6. Why has the use of homeopathic herbal and natural medicines apparently increased in the Western world?

7. What are the characteristics of a good patient from your viewpoint? What does stoicism versus histrionic expression have to do with that assessment?
8. Are you familiar with hot and cold theories of disease and the ubiquitous presence of folk herbal phamacies in Hispanic communities?
9. What forces led to an apparent undertreatment of pain in hospitalized Americans?
10. Explain an apparent correlation in the United States between the use of prescription drugs (psychoactive and nonpsychoactive) and illicit psychoactive drugs.

References

1. Bush, P.J., and M. Osterweis. "Pathways to Medicine Use." *Journal of Health and Social Behavior* 19 (1978):179–189.

2. Gagnon, J.P.; E.J. Salber; and S.B. Greene. "Patterns of Prescription and Nonprescription Use in a Southern Rural Area." *Public Health Reports* 93 (1978):433–437.

3. Murphree, M.A., and M.V. Barrow. "Physician Dependence, Self-Treatment Practices and Folk Remedies in a Rural Area." *Southern Medical Journal* 63 (1970):403–408.

4. Polatin, P., and R.R. Fieve. "Patient Rejection of Lithium Carbonate Prophylaxis." *Journal of the American Medical Association* 218 (1971):864–866.

5. Portelli, A.J., and I. Jones. "Mediterranean Guts Ache." *Medical Journal of Australia* 76 (1969):717–720.

6. Zborowski, J. "Cultural Components in Response to Pain." *Journal of Social Issues* 8 (1952):16–30.

Patterns of Drug Utilization X: Prescribing for Women

Some published studies indicate that women have a higher incidence of depression and, logically enough, that women receive more tricyclic antidepressants than men. Does this indicate an etiological role of estrogens in depression (as some claim), or does it mean that women have received more cultural training in giving up and crying in defeat? Stated differently, do the differences in physician prescribing for women reflect sexism or differences in disease incidence or drug response in women? One difference in prescribing is generated by women seeing physicians more then men. Obviously we are not merely discussing the use of estrogen in ovarian failure. There is a strong case to be made that physicians perceive female patients in a different way than they do men, even if the offered complaints are similar. In fact, the case is so strong that it is difficult not to regard prescribing for women as a prototype of social and cultural effects on the patterns of drug utilization. This unit also yields an opportunity to review briefly the impact of social attitudes on prescription-drug advertising.

Questions

1. What are the indications for postmenopausal use of estrogens? Are there indications that are not specifically cosmetic?
2. A group of physicians was asked to describe a complaining patient. Give an estimate of the sexual breakdown.
3. The weekly AMA news has a cartoon that nearly always reflects hostility to patients. Look at a few and decide how often they are sexist as well.
4. We have used the term *sexism* casually. Would you define it for us?
5. What was the relationship of female to male heroin-dependent humans in 1900? What were the reasons?
6. Physicians are asked to describe the gravity of presenting symptoms offered stoically or histrionically. Which presentation is thought to be more serious?
7. Can you differentiate the style of ad when men present to the physician with anxiety as opposed to women who present with anxiety?
8. Does education and discussion about health-related issues make one more or less likely to receive psychotherapeutic drugs?

9. In ads for drugs that are nonpsychoactive (organic-disease ads), are men under- or overrepresented?
10. Ads apparently seldom depict physicians as women? Can you state some reasons why?

References

1. Jick, H.; R.N. Watkins; and J.R. Hunter. "Replacement Estrogen and Endometrial Cancer." *New England Journal of Medicine* 300 (February 1, 1979):218–222.

2. Linn, L. and M.S. Davis. "The Use of Psychotherapeutic Drugs by Middle-Aged Women." *Journal of Health and Social Behavior* 12 (1971): 331–339.

3. Seidenberg, R. "Drug Advertising and Perception of Mental Illness." *Mental Hygiene* 55 (1971):21.

4. Smith, M.C. and L. Griffin. "Rationality of Appeals Used in the Promotion of Psychotropic Drugs: A Comparison of Male and Female Models." *Social Science and Medicine* 11 (1977):409–414.

5. Usdin, G. "The Coin Needn't Smell: A Response to the Seidenberg Thesis." *Mental Hygiene* 55 (1971):32–34.

Conclusion

We do not know the efficacy of this course although we do know that we have enjoyed developing and teaching it. We are impressed that many criticisms of physician prescribing and of patient use might focus on these issues. Our students usually seem very pleased to have learned about this material, and we are now aware of interest and some similar course development in other schools of medicine.

Notes

1. J.P. Morgan and M. Weintraub, "A Course on the Social Functions of Prescription Drugs: Seminar Syllabus and Bibliography," *Annals of Internal Medicine* 77 (1972):217–222.

2. Available for $10,00 from ARF, 33 Russell St., Toronto M5S 2S1.

3. In recent years, we have produced only a few copies of the reference and filed them in the library.

20 An Analysis of the Impact of Print Advertising on Prescribing

Mickey C. Smith

The advertising of prescription drugs in print, especially in medical journals, has been the subject of critical comment for at least a quarter of a century. This criticism has ranged from expressions of concern for the aesthetics of such promotion to calls for its total elimination. This chapter reviews the criticisms, the evidence used in their support, and some of the remedies proposed. The bases for the chapter include published research and opinion, some of our research at the University of Mississippi, and some modest theorizing on what, if anything, needs to be done.

Leo Bogart, writing of advertising in general, notes that "the striking inconsistency in advertising productivity must lead us to conclude that the yield from advertising is not related significantly to its sheer volume of expenditure or its ratio to sales. Different advertising messages for the same product vary tremendously in persuasive appeal and power."[1]

> (1) It is impossible to conceive of a competitive market economy in which advertising does not play a part. Advertising is one of a variety of forms of selling and promotion. The advantages of size to an advertiser parallel advantages of size in other realms of merchandising, distribution, and sales. There is no logical or reasonable way of restricting one aspect of promotion without restricting all other ways. This would mean the end of competition and the economic advantages and political freedoms that go with it.
>
> (2) In many instances and in many aspects there may be legitimate reason to criticize the economic and social effects of advertising. But these instances must be dealt with on their own specific terms. A knee-jerk defense reaction to any attack on any aspect of advertising is just as witless as knee-jerk hostility. The economic effects of advertising are not subject to universal generalizations.
>
> (3) A growing percentage of all advertising is informational in character. A declining proportion is represented by national advertising in product fields characterized by minor performance differences among brands. This trend should continue as we have increasing product differentiation in the marketplace and more rapid growth in the consumption of services than of goods.

This chapter draws heavily on my article, "Drug Product Advertising and Prescribing," *American Journal of Hospital Pharmacy* 34 (November 1977):1208–1224.

(4) The misallocation of resources that results from overspending by certain advertisers is probably small relative to the misallocation that arises from inadequacies of advertising content and scheduling. The greatest waste in advertising is in the many messages that fall wide of the mark.[2]

In an extensive policy-related analysis of the pharmaceutical industry, Hornbrook has analyzed the interrelationship between promotional intensity and dynamic changes in market structure. Hornbrook's analysis included total promotional expenditures and did not specifically address print advertising. He found, in any case, that promotion has a procompetitive effect—that is, it acts as a means of market entry. In Hornbrook's words, "promotion is not strictly a tool of the large dominant pharmaceutical firms: small firms can do and do use advertising and detailing to make inroads on the market shares of the leaders."[3]

In the context of his policy study, Hornbrook notes two tradeoffs that must be considered if promotional expenditures are to be reduced. If compulsory licensing is chosen, expenditures may (it is by no means sure) be reduced but at the possible cost of reduced drug innovation. If promotional expenditures are reduced arbitrarily, a possible result is a "concomitant reduction in the flow of benefits from the [drug] innovation."[4]

Medical Issues

Perhaps the most damning criticism of advertising, if substantiated, would be that it results in inappropriate prescribing—either too much, too little (hardly likely), or the wrong drug. I have previously published a comprehensive review of the literature on this subject.[5] The weight of published evidence lends little credence to a major effect of journal advertising alone on prescribing, for good or ill.

It is likely that considerable evidence of the effect of advertising on prescribing volume exists in the files of drug manufacturers who certainly have conducted marketing research in this area. For obvious competitive reasons the manufacturers do not publish such research. Consequently, my review was limited to published work.

A further imposed limitation on this review was the inclusion only of studies showing outcomes—that is, either prescribing must be shown to have changed or physicians must have stipulated that the advertisements had such an effect. Not included were studies showing that the physician read the advertisement or remembered the advertisement. While logic supports the view that ads read or recalled affect prescribing behavior, evidence of such an effect was required for the study to be included.

There has been some additional activity since this review. In one of the few published studies linking advertising and prescribing, Walton presents the following summary:

> A sample of 1,000 physicians in private practice, stratified by specialty, made a total of 35,400 observations of 354 ads, which appeared in medical journals, between Autumn 1976 and Winter 1977. The evidence adduced provides reliable support for the postulated linkage between physicians' awareness of medical-journal advertisements and subsequent enhanced prescribing, a linkage that is more than a series of coincidences.
>
> In real terms 95 percent of the ads were associated with positive prescribing behavior patterns. Specifically, within 60 days following a quarterly period of advertising exposure, physicians who recalled ads went on to be prescribers of the products advertised in consistently larger proportions than those who did not recall ads. Moreover, the risk that this behavior was due to change is minute:
>
> For the complete set of observations $p < 0.0001$;
>
> For every subset studied, $p < 0.001$, except in one subset, where $p < 0.004$.
>
> Recognition of ads by physicians appears to be central to intensified prescribing in the postexposure period.[6]

Kalb has reviewed the literature of effects of various influences on prescribing. He notes previous studies that indicate that print advertising serves "principally as a channel of information rather than one of persuasion."[7] In his own research involving 210 physician responses to a questionnaire, 70 percent said they were not influenced to prescribe a product based on reading a medical-journal advertisement.

Two additional points are salient:

1. It should not be surprising to find that advertising does influence prescribing since that is its primary mission.
2. An increase in prescribing of a given drug as a function of advertising is not necessarily bad. Such a judgment requires data on the alternative the physician would have chosen had he not prescribed the drug in question.

Statements like "Drug companies encourage the use of pills as cure-all" are troublesome.[8] First, there is no support for such a statement; indeed, it is indefensible. Second, even if it were true, who is encouraged by the drug companies? The physician, who is either already leaning toward this view or too easily swayed in this direction? Usdin, in a response to Seidenberg, has posed this question: "Are physicians really dullards who await instructions from detailmen and Madison Avenue? If so, blame our medical education system as well as the manufacturers."[9]

Muller maintains that one reason for the vulnerability of the physician to promotional pressures is the relative dearth of pressure to prescribe properly.[10] She points out that effective drug-use review is rare and that even when it exists, the results may not be communicated to the prescriber.

Mason says: "It would be shortsighted to look to the pharmaceutical companies . . . the drug manufacturers cannot be blamed, they're doing their best. If any blame is to be assessed, perhaps we, as physicians, should accept."[11]

Economic and Social Issues

Much has been made of the amount of money spent on advertising, and indeed, it is a great deal of money.

Peltzman has argued persuasively that, at least for conditions that require drug treatment, the costs of not getting the information to the physician may far outweigh the cost of promotion.[12] He suggests the alternative of charging separately for the drugs and for the information but admits that few customers are likely to gamble in advance on the value of the information.

Peltzman's economic argument include the position that the benefits from diffusion of an innovation may rival the benefits from having the innovation in the first place. He also pointed out that the ability of manufacturers to treat promotional expenditures as tax deductions may effectively be a tax subsidy for dissemination of information.

Perhaps the overriding issue with regard to drug advertising revolves around the costs and benefits to the patient since the patient ultimately pays for the advertising—either directly or through taxation. Critics imply or state outright that advertising, in addition to its other shortcomings, is not a cost-effective means of supplying the physician with needed drug information. Less often, critics note that advertising does not provide complete information of the type needed to make a rational choice—either between alternative drugs or between drug and nondrug therapy.

Two concepts are basic to a discussion of this final issue. The first revolves around the agent role of the prescribing physician. The second—the economics of information—follows, and builds upon, the first.

A pedestrian, but widely held view of why the patient visits a physician is so that the physician will do something. A more-enlightened view would describe the physician's role as determining whether or not something should be done and then doing what is appropriate. Because the patient is ill equipped to do so himself, he hires a physician as his agent in the search for, acquisition of, and application of knowledge. Until the point at which the physician performs a physical task (surgery, bone setting, and so forth), the patient is paying for knowledge more than anything else, and that payment includes the three following elements:

1. The core knowledge acquired during medical school,
2. The new knowledge gained following graduation through the information-gathering activities of the physician,
3. The application of that knowledge through discriminatory judgment of alternatives.

The physician is, again, a knowledge or informational agent of the patient, and his fee is based in large part on this function. The patients, individually (as customers) and collectively (as a society), have a right to be concerned with whether or not they are getting the most for their money from the information-gathering activities of these agents.

It is surprising that the economics of the information-search activities of physicians (as patients' agents) has received little formal attention. Indeed, only two authors seem to have made a serious attempt to examine the issue. Schwartzman[13] adapted the economic theories of Stigler[14] and Nelson[15] to an analysis of promotional expenditures by the pharmaceutical industry. Schwartzman concluded that "from the standpoint of the benefits of information to doctors and patients, a reasonable case can be made for the position that the expenditures on promotion by the industry have been inadequate rather than excessive."[16]

In the process of reaching his conclusion, Schwartzman made several other observations that weakened his argument somewhat. He noted, for example, that advertising will not include the advantages of competing products. (He does not note that advertisements will also usually omit the advantage of nondrug therapy.) The physician, therefore, has a complex informational task. Finally, Schwartzman observed that some patients with informed physicians overpay while others underpay for the costs of getting drug information to physicians.[17] He dismissed the problem by stating that there is no way of avoiding it.

A problem with Schwartzman's arguments, which support promotion, as well as with the argument of many negative critics, is that both start from a position of industry responsibility when, in fact, the responsibility for information lies with the information expert—the physician. The heart of the matter may lie in Schwartzman's observation that:

> The elimination of all drug promotion would result in greater demands on doctors to spend time learning about the qualities of drugs and probably in a reduction in the information which they require. Busy practitioners, who are the ones who write a relatively large number of prescriptions, are unlikely to devote the required time to learning about drugs in the event of a reduction in promotional efforts.[18]

Peltzman has prepared the other serious economic evaluation of drug promotion, although he limited his considerations to the benefits, excluding the costs, of what he termed *diffusion* for pharmaceutical innovation.[19]

Further, he did not evaluate the relative efficiency of promotion and other possible methods of increasing the rate of diffusion of drug innovations.

Within the constraints listed, Peltzman presented a strong argument for as rapid as possible (stimulated by promotion if appropriate) adoption of certain pharmaceutical innovations. He used antituberculosis drugs and tranquilizers to illustrate his contention that economic savings could be realized by early adoption. Without the cost analysis, however, one is left only with the potential benefits of promotion, and the magnitude of the potential is cloudy since measures of promotional efficiency and effectiveness, particularly relative to other information sources, are lacking. Similarly, but perhaps less obviously, lacking are considerations of nondrug interventions such as prevention in the case of tuberculosis and psychotherapy or early counseling in the case of the tranquilizers.

Because of their impact on the work of Schwartzman and because it is possible to reach somewhat different conclusions depending upon the context of the argument, a brief look at the Stigler and Nelson work on the economics of information seems in order, even though an in-depth economics treatment is not possible here.

Stigler, noting that "knowledge is power," confined his theoretical treatment to the effort of the buyer to ascertain the most favorable price—a phenomenon he called search.[20] Nevertheless, his arguments apply to searches for other information and to searches on the behalf of others (physician for patient). Adapting freely, and along these lines, Stigler's theories include the following:

> If the dispersion of possibilities is large, it will pay to canvass several sources.
>
> If the cost of search is equated to its expected marginal return, the optimal amount of search will be found. (The cost is largely time, and of course, the time of the physician is valuable to him and his patients. This is not the only cost, however, since subscription rates and other out-of-pocket costs enter into these calculations.)
>
> It is sometimes efficient for searchers to pool their knowledge and thus to reduce the effective cost of search. (This is the function served by Consumers Union for the public and publications such as The Medical Letter for physicians.)
>
> Advertising is one method of easing the difficulties of searching, but it is subject to diseconomies when, for example, a drug is advertised in a journal that has few potential prescribers among its readers.
>
> If selections are repetitive, the frequency of use based upon search must be considered. Thus, a physician may spend more search time econom-

ically on a drug type that will be prescribed frequently than on a drug type that will be prescribed only once or twice a year. (This observation is primarily economic and somewhat lacking in humanitarianism.)

When a physician enters a wholly new market, he will have no idea of the dispersion of drug products and nondrug therapies available and, hence, no idea of the rational amount of search he should make. Based on this observation, the role of the medical school in this regard is to apprise the medical student of the magnitude of the search problem and to instruct him in cost-effective search techniques. (See chapter 22 for such considerations.)

"Advertising is among other things," according to Stigler, "a method of providing potential buyers (or prescribers) with knowledge of the identity of sellers. It is clearly an immensely powerful instrument for the elimination of ignorance."[21]

A common complaint is that the advertising and the commodity are offered together and that the buyer (in this case the patient) must buy both whether or not he wants the advertising. In fact, as Stigler notes, it is possible to search out the seller who advertises little. The evidence, however, shows that the patient's informational agents prefers the advertised, brand-name product, thus in effect, purchasing the advertising for his client.

The presentation of information in an entertaining environment is comprehensible. "The assimilation of information is not an easy or pleasant task for most people, and they may be willing to pay more for the information when supplied in an enjoyable form."[22] This explains a penchant on the part of the physician for a cartoon-laden advertising layout or drug advertisements interspersed with news of his colleagues as is often presented in a medical journal. It does not, however, allow the purchaser/patient an opportunity to determine whether or not he wishes to pay extra so that his physician may be entertained while searching for the optimal drug.

Stigler's thoughtful presentation has been succeeded and elaborated upon by Nelson, who attempted to build product quality as well as price into his analysis; Nelson's assertion that quality information is usually more expensive to buy than price information is complicated for this discussion by the agent relationship described earlier.[23] Indeed, the patient is more likely to obtain price information than his physician-agent, but the patient is ill equipped to evaluate quality information even when it is available to him.

Nelson builds on Stigler's search model by identifying an experience class of goods—"goods it will pay the consumer to evaluate by purchase rather than by search."[24] Schwartzman argues persuasively that drugs fit this latter category better than most goods.[25] He recognizes the agent role of the physician and argues that the special training of the physician strengthens the analogy. (In support of both, let us note that Nelson uses repair expenditures as evidence of experience goods. Surely adverse-reaction rates are good evidence that drugs fit this category).

It is worth noting that if Nelson's and Schwartzman's arguments hold true, then journal advertising would hold little attraction for the physician aside from any value as a dissonance reducer, and the preferred form of promotion would be the drug sample.[26] It is also worth noting that because of the physician's agent role, he is in effect deciding to try drugs on his patients with his only personal cost being patient dissatisfaction (or at its extreme, liability suits). Such dissatisfaction is, of course, a real cost only in a competitive market in which the loss of a customer (patient) is a real concern. In fact, in most medical markets this does not hold true, and (from the point of view of the Nelson model at least) there is no reason for active search efforts. The physician can learn how to use the drugs by trial and error.

What is largely missing from the foregoing discussion is a statement by the patient. At which point does patient input, either individual or collective, become a part of the equation? Since the patient, or a surrogate, ultimately pays the bill, it seems logical to suggest that he have some input into the information-gathering decision—for example, would the patient prefer to pay a higher price for the drug including an information component for advertising and other forms of promotion or (perhaps) a somewhat higher price for the services of a physician who (possibly) must spend more of his time gathering, assessing, and acting upon information gathered?

Latent Effects of Advertising

Crout has stated, "I testify today as a concerned physician who believes that the growing influence of the pharmaceutical industry on medical education is a long-term threat to the integrity of my chosen profession."[27]

In the case of journal advertising, some evidence shows that this concern is justified. In several studies physicians made no distinction between journal advertisements and other journal content in citing medical journals as a major source of drug knowledge.[28]

Another concern that has been expressed more frequently in recent years is the potential influence of the many journal advertisements on physician attitudes aside from the drugs themselves. One of the major criticisms is the possible sexist content of the advertisement.

Kunnes, for example, has noted that advertisements for fixed combination diet pills appear to fit the sexist description.[29] Seidenberg has pointed out that it is possible to use excessively pictures of women as sick or disturbed and thereby to "create the image of women as not only the weaker sex, but the sicker sex."[30] In another paper, Seidenberg referred to a ten-year personal study of psychotropic-drug advertising in which he found that "at least two-thirds to three-quarters of the ads show pictures of women to whom psychoactive drugs are to be given."[31] Unfortunately, the data from this study were not presented.

Mosher has described the portrayal of women in drug advertising as a "medical betrayal." She did not provide data to support her views, but she did provide important medical principles that apply if her charges are valid. She noted that "exaggerated stereotyping appears to minimize the need for complete medical diagnosis, encourages unwarranted drug prescribing, and reduces the status of the person, as a patient and as a consumer.[32] Stimson took a similar position when he reported in a nonquantified fashion on what appear to have been nonrandom, nonsystematic observations of U.K. journal advertising for tranquilizers and oral contraceptives. He concluded that the overall effect "reveals a consistently limited view of women."[33]

Mant and Darroch used content-analysis techniques to study nearly 500 drug advertisements that appeared over a seven year period in two Australian medical journals.[34] Comparisons were made between advertisements for mood-modifying drugs and other categories of drugs, and significant differences were found. Greater use of pictures and use of female models more often than men as well as using sexual stereotypes characterized the advertisements for mood modifiers. Assessment of scientific appeal revealed no significant differences by drug types or sex of the patient.

Unfortunately, this study did not describe adequately the structure of the index of scientific appeal, did not specify whether the aggregate findings were controlled for advertisements that appeared more than once in the sample, and suffered from an apparent need to find sexual discrimination. The researchers, for example, referred to some of the models as seductive, although how this evaluation was made is not clear.

Prather and Fidell concluded that women were shown more often than men in psychotropic-drug advertisements than in those for other types of drugs. In addition to stylistic differences, they found women portrayed as suffering "diffuse emotional symptoms" while men were suffering from "pressure from work or accompanying organic illness."[35] The sample of ads was drawn from one state medical journal and three national journals, one issue randomly selected from each of five successive years.

McRee, Corder, and Haizlip used a mail survey sent to thirty psychiatrists (twenty-three responded) to study whether or not the respondents believed advertisements were sexually biased and the effects of any bias so identified.[36] A majority (70 percent) of male respondents indicated that female models in advertisements were more likely to attract their attention. Several respondents felt that psychiatrists would be less affected by advertisements that implied that more women than men had symptoms of mental illness. Seventy-four percent of respondents believed that nonpsychiatrists might be led by the advertisements to believe that more women than men had symptoms of mental illness requiring medication.

Parish has raised the possibility that drug advertising affects not only prescribing but also diagnosis. He stated, "The pharmaceutical industry is responsible for the way its products are promoted and in so doing it often defines and re-defines indications for the use of drugs and so, not only has the industry influenced treatment, it has influenced diagnosis."[37] No evidence is presented, however.

In a study by Lion and associates, fifty psychiatrists were shown advertisements from two professional journals *(American Journal of Psychiatry* and *Psychiatric News)* in which the names of the products had been deleted.[38] Subjects were queried regarding aesthetic appeal, informational content, and product identification. Eighteen different ads were included.

In spite of frequent criticism of the slickness of drug ads, most respondents did not find the ads aesthetically pleasing. The so-called best ad was liked by only eighteen of the respondents. The respondents also did not find the ads particularly informative (range = 2–28 percent). Finally, the majority could not identify the product being advertised (range = 2–70 percent).

None of the studies cited contains any direct evidence of influence on physician beliefs or behavior.

Research at the University of Mississippi

Over the past several years we have been involved in a series of studies on prescription-drug advertising. Most of these studies also address the latest content of the ads. With one exception, none was aimed at elucidating a link between advertising and prescribing. A brief summary of each study follows.

Humor

A total of 697 ads that appeared to use humor for attention-getting appeal were identified from five medical journals. Among the findings was the close connection between the subject of humor in the ads and subjects of humor generally—diarrhea, sexual problems. The physician or the drug was rarely the target of the humor.[39]

Blacks

In another study we examined all ads in sixty medical journals in a single calendar year (1974). Of 1,465 ads, only 31 portrayed black models. Three black professionals were shown but no black physician. In only one ad was race the message—that is, as a factor in hypertension. No formal followup has been conducted, but our impression is that an appreciable increase has occurred in recent years in the number of blacks in the ads.[40]

Sex Appeal

In yet another study we assessed the degree of sex appeal of models appearing in drug ads as compared with that of pictures of *Playboy* bunnies. As frivolous as this may appear, we had serious intent leading from previous criticisms of the ads in this regard. One clear finding was that the sex of the reader is a determinant of the sex appeal of the ad. It is interesting that female viewers found some ads featuring the female form to be sexy but that men rated the nude male form in an ad very low. In general, the ads were not perceived to be particularly sexy in spite of the fact that they were selected for study on that basis.[41]

The Elderly

In a study using content analysis, we examined all ads in two journals *(Medical Economics* and *Geriatrics)* for the calendar year 1974. Portrayal of both elderly and nonelderly models was assessed. While both types of patients were portrayed in the majority of ads in a negative way, the negative portrayal of the elderly tended to reinforce stereotypes of the elderly.[42]

Psychotropic Drugs

In another investigation of advertising for psychotropic drugs, we examined 329 different ads for anti-anxiety, anti-psychotic, and antidepressant medications.[43, 44] In this study we were interested both in the types of advertising appeals used and their relationship to male and female models portrayed in the ads. We found the headlines and texts of the ads to be almost totally rational (as defined by the study). The illustrations, however, were nonrational in nearly 60 percent of the ads. We found further that male models were associated with rational appeals in a significantly greater portion of the ads than those involving female models.

These studies were interesting to use, but none can be said to predict an effect on prescribing. We feel that the remaining two studies may have more-important implications.

In the first of these studies, an experimental study was undertaken to assess the impact of governmental regulation on the believability of prescription-drug advertising.[45] The specific variables investigated were symbolic impact and fair balance. Mock advertisements were developed for four tricyclic antidepressant drugs. Symbolic impact was operationalized by portraying the advertisements as orginating from U.S. medical journals—that is, regulated—or Mexican medical journals—that is, unregulated. Fair balance was defined operationally as the inclusion of a brief summary in the advertisement. A nonrandom sample of twenty-four physicians saw four advertisements representing the four treatment combinations. On a self-administered questionnaire, they indicated their confidence in the information contained in the advertisement. A two-factor, repeated-measures randomized-block factorial design was employed in the analysis. The results indicated that the presence of fair balance was associated significantly with higher levels of believability; the symbolic-impact factor was associated nonsignificantly with believability. Thus, there appears to be a perception that FDA regulation of drug ads results in more-believable ads.

The second study's results argue, to a degree, against the purported effect of journal advertising on prescribing.[46] Again, however, it is not possible to isolate the effect of advertising from other informational media. In this study, briefly, we selected as a sample the most frequently prescribed brand-name drug in each of twenty major therapeutic classes used by the National Therapeutic Audit. We determined the advertised uses of the drugs from ads for each appearing in medical journals in 1976. We determined the actual uses of the drugs from physician reports in the National Disease and Therapeutic Index. We found that only three of the twenty drugs were used totally as indicated by the advertisements. The largest discrepancies were found among related but unmentioned uses for tranquilizers, antiarrythmics, antidiabetics, and antidiarrheals. These findings, too, are interesting, but only twenty drugs were involved and the effect of the advertising certainly must be viewed as equivocal.

It should be noted that Schwartzman has cited several examples of drugs that, in spite of significant promotional expenditures, were commercial disappointments. He included Vivactil, Edecrin, Tybatran, Serax, and Ponstel in his support for the statement that "a drug must have viable therapeutic claims in order to become a big seller; advertising alone is insufficient for the success of a product.[47]

Remedies

What can or should be done about journal advertising for drugs? The Medical Committee on Human Rights has made, among others, the following recommendations:

> Elimination of all drug advertising and detail men with resultant lowering of the price of medications,
>
> Promulgation of truthful and complete information on all products,
>
> Elimination of trade names, and their replacement by the generic name, followed by the manufacturer's name in parentheses.[48]

I am convinced that it is not that simple.

The degree of complexity in the drug-advertising issue is exemplified in the published conclusions of a panel organized by the National Council of Churches of Christ. One conclusion of the panel was that, "Given no real evidence to the contrary, we are persuaded that there is a link between the promotion of legitimate drugs and drug misuse and abuse."[49] It seems only slightly overdrawn to suggest the following paraphrase: Given no evidence of innocence, we are persuaded that there is guilt. I am convinced that it is not at all overdrawn to suggest that the link, if one exists, clearly must be the prescribing physician.

We have, of course, a regulatory agency charged with monitoring prescription-drug advertising. Jacoby and Small note that the FDA operates under regulations governing *misleading* ads, as opposed to the term *deceptive* used by the Federal Trade Commission. These authors quote a then-under-consideration definition as follows:

> A misleading prescription drug advertisement is one which causes—either through (1) its verbal content, (2) its design, structure, and/or visual artwork, or (3) the context in which it appears—at least n% of a representative group of practicing physicians to have a common impression or belief regarding the advertised drug which is incorrect or unjustified.[50]

Such a definition has intuitive appeal since it is empirically testable and less susceptible to subjective evaluation. As the authors point out, however, each word and phase in the definition requires interpretation. Further, it is patently impossible to conduct the research necessary for a decision on each drug ad. Subjective judgment, therefore, still would be required for selection of ads for study.

Peter Rheinstein, whose job it is to evaluate the proper advertising of prescription drugs, has noted that actions by the FDA include:

About 5 requirements of remedial ads per year,

About 300 required cancellation of ads per year,

Seizure of a drug product about every one or two years.[51]

He does not report and we do not know what the denominator of this regulatory activity is. He does note that thirty-one of the thirty-five medical journals with a 70,000+ circulation are controlled circulation—that is, supported by advertising.

Brown, in a review of European restrictions on promotion, has described proposed rulings in the United Kingdom that would prohibit inter alia the following:

Use of graphic materials that are detrimental to informative value,

Advertising in journals with less than 60 percent editorial content,

Advertising facing editorial material.[52]

The reasoning for these and other restrictions, according to Brown, follows:

There is a limit to public funds.

New drugs are more expensive and tend to replace cheaper drugs.

Acceptance of new drugs depends on promotion.

In one of the most interesting recent papers on drug advertising, Chapman argues that "advertisements have a mythical dimension which parallels aspects of the nature and functions of myth in traditional societies."[53] Using Australian psychotropic-drug ads as case studies, Chapman makes a strong argument for careful regulatory scrutiny of the pictorial and graphic aspects of advertisements. His argued sequence is:

That advertising works on the basis of promises being offered in response to problems or tensions perceived in the reader of advertisements;

That these promises work—that is, appeal or are internalized in association with the product—insofar as they are accurate in their mirroring myths that are meaningful to the group to whom they are being offered (here, doctors);

That successful advertising will, almost by definition, act to reproduce the ideologies of those to whom it appeals to the ongoing commercial benefit of those producing the advertised products.

What is troubling about Chapman's theory is its reliance on problems with the doctor—namely, ads will succeed to the extent that they reinforce the irrationality, biases, and subjectivity in the doctor's mind.

Conclusion

The complexity of the problem may be illustrated by a somewhat farfetched example. Journals that solicit advertising do not promise to influence prescribing. They promise readership. The journal that needs advertising, then, must produce contents that draw readers, and in this sense advertising may act indirectly to improve editorial quality (if readership is a measure of that quality). By the same token, however, the journal that does not accept advertising but that must rely on subscriptions must also produce readership, or logic demands that the number of subscriptions will decrease. (It is recognized that some journals are part of a membership package and thus may or may not be read but do not depend upon readership for survival.)

The concept under consideration in this chapter is that the pharmaceutical industry, through its promotion (and especially journal advertising), is persuading the medical community to prescribe drugs too often or unwisely or both. Based on the evidence, if we were to describe journal advertising in the constrained terminology required for prescription drugs, that description would be *possibly effective.*

Journal advertisements may, and probably do, affect prescribing in the presence of other prior, subsequent, and simultaneous stimuli. Separation of the effects of the advertisements from these other stimuli and separation of the good effects from the bad effects is possible, but unlikely, outside the artificial, experimental situation.

Journal advertisements offer a special kind of promotion for the following reasons:

> They are reasonably easy to regulate—compared to detailment, for example.
>
> They are easy to monitor—anyone can see what they say.
>
> They may, through the support they offer to medical journals, have indirect beneficial effects.

Physicians have some excellent measures available to them as defense against bad advertising: They need not read them, they need not believe them, and they need not do what the advertisement suggests. Physicians who criticize drug advertising as the sole cause of poor prescribing seem similar to the people who complain about the quality or content of television programs that they, nevertheless, watch night after night.

In light of these factors, we are forced to conclude that while the logic and rhetoric is often persuasive, there is little hard evidence that journal advertising alone has affected adversely the quality of prescribing. Conversely, there is no (or little) evidence that such advertising has had any positive effect on that prescribing. Given the age-old medical dictum, *primum non nocere,* and the continuing criticism, it seems appropriate to consider what might be done about the negative effects of journal advertising (even if undocumented). Some possible remedies follow. Restrictions on the advertiser would include the following:

1. Eliminate journal advertising altogether. This "solves" the problem, but probably eliminates several medical journals and certainly raises the subscription cost of others.
2. Attempt to restrict the amount of this advertising. This could take the form of dollar limits, or a tax on advertising.
3. Further restrict the content. In addition to present FDA surveillance, perhaps the advertisements could provide only the package insert, without eye-catching pictures or other devices that are possibly involved in the latent effects of the advertisements.[54]

If one assumes no basic change in journal advertising, perhaps the prescribers could take action. For example:

1. Prescribers could be taught how to read and analyze the contents in a manner similar to that used with some medical students.
2. Viable alternative sources of information could be provided, including, perhaps, free space in the journals for counterinformation.
3. Physicians could be better educated on prescribing in medical school.
4. Better peer-review mechanisms could be developed to make poor prescribing unattractive to the physician. Inclusion of pharmacists in such activities seems logical. In addition, consideration might be given to involving consumers in the review process. Since, after all, the consumer is the one who suffers, he might well hold the answer to the problem. Conger has predicted that consumer participation like this will be routine in the future.[55]

The journal advertising of prescription drugs is a topic for which controversial is not an adequate descriptor. Scientific study of the issues has been sparse, rhetoric has been abundant. Attempting to cut through the latter, what do we really know? Not necessarily in order of importance, we know the following:

A great deal of money is spent in journal advertising.

Some indeterminate amount of this money results in:

More needed information for prescribers from the journals that are supported by the ads,

Some needed information for prescribers from the ads themselves.

Someone, the patient or some third party, pays for the cost of the advertising.

An objective cost-benefit analysis of the above spending has not been conducted and is probably impossible.

The effect of such advertising is more reminder than directly persuasive, but it must play some additive role in the milieu of drug promotion and information.

The advertisements sometimes portray patients in ways that are inconsistent with the realities of practice. This may or may not redound to the benefit of the advertiser.

The ads are sometimes deceptive and/or misleading as evidenced by FDA actions.

Modest regulatory changes excepted, modification of the nature and extent of journal advertising must await major philosophical changes concerning the role and scope of pharmaceutical promotion. Such changes, if indeed they are necessary, should be based on rigid, scientific study.

As a scientist I am not persuaded that the print advertising for prescription medication, considered alone, is nearly the horror that it frequently is made out to be. I do support, however, the strongest possible efforts to assure that it is neither deceptive nor misleading and support, as well, appropriate penalties where such violations occur. This observation is based on the rather sparse published information, reflecting scientific study, on the subject.

Notes

1. L. Bogart, "Is All This Advertising Necessary?" *Journal of Advertising Research* 18 (1978):17–26. Reprinted from the *Journal of Advertising Research* © Copyright 1978, by the Advertising Research Foundation.
2. Ibid.

3. M.C. Hornbrook, "Market Structure and Advertising in the United States Pharmaceutical Industry," *Medical Care* 16 (1978):90–109.

4. Ibid, p. 106.

5. M.C. Smith, "Drug Product Advertising and Prescribing: A Review of the Evidence," *American Journal of Hospital Pharmacy* 34 (1977):1208–1224.

6. H. Walton, "Ad Recognition and Prescribing by Physicians," *Journal of Advertising Research* 20 (1980):39–48. Reprinted from the *Journal of Advertising Research* © Copyright 1980, by the Advertising Research Foundation.

7. C.D. Kalb, "Psychological Motivation in Physician Prescribing Habits," *Medical Marketing and Media* 13 (1978):43–55.

8. R.N. Butler, "Public Interest Report no. 19—The Overuse of Tranquilizers in Older Patients," *International Journal of Aging and Human Development* 7 (1976):185–187.

9. G. Usdin, "The Coin Needn't Smell: A Response to the Seidenberg Thesis," *Mental Hygiene* 55 (1971):32–34.

10. C. Muller, "Economic Aspects of Medical Use of Psychotropic Drugs," in *Social Aspects of the Medical Use of Psychotropic Drugs,* ed. R. Cooperstock (Toronto: Addiction Research Foundation, 1974), p. 42.

11. E. Mason, "Medicines, the Media and the Menace" (letter), *American Journal of Psychiatry* 128 (1971):180–181.

12. S. Peltzman, "The Diffusion of Pharmaceutical Innovation," in *Drug Development and Marketing,* ed. R.B. Helms (Washington, D.C.: American Enterprise Institute for Public Policy Research, 1975), pp. 15–27.

13. D. Schwartzman, *Innovation in the Pharmaceutical Industry* (Baltimore: Johns Hopkins University Press, 1976).

14. G.J. Stigler "The Economics of Information," *Journal of Political Economy* 69 (1961):213–225.

15. P. Nelson, "Information and Consumer Behavior," *Journal of Political Economy* 78 (1970):311–329.

16. Schwartzman, *Innovation,* p. 202.

17. Ibid., p. 188.

18. Ibid., p. 188.

19. Peltzman, "Diffusion of Pharmaceutical Innovation."

20. Stigler, "Economics of Information."

21. Ibid., p. 222.

22. Ibid., p. 214.

23. Nelson, "Information and Consumer Behavior," p. 312.

24. Ibid.

25. Schwartzman, *Innovation,* pp. 184–185.

26. M. Ryan and M.C. Smith, "Are Physicians Dissonant?" *Pharmaceutical Marketing and Media* 4 (1969):14–17.

27. U.S., Senate, Select Committee on Small Business, Subcommittee on Monopoly, *Hearings on Competitive Problems in the Drug Industry,* 24 May 1976, part. 30, p. 14075.

28. R.R. Miller, "Prescribing Habits of Physicians," *Drug Intelligence and Clinical Pharmacy* 7 (December 1973):560.

29. R. Kunnes, "Poly-drug Abuse: Drug Companies and Doctors," *American Journal of Orthopsychiatry* 43 (1973):530–532.

30. R. Seidenberg, "Drug Advertising and Perception of Mental Illness," *Mental Hygiene* 55 (1971):21–31.

31. R. Seidenberg, "Images of Health, Illness and Women in Drug Advertising," *Journal of Drug Issues* 4 (1974):264–267.

32. E.H. Mosher, "Portrayal of Women in Drug Advertising: A Medical Betrayal," *Journal of Drug Issues* 6 (1976):72–78.

33. G. Stimson, "Women in a Doctored World," *New Society* (May 1975), pp. 265–267.

34. A. Mant and D.B. Darroch, "Media Images and Medical Images," *Social Science and Medicine* 9 (1975):613–618.

35. J. Prather and L.S. Fidell, "Sex Differences in the Content and Style of Medical Advertisements," *Social Science and Medicine* 9 (1975): 23–26.

36. C. McRee, B.F. Corder, and T. Haizlip, "Psychiatrists' Responses to Sexual Bias in Pharmaceutical Advertising," *American Journal of Psychiatry* 131 (1974):1273–1275.

37. P.A. Parish, "What Influences Have Led to Increased Prescribing of Psychotropic Drugs?" *Journal Royal College General Practitioner* 23 (1973):49–57.

38. J.R. Lion et al., "Psychiatrists' Opinions of Psychotropic Drug Advertisements," *Social Science and Medicine* 13A (1979):123–125.

39. F.M. Mburu, M.C. Smith, and H. Wetherbee, "Humor in Prescription Drug Advertising," *Medical Marketing and Media* 11 (1976):38.

40. M.C. Smith, "Where Are the Blacks in Prescription Drug Advertising?" *Medical Marketing and Media* 12 (1977):47.

41. M.C. Smith, P. Strecker, and J.F. Hair, "Sex Appeals in Prescription Drug Advertising," *Medical Marketing and Media* 12 (1977):64.

42. M.C. Smith, "Portrayal of the Elderly in Prescription Drug Advertising," *Gerontologist* 16 (1976):329–334.

43. M.C. Smith and L. Griffin, "Rationality of Appeals Used in the Promotion of Psychotropic Drugs: A Comparison of Male and Female Models," *Social Science and Medicine* 11 (1977):409.

44. M.C. Smith, "Appeals Used in Advertisements for Psychotropic Drugs: An Exploratory Study," *American Journal of Public Health* 67 (1977):171.

45. L.N. Larson et al., "Government Regulation and the Believability

of Prescription Drug Advertising,'' *Drug Intelligence and Clinical Pharmacy* 11 (1977):338.

46. S. Usman, C. Marshal, and M.C. Smith, 'Differences between Actual and Advertised Uses of Drugs: A Replicated Study,'' *Journal of Advertising Research* 19 (1979):65.

47. Schwartzman, *Innovation,* p. 194.

48. P. Greenfield and F. Wolff, ''The Pressures of Drug Advertising on Physicians and Patients,'' *Journal of Drug Issues* 4 (1974):254.

49. ''Findings and Conclusions of the NCCC Project on Drug Advertising,'' *Journal of Drug Issues* 4 (1974):310–312.

50. J. Jacoby and C. Small, ''The FDA Approach to Defining Misleading Advertising,'' *Journal of Marketing* 39 (1975):65–73.

51. P.H. Rheinstein, ''Considerations in the Regulation of Prescription Drug Promotion,'' in *Perspectives in Pharmacy,* eds. A.I. Wertheimer and N.L. Suntrup (Minneapolis: University of Minnesota Press, 1980).

52. P.J. Brown, ''Pharmaceutical Promotion in Europe—Regulations and Restricitons,'' *Medical Marketing and Media* 12 (1977):27.

53. S. Chapman, ''Advertising and Psychotropic Drugs: The Place of Myth in Ideological Reproduction,'' *Social Science and Medicine* 13A (1979):751–764. Reprinted with permission.

54. P.D. Stolley, ''Assuring the Safety and Efficacy of Therapies, *International Journal of Health Services* 4 (1974):143.

55. D.S. Conger, *Social Interventions* (Saskatoon, Saskatchewan: Modern Press, 1974), p. 49.

21 The Effect of Prescribing Practices on Drug-Cost Reduction

Peter Temin

The problem of medical costs is on everyone's mind, and medical care is a prime candidate for cost cutting by the current administration. However, while the goal of medical-cost reduction is clear, the mechanism by which this goal is to be attained is less clear. The general approach has been to attack it piecemeal, attempting to reduce the cost of one or another aspect of medical care.

Prominent among the candidates for cost reduction is the cost of drugs. Even though drugs comprise only about 10 percent of personal-health expenditures, they seem to offer a promising area to cut costs. They are very visible since drug costs are insured less than most other medical costs.[1] Also, drug purchases seem to represent a more-normal economic transaction than other medical activities.

This chapter addresses this latter point. It argues that the resemblance between drug purchases and purchases of other, nonmedical commodities is not as close as many people assume, that doctors are not able to learn by prescribing in the way that purchasers of other goods can learn, and consequently, that the opportunities for drug-cost cutting are limited.

How do doctors choose drugs? Doctors cannot and do not exhibit instrumental behavior when prescribing drugs. They are acting instead in a customary way. Persistent references in the literature to prescribing habits show that this attribution is not new, yet its implications have not been explored adequately.[2] Thus, the chapter also explores the implications for reducing the costs of drugs.

Instrumental behavior is goal-seeking behavior—that is, it consists of actions designed to advance an internally consistent goal. People acting instrumentally typically evaluate actions by their efficacy in attaining the goal and interact through a series of explicit exchanges where the value of the exchange in furthering the goal can be evaluated. By contrast, people acting in a customary mode conserve what they think of as historical behavior. They evaluate actions by examination of the actions, not by the consequences of these acts. And social interaction is very important, both for the transmission of custom within the community and for the opportunity for reciprocal actions that it provides. Reciprocity, not exchange, is the dominant form of interpersonal communication.[3]

This chapter describes the physician's behavior to show why the description of prescribing behavior as customary is appropriate. Then it discusses a few implications of this attribution for cost containment in medical care through reductions in drug costs. Three factors inhibiting instrumental actions in drug prescribing need to be described: (1) the relation of doctor to patient, (2) the difficulty of measuring drug costs and benefits, and (3) the absence of learning by doing.

First, in the words of Senator Kefauver, "He who orders does not buy, and he who buys does not order."[4] As a result, the ordering doctor typically does not know that most important of economic data: the price.

How hard would it be for doctors to learn about drug prices? Approximately 1,000 different chemical entities are sold either singly or in combination.[5] The *Physician's Desk Reference* (PDR) lists approximately 2,500 drug products made up from these 1,000 chemical entities. *Drug Topics Red Book,* a standard product and price reference for pharmacists, contains 170,000 entries.

This voluminous information on different drugs, however, contains very little information on costs that is usable by the doctor. The *Red Book* gives wholesale prices, and the consumer must pay retail prices. In addition, within any locality, the retail price of any given drug varies both between pharmacies and over time in any one pharmacy, so the link between wholesale and retail prices is loose.[6] Further, the *Red Book* lists prices but does not identify the chemical composition of brand-name drugs. The *PDR* identifies drugs both by brand name and chemical composition, but it lists only a small fraction of the products in the *Red Book,* and it lacks prices. Thus, price data for drugs simply are not easily available.

As a result, doctors seldom have an accurate sense of drug costs. A 1970 survey of Palo Alto physicians asked them to choose a favored drug for urinary-tract infections and then to estimate its retail price. A correct answer was defined to be one that was in the range of prices in representative retail pharmacies. Only one-third of the doctors polled gave a price ranked as correct by this standard. When asked to identify the more-expensive drug in fifteen different pairs of commonly prescribed anti-infective drugs, half of the doctors chose correctly in eleven or more cases.[7] Since random guessing would yield a correct score of seven, this finding suggests that the doctors polled knew between one-third and one-half of the relative price comparisons. The first test suggests that one-third of doctors knew the price in question, while the second suggests that each doctor knew approximately one-third of the prices asked about. The two tests are consistent. If doctors knew approximately one-third of common drug prices, and if the identity of this one-third was determined more or less randomly, then asking doctors about any specific price should yield approximately one-third correct answers. Doctors are not totally ignorant of drug prices, and we would not expect them to be; but their knowledge is sharply limited. Asked about common drug prices, they reveal ignorance more often than knowledge.

In order to make an instrumental choice between drugs, a doctor needs to know the benefits as well as the costs of using a drug. However, while it is easy to make a choice between broad classes of drugs—say, between analgesics and antibiotics—it is hard to discriminate between the effects of similar drugs. In the extreme, it is particularly hard to distinguish between different brands or manufacturers of the same drug. Yet this is the information that is needed to make the instrumental choice relevant for reducing drug costs. The question for cost reduction is whether or not a given goal—alleviation of a symptom or cure of a disease—is obtainable at lower cost by drug, brand, or manufacturer substitution.

There are several reasons why more information on the comparative effectiveness of drugs does not exist. First, the concept of effectiveness is vague.[8] While it clearly must relate in some way to the ability of a drug to correct some undesirable condition, it can relate to many other drug characteristics as well. The method of administration—oral, parenteral, topical—and the dosage required both can be considered. Speed of action and durability of action are important as well. In addition to a drug's effectiveness against any specific disease, the breadth of conditions treated may be relevant if tests to identify particular problems are difficult. The myriad possible adverse drug reactions are relevant as well. Drugs without adverse side effects are preferable to those with unwanted results, but adverse reactions vary among themselves approximately as much as the beneficial effects and therefore are as difficult to classify and evaluate.

The multidimensional nature of drug effectiveness does not mean that knowledge is absent. It means rather that knowledge is costly to acquire and that different investigators will concentrate on different dimensions. Information is likely to be incomplete, confusing, and sometimes, contradictory.

Epidemiological research is needed to discover comparative effectiveness because the effects of drugs and diseases vary among individuals. However, dramatic the story of one individual may be, there is no way from a single story to know how much, if any, of this story can be extrapolated to other contexts. Norman Cousins checked out of the hospital while suffering from a serious disease and proceeded to recover.[9] Does that mean that we should check out of the hospital only if we have the same disease as Cousins? that we should only check out of the same hospital as Cousins? or that God watches out for children, drunks, and well-known editors? The remarkable story of Norman Cousins does not contain this information.

To find out, it is necessary to analyze the experiences of a variety of people in slightly different circumstances. It is necessary to sample from the populations to which the results will be applied, where the populations are defined according to some relevant characteristics: for example, age, location, symptoms, disease. It is also necessary to analyze the results by formal statistical techniques to find out if the observed variation was due to chance or to some identifiable cause, if the sample was large enough to contain the desired information, or which of two plausible explanations is preferred.

Statistics are not popular among doctors, however; they cut against the grain of medical training and practice. Doctors treat individual patients and write clinical reports. They typically do not learn and do not utilize much statistical knowledge. They are not well qualified to do epidemiological research or to evaluate epidemiological reports in the literature.

Medical journals contain very few reports of randomized clinical trials of competing therapies.[10] Even if the conceptual and professional difficulties were absent, many experiments needed to discriminate between different drugs are expensive and difficult. Small differences between drugs cannot be isolated without large samples. In addition, the payoff from these experiments may not be large: The best and second-best drugs may be almost equivalent. Since current drug regulations do not involve comparative effectiveness, they have not generated research on this question. In fact, it is hard to know if society would benefit from more experiments on comparative effectiveness or not since the gain from knowing that a lower-priced drug will do as well as a more-expensive one must be offset against the cost of the experiment to find out. For similar drugs with similar prices, the expected gain is small and the cost is high. For drugs with a large price difference, it is more likely that the expected gain would offset the cost of acquiring knowledge. In any case, the paucity of comparative experiments at the moment means that doctors and consumers have to make many decisions without experimental evidence on the comparative effect of alternative choices.

Finally, the clinical activities of doctors do not generate useful information on the comparative merits of competing brands of drugs. For the reasons just given, it would be hard for clinical activities to do so. However, it is clear that doctors do not act in a way to generate as much comparative information as they could.

Practicing doctors are engaged in treating patients. They vary treatment according to the patient's condition, and they use the therapy they consider most appropriate; but since the effects of drugs vary from individual to individual, it is necessary to observe a sample of patients to get information that can be applied outside the original clinical situation. To connect the observed effects with the drugs taken—as opposed to some other cause—the patients have to be given randomly or not given the drugs. Thus, the research doctor has to vary his treatment of patients for other than clinical reasons, for reasons uncorrelated with patient's clinical problems.

This method conflicts with the standards of clinical practice, showing that clinical medicine and drug research are separate activities. The doctor treating patients is in no position to construct random samples of patients and to observe the effect of different therapies. It violates his professional relations with his patients, and it raises ethical questions about the role of doctors.[11] He must rely on the research physician or statistician for careful and statistically valid information on drug effectiveness.

The effects of this dichotomy can be seen in the clinical use of drugs by doctors. If it were the case that doctors limited themselves to a small number of drugs, then they might be able to use them with enough care to accumulate useful information on their effects, despite the problems just discussed. However, doctors avail themselves freely of the wide variety of available drugs. With approximately 1,000 chemical entities on the market, sold often under multiple names or by multiple vendors and sometimes in combination, doctors find it hard to restrict themselves to a small number of drugs. No matter how many prescriptions they write, doctors average under a dozen prescriptions a year for each drug product used.[12] (A drug product is a drug or brand of drug but not a dosage unit.)

For example, doctors who used between 50 and 100 different drug products in the year ending in June 1976 wrote an average of 830 new prescriptions during the year. This is only an average of 3 new prescriptions (as opposed to refills) for each of 250 working days; these doctors prescribed far below the average of their colleagues. It is also an average of only 10 prescriptions per drug. Conversely, doctors who used between 400 and 500 different drug products wrote an average of almost 6,000 new prescriptions during the year, or an average of just under 24 new prescriptions on each of 250 working days; but they used each drug, on average, only thirteen times during the year. Despite the difference in the volume of prescriptions between the two groups, the frequency with which they used any single drug product was remarkably constant. This constancy was preserved throughout almost the full range of doctors.

It is worth noting that this finding—that doctors do not repeatedly use a small number of drugs—does not depend upon the method of derivation. I have distinguished doctors by the number of prescriptions they wrote and have found that the number of times they used a given drug product on average did not vary. If instead doctors are distinguished by medical specialty, the same result is obtained. Dermatologists appear to use individual drug products about twice as often as the average doctor, while internists appear to use each given drug product about half as often as average. However, these comparatively minor variations are the extremes of the distribution, and cross classifying by specialty and type of drug reveals that even within therapeutic classes doctors typically do not use individual drug products more than once a month.[13] Doctors, faced with an abundance of drugs and sources of drugs on the market, range widely as they choose which drugs to prescribe.

Any doctor who used a drug a dozen times in the course of the year could not evaluate the benefits and risks of using this drug relative to the benefits and costs of other drugs even if he tried. While the rate of a dozen prescriptions a year is only an average, deviations to one side are matched by deviations on the other. For example, the finding that doctors average a dozen prescriptions a year for each different drug used does not mean that each doctor prescribes each drug a dozen times a year. Some drugs undoubtedly are used more—maybe much more—than that, while others are used less. To see how this might work out, consider a doctor who uses 200 different drug products and writes 2,000 new prescriptions a year. (He is near the median doctor in 1976). If he uses 30 drugs most of the time—say, once a week—he would use these 30 drugs in 1,500 of his new prescriptions. This leaves 500 other new prescriptions spread among 170 other drugs. Each of these other drugs, therefore, is used an average of only three times a year, hardly enough to gather information on patient reactions at all. Acknowledging that physicians use some drugs more than others only emphasizes the point that doctors have very limited experience with most of the drugs they use.

In addition, doctors are not loyal to specific drug companies. For example, doctors who write more prescriptions for antibiotics use antibiotics from more different drug manufacturers. Larger prescribers write more prescriptions for the products of each manufacturer, but they do not confine themselves to a small group of manufacturers, even within a single therapeutic classification. Almost three-quarters of the doctors surveyed in 1976 prescribed antibiotics from more than five different drug firms.[14]

As with the diversity with which different drugs are used, this pattern is evident at any level of detail. Consider tetracycline. A doctor who writes as few as five new tetracycline prescriptions a month typically uses two different kinds of tetracycline, and those few doctors who write close to one new tetracycline prescription a day use five or more different kinds.[15] Doctors do not choose a best tetracycline and stick with it. Given the assurances of rough equality between them, doctors who prescribe this drug repeatedly use several different brands or alternate between brand-name and generic tetracycline.

The prescribing habits of doctors therefore are dominated by diversity. Doctors use many different drugs in the course of the year, including similar drugs from many different manufacturers and different drugs for the same diseases. They use far too many drugs to have accurate information on the comparative costs and benefits of these drugs even if this information existed, which in most cases it does not. Consequently, doctors follow the customs of the medical community in choosing drugs to prescribe. Like all customs, they are sustained by the institutions of the community; and like most customs, they are also functional. Nevertheless, the prevalence of customary behavior indicates that the link between prescribing habits and the cost-effectiveness of drugs is weak.

It follows, therefore, that efforts to increase the cost-effectiveness of drug prescribing will be less successful than might have been imagined. It is not the case that there is a simple barrier to entry that keeps prices high and that once this barrier is removed, the press of competition will force drug prices down. It is rather that the drug market operates in a cloud of uncertainty that renders the demand considerably less responsive to price than it is in many other markets.

This can be seen in the results—still only imperfectly known—of the government's two programs to reduce drug costs. Two programs are needed because drug purchases are financed in two different ways. Most drug purchases are financed by individuals, but some are financed by the federal and state governments under Medicare and Medicaid. For the private purchases, policymakers have tried to give competition a chance by repealing nonsubstitution laws. For the public purchases, policymakers have tried to set a ceiling on what they would pay.

State substitution laws proliferated after World War II as the flood of new drugs hit the market (see chapter 9). Drug companies wanted laws to make sure that their advertising to doctors was reflected in consumer purchases, and pharmacies wanted them to limit their liability in filling prescriptions. During the 1960s, the patents on the initial wave of new drugs began to expire and generic drugs appeared on the market. In order to make it easier to purchase the lower-priced generics, almost all states have repealed their antisubstitution laws or replaced them with laws defining the allowable range of substitution. Although it seems clear that this legal change should work to lower drug prices, preliminary assessments of its impact have not revealed a powerful effect.[16] In light of the conditions of competition in the drug industry just described, this is not surprising.

The federal government has introduced its maximum-allowable-cost program to reduce its drug costs. The plan was for the government to designate the maximum amount for which it would reimburse pharmacies for filling prescriptions of each drug. Drugs were identified by generic name in this program, and the aim was to set the maximum allowable cost equal to the price of the representative generic drug. This program, however, has been mired in administrative delays, so that the number of drugs under the program is still quite small, and it is not clear that the cost savings from the program exceed the costs of administering it.

In short, it is proving difficult to reduce medical costs even in this most promising area of drug purchases. True, drug costs are a minor part of total health expenditures, but a dollar is a dollar, and drugs looked like a good place to start. For the reasons I have given here, however, the drug market lacks the feedback that is an essential part of well-functioning economic markets, and the possibilities of cost reduction are fewer than they might appear.

If this is true for drugs, how much truer is it for other aspects of medical care? Medical costs will not be cut by marginal changes in the way medical care is provided. The problem of excessive medical costs cannot be solved by growling around its edges.

Notes

1. R. Gibson, "National Health Expenditures, 1979," *Health Care Financing Review* 2 (Summer 1980):1–36.

2. M.C. Smith, *Principles of Pharmaceutical Marketing* (Philadelphia: Lea & Febiger, 1968), p. 74.

3. P. Temin, *Taking Your Medicine: Drug Regulation in the United States* (Cambridge: Harvard University Press, 1980), p. 14.

4. E. Kefauver, *In a Few Hands: Monopoly Power in America* (New York: Pantheon Books, 1965), p. 8.

5. U.S., FDA, Drug Listing Branch, Bureau of Drugs, *National Drug Code Directory.* (Washington, D.C.: Department of Health, Education and Welfare, 1969).

6. S.E. Berki, J.W. Richards, and H.A. Weeks, "The Mysteries of Prescription Pricing in Retail Pharmacies," *Medical Care* 15 (March 1977): 241–250.

7. D.R. Lowy, L. Lowy, and R.S. Warner, "A Survey of Physicians' Awareness of Drug Costs," *Journal of Medical Education* 47 (May 1972): 349–351.

8. S. Goodman, "The Problem of Drug Efficacy: An Exercise in Dissection," in *Drugs in Our Society,* ed. Paul Talalay (Baltimore, Johns Hopkins University Press, 1964), pp. 49–54.

9. N. Cousins, *Anatomy of an Illness as Perceived by the Patient* (New York: W.W. Norton, 1979).

10. E. Juhl, E. Christensen, and N. Tygstrup, "The Epidemiology of the Gastrointestinal Randomized Clinical Trial," *New England Journal of Medicine* 269 (6 January 1977):20–22.

11. S. Bok, "The Ethics of Giving Placebos," *Scientific American* 231 (November 1974):17–23.

12. Temin, *Taking Your Medicine.*

13. P. Temin, "Physician Prescribing Behavior: Is There Learning by Doing?," in *Drugs and Health,* ed. American Enterprise Institute (Washington, D.C., 1981), pp. 173–182.

14. Temin, *Taking Your Medicine.*

15. Ibid.

16. R.A. Horvitz, J.P. Morgan, and L. Fleckenstein, "Savings from Generic Prescriptions: A Study of 33 Pharmacies in Rochester, New York," *Annals of Internal Medicine* 82 (May 1975):601–607.

22 A Drug-Information Project for Medical Students

Marlin Demlinger, Doreen V. Kagan, Stephen Janofsky, and *John P. Morgan*

The academic library is becoming more and more complicated as technology gradually changes methods and services. Computerized circulation and cataloguing records, online searching, and new techniques in microform are now common. Libraries not only are vast storehouses of information but also the bibliographic apparatus that provides the key to that information has become more complex. The uninvolved student cannot use the sophisticated indexes and abstract services without proper guidances and instruction.

Library, or bibliographic, instruction has grown into a discipline itself and should be a major part of every library's public service.[1] The basic objective of bibliographic instruction is to train students to use library resources effectively so they will be independent searchers in the future. The goal, phrased fashionably, is *library literacy:*

> Thus the concept of library literacy helps us to identify user instruction as not only a specific basic educational skill, but also as being central to the goals of education generally.[2]

Library staff members develop, implement, and perform bibliographic instruction. Librarians discover through the questions asked them at reference and information desks that a need for information exists. If these questions are course related, as they often are, the librarian may bring this matter to the attention of the faculty and propose a formal session in library instruction.

Ideally, any course-related instruction is best given jointly by the library and course teachers, but for various reasons, cooperation on this level is not a reality.[3] In practice, the library staff must promote this service to persuade the faculty that bibliographic instruction is beneficial. Rarely, the faculty instructs students in methods of library research without the guidance or help of the library staff.

Methods

A variety of instructional techniques have been developed. In the simplest case, no formal instruction exists. Students are guided by signs telling them where things are, by instruction sheets telling them how to use a specific reference tool, and by handbooks giving them a detailed explanation of the library and its resources.[4] A much more-sophisticated version of this procedure has come to be known as the point-of-use approach, developed most prominently at Massachusetts Institute of Technology (MIT) in its Intrex Project.[5] Here, audiovisual equipment is strategically located in the library. Slides, tapes, and filmstrips instruct the student where to find material or how to use a particular index. Another form more commonly used is a workbook containing library problems for the student to solve.[6] Programmed instruction is also used, either in textual or computer form.[7]

Library-orientation tours are still widely practiced, probably because they are relatively easy to implement. Students are herded into the library and led around from point to point. Evidence exists that students retain very little of what they are told during these tours. They are seldom strongly interested, and the orientation is usually too general to be of immediate use to them. Later, when they begin to do projects, they have lost what little they learned and need re-instruction.[8]

Course-related bibliographic instruction varies greatly. Often the librarian enters the class and lectures on specific pertinent library resources. Other times the class attends at the library. This lecture may be recorded on videotape.[9] In rarer cases there is cooperation between the faculty and the library. We believe that good bibliographic instruction may occur when the course instructor and the librarian teach together.

The course-related instruction should take place as part of the classroom instruction. In some institutions the library designs its own courses that are offered as credit courses; however, usually they are optional.[10] Where the library has sufficient staff, seminars on specific course material may be offered. In these courses, students are not taught general library research methods but methods focused on the characteristics of their subject.[11]

Library Methods in Drug Information

Information in the field of biomedicine, as elsewhere, continues to grow rapidly. A report to NATO, published in 1974, estimated that a new medical publication appears about every half-hour.[12] Some 60,000 drug products are marketed worldwide. New drugs appear every year. There are about 16,000 biomedical journals. Those undertaking drug research may spend up to 60 percent of their time finding information, but at best they cannot read more than about 5 percent of the original literature in the field.[13]

Confronted by this profusion, even the experienced physician or medical researcher will find it difficult to cope. Tools to search out the literature are not very complex structurally, but the vastness of material may make it seem so.

The project herein described focuses on teaching drug-information skills. Medical students are joining a profession whose practitioners are known to have consulted questionable informational sources for new drug products and drug prescribing. Studies done between 1952 and 1974 indicated a reliance upon three major drug-information sources: detail men,[14] direct-mail ads,[15] and journal advertising.[16] A 1974 FDA survey indicated that the *PDR* had replaced these sources as the practitioner's preferred reference.[17] A more-recent study identified colleagues as important informal drug advisors.[18]

Despite little evidence that physicians desire them, more and more published guides appear to meet the practitioner's need for answers. Some authors have attempted to evaluate these critically.[19] For medical students, finding drug facts in this mass may be difficult and unmanageable.

Methods of Bibliographic Instruction for the Sophie Davis School of Biomedical Education

We now describe the library-instruction program developed for the fourth-year medical students in the pharmacology course at the Sophie Davis School of Biomedical Education.[20] The project evolved into its present form from the joint efforts of Stephen Janofsky, the medical librarian, and John P. Morgan, director of the pharmacology program in the school.

In its first year the library project was informational in nature—that is, Dr. Morgan assigned his students drug-information problems to solve. Mr. Janofsky had already developed a library guide that each student received. With its circulation Mr. Janofsky offered to provide guidance for any student needing help with the assignment.

Dr. Morgan was disappointed in the student papers because of an obvious deficiency in student library skills. He and Mr. Janofsky redesigned the project, submitted a proposal for funding, and received a small grant for a drug-information project from the Ruth W. Dolan Foundation in New York City.

The current library project has taken the following form. Each student in the pharmacology class selects a drug topic from a limited list, uses at least four required abstract/index medical tools, writes a final paper, and defends it orally. The final paper is not a substantive essay but rather describes the search strategy and methodology and ends with a selective bibliography.

The pharmacology-class syllabus contains a description of the library project: assignment requirements, educational objectives, descriptions of the four major library tools, and a sample library search. A designated class session is devoted to discussion of the project. Topics are posted from which students choose, or rarely, they propose their own. The course director generates topics that interest him and occasionally that constitute his research interests. The following are some examples of topics, covering a wide range of drug-related areas:

Categories	*Topics*
New drugs	Domiperidone, nifedipine, ranitidine.
Old drugs with new uses	Clonidine, propranolol, thalidomide.
Controversial topics	Do estrogens cause endometrial adenocarcinoma? Why was ticrynafen withdrawn from the U.S. market? Is dextropropoxyphene (Darvon) and drug-related death a real association? Is DMSO good for anything? Does reserpine cause breast cancer?
Therapeutic dilemmas	Should iron be added to flour? Does physical dependence to benzodiazepines occur in humans? Should myocardial infarction be treated routinely with beta blockade?
Social problems and pharmacology	Societal response to the introduction of caffeine into North America, Beta blockers and the anxiety of musical performance.
Drug information	Do any empirical studies illustrate the effect of pharmaceutical advertising on doctors? What do patients understand about patient package inserts?
Drug abuse	What is the toxicity of combusted free-base cocaine? What is the treatment for phencyclidine toxicity?

Mr Janofsky developed a four-hour seminar/workshop for three to six students. He discussed searching strategies, concentrating on the four major bibliographic tools: *Index Medicus,*[21] *Excerpta Medica,*[22] *Biological Abstracts,*[23] and *Biological Abstracts RRM*[24] (Reports, Reviews, Meetings), *Science Citation Index*[25]. Students learned distinctions between primary, secondary, and tertiary literature and the utility of abstracting. They learned differences between available indexes and abstracts and their formats, coverage, and systems. Some students learned about other bibliographic tools when they sought individual help. Mr. Janofsky focused on the required student research topics, emphasizing that no single research route existed since the subjects varied widely and that no two searches would be identical.

Those who did not attend the seminar workshops read a library guide or struck out on their own. Resistance to the project is appreciable because students feel that the course material is already too dense; however, the project is graded, and that provides significant motivation.

Both Mr. Janofsky and Ms. Doreen Kagan, research associate in pharmacology, are available for planning strategy and solving individual problems. They are also the two assigned faculty members who evaluate both the papers and an oral presentation, then award a grade. Facility in the use of the four major bibliographic tools earns students a 90 percent grade. Additional points are granted when other bibliographic tools are used or when creativity is displayed. The project grade is ranked equal to one of five examination grades. The final examination counts for two examination grades. The final class grade is based on the average of eight scores.

Subjects were chosen for inherent interest, and the topics varied widely in their utility as search problems. The following examples illustrate.

Subject: The clinical pharmacology of sodium valproate. This subject revealed a common problem in single-subject topics of current interest. In *Index Medicus* alone, this student, like many others, found so many citations that she was no longer active in compiling a selective bibliography.

Subject: What is "china white?" This student could not begin his search with the four major library tools. After he learned that this phrase was street slang, he consulted *Narcotics and Drug Abuse A to Z,*[26] and found the term defined as high-grade heroin. *The New York Times Index*[27] led him to an article expanding the reference to a variety of drugs substituted for heroin, particularly methylfentanyl. He then used the Permuterm Index of the *Science Citation Index* and found more citations.

Subject: The clinical pharmacology of ranitidine. This search was initially difficult because the professor had misspelled the new drug's name. As a new drug, it was not yet listed in the closed vocabulary of *Index Medicus. Inpharma,*[28] a drug-literature-indexing periodical, provided an important start. The more-fluid subject listings of *Biological Abstracts* and the Permuterm Index of *SCI* listed the term; *Excerpta Medica* listed it under *antihistaminic agent.*

Subject: The impact of lithium carbonate on renal function. Again, this was not easily found in the *Index Medicus* major/minor listings. The student consulted the four required tools, *Martindale's Extra Pharmacopoeia,*[29] *Merck Index,*[30] *PDR,*[31] Jablonski's *Illustrated Dictionary of Eponymic Syndromes and Diseases and Their Synonyms,*[32] *Ulrich's International Periodicals Directory,*[33] *International Pharmaceutical Abstracts,*[34] and *Toxicity Bibliography*[35] and produced one of the best bibliographies we have seen.

Subject: Doping in horse racing: What agents are used? The first year this topic was used, the student author composed a fanciful short story about the criminal world of doping horses. He utilized the genus index (equine) of *Biological Abstracts* successfully, an unusual event in this project. The second year a student found articles through the *Reader's Guide to Periodical Literature.*[36]

Subject: The physical-dependency liability of benzodiazepines. The student started his research by writing Roche Laboratories for information on the topic. The company sent materials not found elsewhere and also called the pharmacology professor to let him know of this student's interest.

Subject: Does colchicine treatment of cannabis constitute a potential hazard? The student had learned from a television drama that colchicine added to the cannabis plant putatively increased its growth and psychoactivity but that it might cause toxicity. A counterculture journal, *High Times,*[37] advertised the availability of colchicine-detection kits. The student searched for information, using every required library tool and several indexes for popular journals and even called California to speak with the producer of the television drama. The student did not obtain a single citation but surely earned his 95 grade.

Subject: What is the "United States Pharmacopoeia?" Most physicians know nothing of the important function this organization fulfills. The student researcher consulted various historical sources including the *U.S. Surgeon General's Catalogue.*[38] She learned of this unusual governmental-private cooperative organization in establishing pharmaceutical-quality standards for drugs.

Conclusion

The evaluation of bibliographic instruction has been of much concern to librarians over the past few years, and the literature on the subject has grown extensively.[39] Because most instructional programs are not closely integrated with course work, and because communication between the librarian and the teaching faculty often is poor or nonexistent, the evaluators must rely on indirect techniques such as the questionnaire or the quiz. In this program, success of the instruction at one level can be evaluated directly when the research projects and oral presentations are graded.

After five repetitions we believe the project is successful. Approximately 325 students have completed it. Each has had a practical experience with the major medical-library tools. Each has written and defended a paper on the searching process. Each has received a passing grade. The bibliographies they compiled have been useful to the professor and have been used by later students—an unusual and effective testimony for an educational project.

Notes

1. For discussion of bibliographic instruction, see C.A. Kirkendall, ed., *Directions for the Decade: Library Instruction in the 1980's,* (Ann Arbor, Mich.: Pierian Press, 1981); J. Lubens, Jr., ed., *Educating the Library User* (New York: Bowker, 1974); J. Lubens, Jr., ed., *Progress in Educating the Library User* (New York: Bowker, 1978); and H. Rader, *Academic Library Instruction* (Ann Arbor, Mich.: Pierian Press, 1975).

2. J. Lindgren, "Toward Library Literacy," *RQ* (Spring 1981), p. 233.

3. E. Farber, "Librarian-Faculty Communication Techniques," in *Southeastern Conference on Approaches to Bibliographic Instruction,* ed. C. Oberman-Soroka (Charleston, S.C.: College of Charleston, 1978), pp. 71–86; J. Lee, "Instruction, Communication, and the Faculty," in *Reform and Renewal in Higher Education* (Ann Arbor, Mich.: Pierian Press, 1980), pp. 29–38; and J. Lubens, Jr., "Seeking a Partnership between the Teacher and the Librarian," in *Progress in Educating the Library User* (New York: Bowker, 1978), pp. 1–12.

4. M. McCormick, "Library Handbooks and other Printed Bibliographic Aids," in *Educating the Library User,* ed. J. Lubens (New York: Bowker, 1974), pp. 307–317; P. Olevnik, "Non-formalized Point of Use Library Instruction: A Survey," *Catholic Library World* 50 (December 1978):218–222; and C. Stevens, "Library Pathfinders," *College and Research Libraries* 34 (January 1973):40–46.

5. K. Cipolla, "M.I.T.'s Point-of-Use Concept: A Five-year Update," *Journal of Academic Librarianship* 5 (January 1980):326–328; C. Stevens and J. Gardner, "Point-of-Use Library Instruction," in *Educating the Library User,* ed. J. Lubens (New York: Bowker, 1974), pp. 269–278; and L. Hardesty, "Use of Slide/Tape Presentations in Academic Libraries," *Journal of Academic Librarianship* 9 (1977):83–95.

6. P.A. Berge, J. Pryor, and C. Stoffler, "A Workbook Approach to Teaching Library Research Skills," *Urban Academic Librarian* 1 (Spring

1981):19–24; S. Phipps and R. Dickstein, "The Library Skills Program at the University of Arizona," *Journal of Academic Librarianship* 5 (September 1979):205–214; and B.L. Renford, "A Self-Paced Workbook Program for Library College Students," *Journal of Academic Librarianship* 4 (September 1978):200–203.

7. A. Clark, "Computer-Assisted Library Instruction," in *Educating the Library User,* ed. J. Lubens (New York: Bowker, 1974), pp. 336–349; P. Culkin, "Evaluation of Computer-Assisted Library Use Instruction," in *Evaluating Library Use Instruction,* ed. R. Beeler (Ann Arbor, Mich.: Pierian Press, 1975), pp. 43–49; and M. Williams and E. Davis, "Evaluation of PLATO Library Instruction Sessions," *Journal of Academic Librarianship* 5 (March 1979):14–19.

8. R. Frederick, "Library Orientation," *Improving College & University Teaching* 26 (Summer 1978):200; J.M. Hughes, "A Tour of the Library by Audiotape," *Special Lib* (July 1974), pp. 288–290; J. Rosenblum, "Toward an Alternative to the In-House Tour," *Southeastern Lib* 28 (Winter 1978):235–238; and R. Vuturo, "Beyond the Library Tour," *Wilson Library Bulletin* 51 (May 1977):736–740.

9. M.B. Binder, A. Mathai and M. Wiegmann, "Library Instruction by Videotape and Lecture: A Case Study," *Urban Academic Librarian* 1 (Spring 1981):16–18; J. Kennedy and T. Kirk, "Course-Related Library Instruction," *Drexel Library Quarterly* 7 (1971):277–297; T. Kirk, comp., *Course-Related Library Instruction* (New York: Jeffrey Norton Pub., 1978); J. MacGregor and R. McInnis, "Integrating Classroom Instruction and Library Resources," *Journal of Higher Education* 48 (January–February 1977):17–38; Superenant, "A Comparison of Lecture and Programmed Instruction," pp. 54–66; and P. Walsh, "Videotape: A Case Study," in *Educating the Library User,* ed. J. Lubens (New York: Bowker, 1974), pp. 376–382.

10. For discussion of credits earned for library courses, see C. Bodien and M.K. Smith, "Developing Library Skills: How to Use the University Library. A One Credit Course," ERIC Document no. ED 153 656, 1978; M. Dudley, "The State of Library Instruction Credit Courses and the State of Use of Library Skills Workbooks," in *Library Instruction in the Seventies,* ed. H. Rader (Ann Arbor, Mich.: Pierian Press, 1977), pp. 79–84; A. Reveal, "Library Instruction and Team Teaching," ERIC Document no. 144 604, 1976; and A. Roberts, "A Study of Ten SUNY Campuses Offering an Undergraduate Credit Course in Library Instruction," ERIC Document no. 157 529 (Albany: SUNY, 1978).

11. For discussion of seminar/workshop-style library instruction, see M. Blum and S. Spangehl, "Introducing the College Student to Academic Inquiry: An Individualized Course in Library Research Skills," ERIC Document no. 152 315, 1978; E. Dubin, "An In-Depth Analysis of a Term

Paper Clinic,'' *Illinois Libraries* 60 (March 1978):324–333; and J. Hobbins, ''Seminars and Assignments,'' in *Academic Library Instruction,* ed. H. Rader (Ann Arbor, Mich.: Pierian Press, 1975), pp. 65–68.

12. G. Unger, ''International Medical Information Systems,'' in *How to Obtain Information in Different Fields of Science and Technology: A User's Guide,* AGAARD Lecture Series, no. 69, AD 780 061, ed. Advisory Group on Aerospace Research and Development, p. 3–2.

13. Ibid.

14. A. Bauer and L. Wortzel, ''Doctor's Choice: The Physician and His Sources of Information about Drugs,'' *Journal of Marketing Research* 3 (February 1966):40–47.

15. M. Reilly, *Drug Information: Literature Review of Needs, Resources and Services* (Rockville, Md.: DHEW, March 1972), pp. 16–25.

16. R.F. Palmer, ''Drug Misuse and Physician Education,'' *Clinical Pharmacology and Therapeutics* 10 (January–February 1969):1–4.

17. A. Ruskin, *Survey of Drug Information Needs and Problems Associated with Communications Directed to Practicing Physicians. Part I: Physician Information Survey* (Rockville, Md.: FDA, 1974).

18. D.B. Christensen and A.I. Wertheimer, ''Sources of Information and Influence of New Drug Prescribing among Physicians in an HMO,'' *Social Science and Medicine* 13A (1979):313–322.

19. J.R. DiPalma, ''Sources of Prescribing Information,'' *American Family Physician* 18 (October 1978):188–191; and A.B. Amerson, ''Drug Information Needs and Solutions for General Family Practitioners,'' *Journal of Clinical Pharmacology* 21 (May–June 1981):260–262.

20. The Sophie Davis School of Biomedical Education at City College, the City University of New York, is a seven-year integrated BS-MD degree program whose graduates are obligated contractually to serve as primary-care physicians in underserved urban areas.

21. *Index Medicus,* National Library of Medicine, Bethesda, Md.

22. *Excerpta Medica,* Sections 1–51 (Amsterdam, Netherlands: Excerpta Medica).

23. *Biological Abstracts* (Philadelphia: Bioscience Information Service).

24. *Biological Abstracts, RRM* (Reports, Reviews, Meetings) (Philadelphia: Bioscience Information Service).

25. *Science Citation Index* (Philadelphia: Institute for Scientific Information).

26. K.J. Guggenheimer, E. Bartlett, and M. Klebl, comps. *Narcotics and Drug Abuse A to Z* (Queens Village, N.Y.: Social Service Publications, 1971).

27. *The New York Times Index* (Sanford, North Carolina, Microfilming Corporation of America).

28. *Inpharma* (Birkenhead Auckland, New Zealand: Adis Press Ltd.).

29. *Martindale The Extra Pharmacopoeia* (London: The Pharmaceutical Press).

30. *The Merck Index* (Rahway, N.J.: Merck & Co., Inc.).

31. *Physician's Desk Reference* (Oradell, N.J.: Medical Economics Co.).

32. S. Jablonski, *Illustrated Dictionary of Eponymic Syndromes and Diseases and Their Synonyms* (Philadelphia: W.B. Saunders Company).

33. *Uhlrich's International Periodicals Directory* (New York: R.R. Bowker Company).

34. *International Pharmaceutical Abstracts* (Washington, D.C.: American Society of Hospital Pharmacists).

35. *Toxicity Bibliography* (Bethesda, Md.: National Library of Medicine).

36. *Reader's Guide to Periodical Literature* (Bronx, N.Y.: H.W. Wilson, Co.).

37. *High Times* (New York: Trans-High Corporation).

38. *Index Catalogue of the Library of the Surgeon General's Office,* Superintendent of Documents (Washington, D.C.: Government Printing Office).

39. For discussion of evaluating library instruction, see: R. Beeler, ed., *Evaluating Library Use Instruction* (Ann Arbor, Mich.: Pierian Press, 1975); S. Burton, "Objective Tests as an Evaluation Tool: Problems in Construction and Use" in *Library Instruction in the Seventies: State of the Art,* ed. H. Rader (Ann Arbor, Mich.: Pierian Press, 1977), pp. 99–104; D. King and J. Ory, "Effects of Library Instruction on Student Research: A Case Study," *College and Research Libraries* 42 (January 1981):31–41; and L.A. Magy and M.L. Thomas, "An Evaluation of the Teaching Effectiveness of Two Library Instructional Video Tapes," *College and Research Libraries* 42 (January 1981):26–30.

Part VII
Characterizing and Modifying Prescriber Behavior

23 Psychosocial Issues in Prescribing

Patricia J. Bush

A number of psychological and social issues exist in the drug-use process, but one issue overrides the others: How can we use what we know about psychological and social factors to increase drug effectiveness and to decrease their influence on drug selection? I believe that these factors should be less influential than they are at the point of prescribing and more influential at the point of patient use.

Psychological and social factors—for example, physician's specialty, education, and sources of drug information—have a greater influence on selection of specific drugs than the morbidity of patients.[1] Even lay persons recognize that the particular medicine they get depends upon the physician they see. Yet most of the emphasis in medical education is on pharmacology—the action of drugs in the body once they are taken.[2] There is a tacit belief that if physicians learn pharmacology and keep up with the medical literature, they may ignore psychological and social influences on their prescribing. This situation may exist for several reasons: Physicians are usually uncomfortable with the uncertainties offered by the social sciences, and the social sciences have failed to provide them with practical, behavior-oriented guidance. Social scientists have documented psychological and social correlates of prescribing behavior in terms of its quantity and quality but have not helped physicians to improve their prescribing quality.[3] They have not helped physicians to learn how to be good prescribers.

There is a difference in focus between medical sociologists and practitioners. Sociologists believe their purpose is to identify and explain social relationships in medicine. Practitioners ask: How does that help us when we have patients in front of us? Sociologists focus on the sociology of medicine, answering the question What is going on here and why?, while practitioners would prefer sociology in medicine to answer the question How can I use sociology to help particular patients? Also, sociology deals in aggregates, while patients must be treated one at a time. Psychologists might be thought to offer the physician more help, but to date, sociologists have performed most of the work in doctor-patients relationships except, perhaps, in explaining the placebo effect.[4]

To improve the quality of the medicine-use process from prescribing to taking, it is necessary but not sufficient to consider the of level. Knowledge of the medicine-use process needs to be translated into actions that can be taken by regulators, educators, physicians, and patients.

This chapter reviews some of what is known about psychological and social influences on the drug-use process and suggests how we can use that knowledge to improve prescribing quality and drug effectiveness. First is a discussion of the general types of prescribing-control strategies.

Prescribing Influences

Prescribing-Control Strategies

There are two basic ways to attempt to control prescribing patterns. One type coerces prescribers through a structural change in the organization of care, and the other relies on the cooperation of prescribers.[5] Most coercive mechanisms are not focused directly on physicians but on manufacturers—for example, quality control, advertising, and labeling regulations. Coercive mechanisms also are directed at pharmacists—the maximum-allowable-cost program is an example—and at patients—copayments and deductibles for prescription purchases are examples. An example of a coercive mechanism focused on physicians is a drug formulary, a list of permitted or prohibited drugs with perhaps quantity limitations.

Most physician-focused mechanisms to improve prescribing quality rely on their cooperation, their voluntary compliance. Among these are educational programs, drug-therapy protocols, and provision of drug-price information.[6] The patient package insert is a voluntary mechanism ostensibly directed at patients but one that many observers recognize to be directed at pharmacists and physicians as well.[7]

A problem is to find prescribing quality-control mechanisms that can achieve their goals without adverse consequences. If we knew what satisfied and dissatisfied physicians, this knowledge could be used to encourage prescribing-control mechanisms that are congruent with physicians' value systems and to discourage those that are not. Moreover, knowledge of psychological and social aspects of patients' medicine use might be used to improve the effectiveness of drug therapy.[8]

Psychosocial Influences on Physicians

What is known about the psychosocial influences on physicians when they are prescribing? First, at any occasion of prescribing, a physician has one propensity to prescribe and another to prescribe certain drugs instead of others. These propensities may be seen as the result of past experience with prescribing and response to present psychological needs. The influence of the past may be viewed as an appraisal of the therapeutic outcome of prescribing a drug—that is, as an appraisal of the expected net benefit.

A model of cognitive decision making that takes account of risks-to-benefits appraisal was tested by Knapp and Oeltjen, who evaluated the relative weights given to expected beneficial and harmful effects when physicians selected drugs for hypothetical cases of hypertension.[9] A number of physician characteristics such as prescribing rate, practice site, age, and status and physician specialty were correlated with the relative weighting given to the hypothetical drugs. Although hypothetical situations may not reflect reality accurately, the results suggested that some physician social characteristics influence prescribing decisions.

A benefits-to-risks model of prescribing has a great deal of intuitive appeal, being apparently grounded in the rational approach to therapy as exemplified by the following opening statement in a medical-journal article: "The physician's first substantive step in treating a patient is to compile the pertinent signs, symptoms, and laboratory findings in order to make a correct diagnosis. Having done this, he correlates what he knows about the disease with what he knows about the particular patient in order to arrive at therapy and prognosis."[10]

The risks-to-benefits appraisal model also seems capable of accounting for the rapid initial adoption of new drugs for life-threatening medical problems. A desperation-reaction model of drug diffusion has been proposed by Warner, who argued that a major influence on a physician's decision to prescribe a new drug is an appraisal of the patient's disease.[11] If the prognosis is desperate, the risk of prescribing a new drug or an old one for an unlabeled indication is virtually nil. If the drug does not help, things are simply not better. If the prognosis is relatively optimistic, standard therapies carrying known risks are more likely to be used. Warner's desperation-reaction model also acknowledges the influence of patient characteristics on a physician's decisions to try new therapies. Tracing the use of antineoplastic drugs for leukemia, he found that proportionately more children than adults were given these drugs. He suggested that the more-rapid diffusion of antineoplastics for children reflected a greater sense of loss and thus greater desperation associated with children's as compared to adults' terminal illness. If Warner's theory is correct, one should also find that higher-status patients are more likely to be the recipients of innovative drug-use technologies.

The risks-to-benefits appraisal model, with or without desperation reaction, is assumed to describe the physician's appraisal of the risks (or costs) and benefits to the patient, but the model would be more comprehensive if the risks and the benefits encompassed those to the prescriber as well. Prescribers have needs to maximixe benefits and minimize risks to themselves as well as patients (avoiding litigation being only one), and these needs may be met in part by writing prescriptions.

Physicians need to earn the approval of self, colleagues, and patients.[12] Approval of self and colleagues is earned by working in conformity with the values esteemed by the medical profession. Among these are values for autonomy (ability to work and make decisions independently) and giving good patient care. Physicians also have economic needs—that is, to spend time efficiently and to attract, satisfy, and thereby retain patients.

Competence in diagnosis is a highly valued skill in the medical profession.[13] Physicians also understand that patients demand diagnoses from them despite the uncertainties that frequently accompany patients' complaints. The act of prescribing has considerable value both in helping the physician to arrive at a diagnosis and by tangibly demonstrating to the patient that a diagnosis has been achieved.

A British researcher recently has suggested that some drug prescribing is used to help physicians to make diagnoses. According to Raynes, physicians tend to develop diagnostic routines that are initiated by patients' responses to questions asked by the physician.[14] When the responses and other diagnostic procedures leave the diagnosis uncertain, a situation that occurs in much of ambulatory care, a medicine may be tried out and the patient asked to make a return visit to evaluate the success of the therapy. For example, the patient may complain of a rash and may say that he has had the problem for two weeks. He remembers it because that was the day he was sent to a new department at work. In such a case, the physician may treat the patient's psyche, the patient's soma, or both. Certainly the rash may be due to an environmental agent, or it may be due to situational stress. If the physician treats both of these, then achievement of the valued diagnosis may never be achieved. If only one of the possibilities is treated by a drug and the patient later reports success, the patient's diagnosis may be identified. If the drug is reported by the patient not to have worked, then a drug for the alternative hypothesis may be employed. Thus, a physician may move from less-serious to more-serious alternatives and from less- to more-vigorous therapy.

The prescription, evidence of the physician's ability to act, has symbolic value as well, whether deriving from a diagnostic routine or as the treatment for a diagnosis. The prescription serves as a tangible evidence to the physician that he or she is able to act, to provide health care to the patient.[15] A secondary psychological gain may be earned by prescribing a drug known to be prescribed by an esteemed colleague, recommended in a prestigious medical journal, or even one that is widely advertised and vigorously promoted by the manufacturer's representative. The prescription also benefits the physician when it meets patients' needs and expectations. Satisfying patients is part of the physician value system.

In addition to needs to earn the rewards deriving from conforming to professional values, physicians have needs deriving from the economics of medical practice. Although some researchers found that less-busy practices were associated with more prescriptions per visit, suggesting that more time leads to finding more problems and thus more therapy,[16] a recent study in an HMO found that physicians with the largest patient panels and the highest rates of patient visits prescribed more drugs per patient.[17] This suggests that prescriptions may substitute for other, more-time-consuming forms of therapy and diagnostic procedures and may function to help the physician meet time constraints imposed by the organization of practice and pressures to see many patients. The act of writing and handing a prescription to a patient also may signal the patient that the interview is at an end and that the patient should leave the office so that the physician can move on to the next patient.[18] Moveover, patients who receive prescriptions are more likely than others to return to the physician, thus increasing the probability that the patient will become a member of the physician's stable patient population.[19]

To summarize, prescriptions serve the psychological and social needs of physicians that derive from the physician value system, patient expectations, and the organization of care. This suggests that strategies to control prescribing would be more likely to succeed if they took advantage of these needs.

Psychosocial Influences on Patients

Prescriptions have symbolic functions for patients as well as physicians. Also, aspects of the prescribing process have a strong influence on the ability of the prescribed drugs to help the patient because of their influence on compliance and the placebo effect.

The prescription confirms that the patient behaved correctly in coming to the physician. Here is tangible evidence from an expert that the patient did indeed have a medical problem. Once obtained, the medicine is a signal to others—household members, friends, fellow workers—that the patient is ill and is justified in assuming the sick role. Sackett and Haynes found that after Canadian steel workers were told they were hypertensive, they took more sick days.[20] It seems likely that taking medicines would contribute to this kind of sick-role behavior.

Complaint behavior relative to taking prescribed medicine also fulfills one of the obligations of the sick role. According to Parsons, a patient has a duty to want to get well, to seek out competent help, and to comply with prescribed therapy.[21]

A prescribed drug cannot help a patient unless the patient obtains it and takes it according to directions. Compliance with prescribed therapy has been shown to be influenced by aspects of the physician-patient relationship. The patient comes to the physician with a history of drug use, an opinion about the usual effectiveness of medicines, a propensity to take medicines, and expectations about whether or not the physician should prescribe. During the encounter, these expectations may be met, left unmet, or modified. If patients are dissatisfied with their medical visit, if they are not convinced of the seriousness of their problem, or if they do not have faith in the ability of the medicine to help them, they are likely to be noncompliant with therapy.[22]

As patients take doses of their medicine, they are reminded of the physicians who are taking care of them and who have assumed some responsibility for their lives. These relationships may recall child-parent dependency relationships. It has been suggested that these feelings also may account for some noncompliance with drug therapy—the adult patient using noncompliance to rebel against the physician who is perceived as an authoritarian parentlike figure.[23]

Many health providers may not fully appreciate that expectations about taking medicines begin to be formed in childhood and that most young children take some responsibility for their own medicine use. In a study of urban children's orientations toward medicines, Bush and Davidson found that nearly three-fourths of children in grades Kindergarten through six said they sometimes asked for medicines and that nearly as many said they sometimes got medicines by themselves.[24] Nearly a fifth of children said they bought medicines by themselves. Most children in the study were able to name and to state the probabilities of taking medicines for a set of common illnesses. These results suggested that physicians' remarks about medicines they are prescribing for children should be addressed not only to the parents who are assumed to have the entire responsibility for their children's compliance with medicine use but also to the children. When children are of school age, compliance with medicines may depend more on children's health beliefs than their mothers'. By the time persons are adults, they are likely to have well-formed expectations and beliefs about medicines that may differ from those of their physicians and that may be difficult to change.

In addition to its effect on compliance with drug therapy, the prescribing process may contribute to a positive or a negative placebo response.[25] The placebo response has been found to be associated with the context of the treatment, the personality and communications of the physician, and the form and color of the medicine. Illness states in which anxiety or pain are associated are more likely to be benefited by the placebo response. The exact mechanism of the placebo response is unknown, but some characteristics of the prescribing process are more likely to produce it. For example, the more faith and enthusiasm exhibited by the physician in the treatment and the greater the physician's success in reducing the patient's anxiety, the more likely the physician is to succeed in mobilizing the patient's expectations of help and the greater assistance the physician will have from the placebo response. Some physicians, knowing that the placebo response cannot be predicted, are suspicious of it, regarding it as a psychological aberration of the patient or a response that distinguishes between real and psychological problems. These physicians miss the point. The placebo response cannot be avoided; it may result from any aspect of the therapeutic encounter. Physicians should recognize that they cause placebo effects that may be negative or positive. Physicians may help or hinder the ability of the medicines they prescribe to succeed. There is an opportunity cost in not taking advantage of what is known to maximize the probability that a positive placebo effect will result from the prescribing process.

To summarize, prescriptions have symbolic roles for patients, and the prescribing process affects therapeutic effectiveness through patient compliance and the placebo effect. One reason that physicians fail to achieve the level of compliance they desire is that they may fail to recognize that patients' orientations toward medicines begin to develop in early childhood and that they may be relatively rigid and difficult to change in adulthood.

From Theories to Action

There is little value in knowing about psychosocial aspects of the drug process if that knowledge is not used to guide changes that improve prescribing and help patients to receive more benefit from their drug therapies. Occasionally, of course, such knowledge may tell us to leave a prescribing pattern be.

It is generally known that structural changes are efficient change mechanisms. Because they are usually coercive, they work quickly and their primary effects are usually easy to monitor. Examples of structural changes are safety caps on medicine containers, fluoridated water, unit-dose systems, drug formularies, and claims denial for unauthorized medicines.

The problem with coercive drug-control mechanisms is that they may have unanticipated adverse consequences. To the extent they are perceived by physicians to interfere with their professional values—those they hold for autonomy and giving good patient care—coercive mechanisms tend to make physicians uncooperative. Drug-control mechanisms that interfere with physicians' prescribing freedom provide incentives for physicians to opt out. States that publish restrictive drug formularies and that review and deny claims provide disincentives for physicians to participate in public programs. Organizations like HMOs that review physicians' prescribing or that have tried other prescribing-control mechanisms like drug-therapy protocols have recognized that restrictions on prescribing are viewed by most physicians as interference in their clinical freedom.[26] These physicians have taken steps to counteract the negative effects, usually by putting physicians in charge of prescribing-control mechanisms. For example, physicians are usually in charge of selecting the drugs and setting the rules for drug formularies in HMOs. Where compliance with the prescribing guidelines is voluntary, those physicians directly involved with the development of the guidelines are most likely to follow them.[27] It seems probable, ceteris paribus, that a physician would prefer to work in organizations without prescribing restrictions. Thus, although structural prescribing-control mechanisms may achieve their goals quickly, they are likely to have some adverse consequences on the job satisfaction of physicians unless the physicians can be convinced that the mechanism helps them to give better patient care or unless physicians personally can be involved in development and administration so that de facto coercive mechanisms are perceived as voluntary.

Learning to Prescribe

Physician education is the traditional approach to improve prescribing quality, probably because of the reluctance of physicians to propose or participate in programs that may limit their own or the clinical autonomy of other physicians. In its formal undergraduate years, an education in therapeutics concentrates on the mechanisms of action of drugs in the body. After a drug is ingested, where does it go, how does it get there, what does it do, how does it do it, what happens to it then, and how long does it take? This necessary but insufficient education does not provide a physician with enough information to select the drug of choice from among a number of so-called equivalent products. It also does not provide a physician with the skills needed to maintain prescribing proficiency in the face of an ever-changing market of drugs. Once in the clinical area, a physician learns which drug to use by observing what is used. Recently, a family-practice resident said to me, "I want to know about drugs, but I just don't have time when I'm on the floor to look it up. I just turn and ask someone." Other residents have said they play what Stein has called the doctor-nurse game. Nurse Jones, what did Mr. Smith take for that problem last time? Ah, yes, well give him some of that—2 mg. Oh, Dr. Johnson always gives 4 mg., did you say? The order, Nurse Jones, is Drug X, 4 mg. by mouth, and call me again if you have any more problems with Mr. Smith.[28]

Of course, junior house staff also learn what drugs to use from senior staff and admitting private physicians. Manufacturers' representatives are well acquainted with the ripple effect that occurs when a prestigious specialist begins to use their recently detailed product.

Learning what to prescribe in ambulatory care, as well as the diagnostic routines leading to prescribing, is more difficult. There is simply less opportunity to learn through observation. In ambulatory care, the manufacturer's representative, an inherently biased source however well informed about his or her product, has the most influence over the development of many physicians' personal armamentarium. Over time, the drugs prescribed by an individual are adopted and relinquished through a number of mechanisms including professional journals and meetings, colleagues, patients, advertisements, manufacturers' representatives, and trial and error.[29] Few formal educational programs teach medical students or physicians how to be good prescribers—that is, teach the information and the behaviors that lead to and maintain good prescribing over time.

As noted, there is a strong value in the medical profession for providing high-quality care. Such ability is a major source of physician satisfaction. It follows that physicians want to be good prescribers but prefer not to have prescribing controls limiting their clinical freedom. This implies that education focusing on the prescribing process should remain as the quality-control strategy of choice. Education should take an action orientation to teach students how to be good prescribers and how to interact with patients to increase the effectiveness of therapy.

The educational approach does not necessarily rule out coercive prescribing-control strategies. The key is what physicians perceive. If physicians can be convinced that prescribing-control strategies, even coercive ones, help them to prescribe better and to give better patient care, then they might become more receptive to prescribing controls.

When and What to Teach

Little guidance exists for medical educators who wish to develop curriculums for teaching medical students how to be good prescribers. Literature does exist on the social correlates of the drug-use process, and a (very) few medical schools are experimenting with courses on the nonpharmacologic aspects of prescribing. What seems to be needed is for interested educators to come together to plan curriculum content and to determine the appropriate place in the curriculum, amount of curriculum time, faculty qualifications, and teaching methods. These educators should consider some of the following areas that might be in a curriculum whose goal is to provide medical students with a set of behaviors for attaining and maintaining high levels of prescribing quality and increasing the effectiveness of prescribed drugs.

Necessary to the acquisition of good prescribing skills are knowledge, critical abilities, and sensitivity. This suggests that potential prescribers should know facts, be acquainted with issues, and learn to interact with patients in ways that will increase drug effectiveness. One approach to imparting information and sensitivity to issues is to proceed through the three major influences on prescribing: drug manufacturers, regulators, and patients. Prospective prescribers also should be acquainted with and able to evaluate drug-information sources. They should be acquainted with various prescribing-control mechanisms and their effects, both positive and negative. For increasing drug effectiveness, physicians need to understand the social roles of prescriptions, and most important, physicians need excellent communication skills. A thorough discussion of what to teach is beyond the scope of this chapter, but as examples, a few areas are touched upon briefly.

One of the most important skills physicians can learn is how to use drug-information sources—books, journals, libraries, computers, and most important, people—to obtain the information they should have to select the drug of choice for the problem at hand and to prescribe it appropriately (see chapter 22). This is no easy skill to acquire. No reference contains more than a few items of such information. Most drug references are organized according to the drug, whereas physicians are faced with a problem and need to find the most appropriate drug to treat it. Having selected a drug, it is another problem to find all of the prescribing information such as side effects, dose sizes and forms, prices, brands, and pharmacokinetics. Special groups such as pediatric and geriatric patients, pose special problems. Clinical pharmacists and drug-information services are available increasingly in hospitals, but no complete, easily accessible, unbiased source of drug information is available to physicians in ambulatory care, who write the majority of prescriptions. Techniques are needed to teach medical students and practicing physicians how to use information sources efficiently, and physicians need to be sensitized to their needs for better drug information.

Sexism in prescribing is one issue that can test students' critical abilities and that can be used to demonstrate subtle patient influences on prescribing. Students can be sensitized to the possibilities that they have sex biases and convinced that sex bias has no place in medical care. These goals may be accomplished by discussing research results and possible explanations. For example, women receive more prescriptions than men,[30] and they receive more psychotropic drugs[31]; physicians may be inordinately influenced by drug advertising,[32] stereotypical cultural images,[33] and differences in male and female patient behavior.[34]

The communication skills that are needed to improve the effectiveness of medicines may be taught through a combination of information and behavior—that is, action-oriented skills, Students can be sensitized to the correlates and rates of noncompliance with drug therapy and taught to use mechanisms that may increase patient compliance. Students can be sensitized to the power and factors associated with the placebo response and can learn how they may contribute to a positive response. Students can learn how they can enlist other health professionals and family members to help, especially with compliance efforts.

Acquiring prescribing skills may require innovative educational techniques, perhaps videotaped sessions or self-learning modules such as slides, tapes, or interactive computer programs. This education in prescribing should be begun before prescribing routines are established, presumably early in medical school, with follow-up coursework during clinical years. A demonstration of prescribing proficiency that goes beyond selection of a chemical entity should be required for recertification. This suggests that continuing education as well as undergraduate curriculums in prescribing need to be developed.

Throughout prescribing-skills curriculums, an appeal to the physician value for providing good patient care should be stressed. Physicians and medical students are relatively disinterested in cost-control mechanisms or the poor quality of prescribing of other physicians at other times and other places. However, physicians may trade off considerable clinical freedom if they are convinced that a control mechanism gives better patient care and particularly if they can be involved in the development and administration of the control mechanism.

Summary

Physician- and patient-related psychosocial factors affect prescribing and the effectiveness of drug therapy, the former through drug manufacturers and regulators as well as personal characteristics and physician-patient relationships, and the latter through compliance and the placebo effect. Physicians value clinical freedom and tend to avoid coercive prescribing-control mechanisms. Appealing to the physician value for providing good patient care may facilitate acquisition of prescribing skills. Prescribing-skills curriculums that include information, sensitizing issues, and drug-information sources and that have a behavior orientation are needed.

Notes

1. For discussions of psychosocial issues in drug prescribing, see, for example, M. Balint, *The Doctor, His Patient, and the Illness,* 2d ed. (London: Pitman Medical, 1971); H.L. Lennard, *Mystification and Drug Misuse* (San Francisco: Jossey-Bass, 1971); P.J. Bush, "Psychosocial Aspects of Medicine Use," in *Perspectives on Medicines in Society,* eds. A.I. Wert-

heimer and P.J. Bush (Hamilton, Ill.: Drug Intelligence, 1977); P.J. Bush, "Prescribing Is a Social Process," *Pharmacy International* 1 (1980):viii–x; and J.J. Strain, "Meaning of Medication," *Art of Medication* 1 (1980): 19–24.

2. J.P. Morgan and M. Weintraub, "A Course on the Social Functions of Prescription Drugs," *Annals of Internal Medicine* 77 (1972):217–222.

3. For review articles on the social and psychological correlates of prescribing, see R.R. Miller, "Prescribing Habits of Physicians: A Review of Studies on Prescribing of Drugs, Parts 1–3," *Drug Intelligence and Clinical Pharmacy* 7 (1973):492–500; Ibid., "Parts 4–6" 7 (1973):557–564; Ibid., "Parts 7–8" 8 (1974):81–91; E. Hemminki, "Review of Literature on the Factors Affecting Drug Prescribing," *Social Science and Medicine* (1975):111; D.B. Worthen, "Prescribing Influences: An Overview," *British Journal of Medical Education* 7 (1973):109; and C.M. Herman and C.A. Rodowskas, "Communicating Drug Information to Physicians," *Journal of Medical Education* 51 (1976):189. For examples, see M. Hayman and R. Ditman, "Influence of Age and Orientation of Psychiatrists on Their Use of Drugs," *Comprehensive Psychiatry* 7 (1966):152; M.H. Becker et al., "Characteristics and Attitudes of Physicians Associated with the Prescribing of Chloramphenicol," *HSMH Health Report* 86 (1971):993; and A. Melville, "Job Satisfaction in General Practice: Implications for Prescribing," *Social Science and Medicine* 14A (1980):495–499.

4. For discussions of the differences between sociology of and sociology in medicine, see R. Straus, "The Nature and Status of Medical Sociology," *American Sociological Review* 22 (1957):200–204; and D. Mechanic, *Medical Sociology* (Glencoe, Ill.: Free Press, 1968):408–411.

5. D.B. Christensen and P.J. Bush, "Drug Prescribing: Patterns, Problems, and Proposals," *Social Science and Medicine* 15A (1981):343–355.

6. R.J. Bertin, *The Evaluation of a Cost Containment Role for Institutional Pharmacists* (Ph.D. dissertation, University of Minnesota, 1976); R.E. Johnson et al., "Studying the Impact of Patient Drug Profiles in an HMO," *Medical Care* 14 (1976):79; and P.J. Bush, D.L. Rabin, and K.K. Spector, "Evaluation of a Drug Therapy Protocol in an HMO," *Medical Care* 17 (1979):566.

7. U.S. DHHS, FDA, "Prescription Drug Products: Patient Package Inserts Requirements," *Federal Register* 12 September 1980, pt. 5, pp. 60754–60817.

8. We are indebted to Sackett and Haynes for pointing out the differences between drug efficacy and the compliance-dependent drug effectiveness. See D.L. Sackett and R.B. Haynes, "Compliance with Therapeutic Regimens," in *Perspectives on Medicines in Society,* eds. A.I. Wertheimer and P.J. Bush (Hamilton, Ill.: Drug Intelligence, 1977), pp. 335–357.

9. D.E. Knapp and P.D. Oeltjen, "Benefit to Risks in Physician Drug Selection," *American Journal of Public Health* 62 (1972):1136.

10. T.S. Linn, M.W. Linn, and L. Gurel, "Correlates to Prognosis: A Study of the Physician's Clinical Judgment," *Medical Care* 11 (1973):430.

11. K.E. Warner, "A Desperation-Reaction Model of Medical Diffusion," *Health Services Research* 10 (1975):369.

12. For a discussion of physicians' job satisfactions, see M. Osterweis and P.J. Bush, "The Satisfaction Continuum in Health Care: Consumer and Provider Preferences," in *Consumer Incentives for Health Care* ed. S.J. Mushkin (New York: Prodist, 1974), pp. 304–332.

13. Ibid.

14. N.V. Raynes, "What Can I Do for You?," in *Prescribing Practice and Drug Usage,* ed. R. Mapes (London: Croom Helm, 1980), p. 83.

15. P.J. Bush, "Psychosocial Aspects of Medicine Use."

16. K. Dunnell and A. Cartwright, *Medicine Takers, Prescribers and Hoarders* (London: Routledge & Kegan Paul, 1972). pp. 75–77.

17. A.G. Hartzema and D.B. Christensen, "Nonmedical Factors Associated with Prescribing Volume among Physicians in an HMO," (Unpublished paper, University of North Carolina, 1980).

18. C. Muller, "The Overmedicated Society: Forces in the Marketplace for Medical Care," *Science* 16 (1972):488–492.

19. D.M. Tagliacozzo, K. Ima, and J.C. Lashoff, "Influencing the Chronically Ill: The Role of Prescriptions in Premature Terminators of Out-Patient Care," *Medical Care* 12 (1973):21.

20. D.L. Sackett and R.B. Haynes, "Is There a Patient Compliance Problem?," in *Controversies in Therapeutics,* ed. L. Lasagna (Philadelphia: W.B. Saunders, 1980), p. 552.

21. T. Parsons, *The Social System* (New York: Free Press, 1964), pp. 439–447.

22. Sackett and Haynes, "Is There a Patient Compliance Problem?;" and V. Francis, V.M. Korsch, and M.J. Morris, "Gaps in Doctor-Patient Communication," *New England Journal of Medicine,* 280 (1969):535; B.L. Svarstad, "Physician-Patient Communication and Patient Conformity with Medical Advice," in *The Growth of Bureaucratic Medicine: An Inquiry into the Dynamics of Patient Behavior and the Organization of Medical Care,* ed. D. Mechanic (New York: Wiley & Sons, 1976), p. 220. and D.B. Christensen, "Drug Compliance: A Review and Synthesis," *Health Services Research* 13 (1978):171.

23. P.J. Bush, "Psychosocial Aspects of Medicine Use."

24. P.J. Bush and F.R. Davidson, "Medicines and Drugs: What Do Children Think?" *Health Education Quarterly* nos. 2 and 3 (1982):113–128.

25. For a review of factors associated with the placebo effect, see P.J. Bush "The Placebo Effect," *Journal of the American Pharmaceutical Association* NS14 (1974):671.

26. Bush, Rabin, and Spector, "Evaluation of Drug Therapy Protocol."

27. Ibid.

28. L.I. Stein, "The Doctor-Nurse Game," *Archives of General Psychiatry* 16 (1967):699.

29. J.S. Coleman, E. Katz, and H. Menzel, "Social Processes in Physicians Adoption of a New Drug," *Journal of Chronic Diseases* 9 (1959):1; and D.B. Christensen and A.I. Wertheimer, "Sources of Information and Influence of New Drug Prescribing among Physicians in an HMO," *Social Science and Medicine* 13A (1979):313.

30. L.M. Verbrugge and R.P. Steiner, "Physician Treatment of Men and Women Patients—Sex Bias or Appropriate Care?" *Medical Care* 19 (1981):609–632; and P. Bush and D.L. Rabin, "Who's Using Prescribed Medicines?" *Drugs and Health Care* 3 (1976):89.

31. H.J. Parry et al., "National Patterns of Psychotherapeutic Drug Use," *Archives of General Psychiatry* 28 (1973):769–784; and J.W. Milliren, "Some Contingencies Affecting the Utilization of Tranquilizers in Long Term Care of the Elderly," *Journal of Health and Social Behavior* 18 (1977):206.

32. Milliren, "Contingencies Affecting Utilization"; and J. Prather and L.F. Fidell, "Sex Differences in the Content and Style of Medical Advertisements," *Social Science and Medicine* 9 (1975):23.

33. R. Cooperstock, "Sex Differences in Psychotropic Drug Use," *Social Science and Medicine* 12B (1978):179.

34. Verbrugge and Steiner, "Physician Treatment."

24 Opiophobia in the United States: The Undertreatment of Severe Pain

John P. Morgan and
David L. Pleet

Pain is the most common presenting complaint of patients, and its relief may take precedence over all other considerations.[1] The contemporary physician may choose between 140 analgesic products including combinations and 50 distinct opioid analgesics. Jaffe quotes Sydenham:

> Among the remedies which it has pleased . . . God to give to man to relieve his suffering, none is so efficacious as opium.[2]

Despite this venerable statement of divine analgesic gifts, there is evidence that patients are undertreated with opioids and suffer apparently unnecessary pain.

We based this study in part on the 1973 publication of Marks and Sacher to assess any change in opioid use in the ensuing six years (the data for this project were gathered in 1979).[3] Marks and Sacher, both psychiatrists, initiated their critical review of opioid analgesic use after realizing that many of the inpatients they were asked to see were indeed in emotional stress—an appropriate response to unrelieved pain. They decided that undertreatment was the characteristic treatment. Meperidine was used in doses of 50 mg. every three to four hours or less in 63 percent of their patients and rarely used in doses greater than 75 mg. They assessed patient response and discovered that 73 percent of evaluated patients continued to experience moderate to severe distress.

Their study also gathered questionnaire data in which house staff:

Overestimated addiction liability,

Overestimated the duration of action of opioids,

Underestimated effective dosage.

Note: The initial coinage *narcophobia* seemed to mean fear of sleep. *Opiophobia* seems better to convey U.S. physician fear of use of opioid drugs.

Marks and Sacher speculated that physician fear of addiction was excessive and unrealistic and served as a major barrier to proper opioid analgesia.

The current study reassesses some of these findings and concentrates on the potential for increased use of oral therapy for severe pain.[4]

Methodology

We gathered data in two ways. We gave a questionnaire to the house staff that was designed to assess knowledge and elicit attitudes about opioids. We also reviewed the medical inpatient charts to assess actual prescription habits of these house officers. We did not assess directly the efficacy of analgesic therapy in these patients. Since the questionnaire was completed anonymously, we did not compare individual prescribing with individual knowledge.

We distributed a questionnaire to the internal-medicine and general-surgery house staff at the Mount Sinai Hospital, New York City, in 1979, asking for responses to thirty-three questions. The questionnaire was handed to sixty (of eighty-two) physicians in training, and forty-five (77 percent) completed all or a major portion and returned it. Completion of the items required fifteen to twenty-five minutes and physician's names were not collected. Several of the questions were discarded later because of unanticipated ambiguity.

We also assessed the medical charts of 110 patients who were given opioids for analgesia on the medical and general surgical floors for a forty-eight-hour period. Of the fifty-six surgical and fifty-four medical patients, 52 were men and 58 were women. We excluded patients who had received opioids for only one day prior to the survey and those who had received the opioid solely for cough. We tabulated drug dosage, route of administration, and the patient's diet.

Results

Questionnaire: General Approach

A copy of the questionnaire with a distribution of choices appears in appendix 24–A.

Although 80 percent of respondents felt that their personal knowledge of opioids was adequate, 52 percent felt that most hospitalized patients were undertreated and 23 percent felt that most patients were overtreated. Although 80 percent would attempt to relieve pain completely, 18 percent would allow distressing pain to exist, and four physicians stated that they wished to relieve pain only during the peak action of the narcotic.

Regimens and Drug Choices. Given that a patient who was receiving 75 mg. of meperidine intramuscularly every four hours reported a return of pain after three hours, eight of forty-five physicians (18 percent) would not change dose or interval. Thirty-three percent of those responding predicted that 90 percent of severe pain would be relieved by 75 mg. of meperidine; further, 70 percent thought there was no additional analgesic effect of meperidine in doses greater than 100 mg.

In treating two patients with severe pain (sickle-cell crisis and non-life-threatening gunshot wound), 74 percent chose meperidine, 13 percent chose morphine, and 10 percent chose oral codeine. Forty-one percent believed that codeine could be as effective as morphine or meperidine if the dose were large enough. If the patient in severe pain were to be treated with intramuscular morphine, 72 percent of our respondents would give doses between 1 and 6 mg.

Orally Administered Opioids. When presented with the clinical descriptions of severe pain, 13 percent of physicians selected oral narcotics and most named oral codeine. Other drugs mentioned included meperidine and morphine. Fully 67 percent thought morphine to be ineffective when given orally. When given a chance to select an effective oral dose of morphine, 78 percent underestimated it. Forty-one percent thought meperidine to be ineffective orally, and when given a chance to select an oral dose, 60 percent underestimated it. When questioned further, 81 percent of respondents felt oral opioids to be inferior because absorption was erratic. Sixteen percent thought that the effect of oral opioids might be prolonged advantageously, and 88 percent felt that the onset of action was delayed significantly.

Methadone. Sixty-nine percent of respondents overestimated the duration of action of methadone (four to eight hours) by more than six hours, and 77 percent significantly overestimated the time of the peak effect of oral methadone (one hour). One-quarter of our sample thought methadone's effect peaked at eight hours. Seventy-six percent of those answering stated that, milligram for milligram, intramuscular methadone was of equal or less potency than intramuscular morphine.

Addiction Liability. More than half of our respondents thought that a ten-day course of 100 mg. of meperidine (every four hours) was attended with an addiction rate of more than 6 percent. Three respondents thought the rate to be greater than 25 percent. Thirty percent of our respondents felt that greater than 6 percent of addicts initially became addicted in a hospital setting. Only 16 percent of these physicians correctly realized that a ten-day course of full dosage with an opioid will result in withdrawal symptoms in a majority of patients.

Chart Review

Of the 100 patients receiving opioids, nearly 60 percent were given meperidine. In 11 percent of instances meperidine was given at a dosage interval of greater than every five hours. All of these patients treated with prolonged intervals were on 50 mg. of meperidine or less. Nearly 60 percent of patients receiving this drug got 50 mg. or less. No patient received a single intramuscular dose greater than 100 mg.

Of the patients receiving oral meperidine, none got a dose greater than 100 mg. Eleven percent of meperidine orders were written with the direction oral or intramuscular, leaving to the nursing staff the choice of the route of administration. All sixty-three patients on meperidine were given the drug on a when-needed basis.

Codeine was used in thirty-two patients. All received (orally) 60 mg. or less—all on a when-needed basis.

Only twenty-five patients received oral opioids other than codeine. Other than the seventeen patients who received meperidine, three received hydromorphone in 4 mg. doses, two received methadone, two received morphine via an alcohol elixir (Brompton's Solution), and one received oxycodone plus aspirin (Percodan).

Seventy-six percent of patients receiving strong opioids (this excludes codeine) were given the drug intramuscularly although 80 percent of studied patients were on oral diets.

Discussion

The Marks and Sacher study of 1973 has received much attention. Indeed, by 1979, it had been cited forty-seven times in the medical literature according to the *Science Citation Index.* They described the need for physician education in this area as critical. We interpret our study's results pessimistically. There is minimal evidence of improvement, and patients with severe pain are still markedly undertreated.

Our study physicians chose meperidine as their favorite strong narcotic, and yet nearly 20 percent would not alter their initial dose regimen in the face of unresponsiveness. Thirty-three percent of our respondents felt that 90 percent of patients in severe pain would achieve relief with 75 mg. of meperidine, and 70 percent thought that there would be no additional analgesia with doses greater than 100 mg. These beliefs apparently were reflected by the fact that only five of sixty-three patients receiving meperidine in this study got a dose greater than 75 mg. intramuscularly. In truth, doses of 125 mg. are easily within the therapeutic range,[5] and in one standard text, 150 mg. intramuscularly is the recommended highest dose.[6] Add to this the depressing fact that 60 percent of the patients were treated with 50 mg. of meperidine or less, an inadequate dose according to the pharmacological text most of these physicians used in medical school.[7] Meperidine, despite its hospital popularity, probably offers no advantages over morphine; yet almost no patients received morphine by injection. If they had, more than 70 percent of those young physicians would have given doses much less than the standard of 8–16 mg. recommended in the standard sources cited here.[8]

We were very interested in the issue of oral use of opioids. We had hoped that an interest in the effective oral use of opioids in the treatment of cancer patients had affected our prescribers.[9] There are many reasons why oral use makes sense. The pain, inconvenience, and increased cost of injection are obviated. The duration of efficacy with adequate dosage is prolonged, and we assumed that our prescribers might have learned that all opioids are effective orally if the dose is large enough. Recent studies indicate that morphine is a perfectly useful substitute for heroin in Brompton's mixture.[10] The lack of appropriate oral use here attends quite logically on a failure of knowledge. Since most of the study physicians simply did not know that morphine is useful orally, it would not be used. Oral meperidine poses an interesting dilemma. The oral/parenteral-efficacy ratio for meperidine is well known and is usually estimated to be 3:1.[11] In a published clinical trial, 200 mg. of oral meperidine was significantly superior to 650 mg. of aspirin.[12] The maximum dose used here, 100 mg. of meperidine, is inferior to two aspirin tablets—a fact widely published. As noted, most patients receiving opioids intramuscularly were taking full oral diets, and physicians might be encouraged to utilize oral opioids, including methadone, but we do not know how to convey to them the appropriate dosage.

This poor prescribing may have its genesis in the U.S. phenomenon of opiophobia, our national preoccupation with narcotic addiction. Porter and Jick surveyed more than 11,000 patients who received strong opioids in the hospital to see if any subsequently were readmitted for the diagnosis of narcotic dependence. To our surprise, this survey found three such patients (an incidence of .003 percent).[13] An important myth in the United States is to believe that individuals are attracted to the social malfunction of addiction by legitimate exposure to the pharmacological agent. These physicians may know that social, economic, moral, and personal issues must interplay with the pharmacological to yield a rare life in which drug use becomes the cardinal event. Still, the myth has more power than the analgesia offered to contemporary U.S. patients with severe pain.

Notes

1. C.G. Moertel, "Relief of Pain with Oral Medications," *Australian and New Zealand Journal of Medicine* 6 (1976):1.

2. J. Jaffe, "Narcotic Analgesics," in *The Pharmacological Basis of Therapeutics,* 6th ed., eds. L.S. Goodman and A. Gilman (New York: Macmillan, 1980), p. 494.

3. R.M. Marks and E.J. Sacher, "Undertreatment of Medical Inpatients with Narcotic Analgesics," *Annals of Internal Medicine* 78 (1973):173.

4. R. Melzack, J.G. Ofiesh, and B.M. Mount, "The Brompton Mixture: Effects on Pain in Cancer Patients," *Canadian Medical Association Journal* 115 (1976):125; Moertel, "Relief of Pain," p. 1; J.P. Morgan and P. Penovich, "Methadone: Still an Analgesic," *Drug Therapy,* Hosp. Ed. 2 (1977):18; and B.M. Mount and S. Ajenian, "Use of the Brompton Mixture in Treating Chronic Pain of Malignant Disease," *Canadian Medical Association Journal* 115 (1976):122.

5. G. Avery, *Principles and Practice of Clinical Pharmacology and Therapeutics* (Sydney: Adis Press, 1976).

6. W. Modell, ed., *Drugs of Choice 1976–1977* (New York: C.V. Mosby, 1977), pp. 195–233.

7. Jaffe, "Narcotic Analgesics," p. 494.

8. Avery, "Principles and Practice"; Modell, *Drugs of Choice;* and Jaffe, "Narcotic Analgesics."

9. Mount and Ajenian, "Use of Brompton Mixture."

10. R. Twycross, "Clinical Experience with Diamorphine in Advanced Malignant Disease." *International Journal of Clinical Pharmacology* 9:184.

11. Moertel, "Relief of Pain."

12. W.T. Beaver, "The Pharmacologic Basis for a Choice of An Analgesic," *Pharmacology for Physicians* 4 (1970):1.

13. J. Porter and H. Jick, "Addiction Rate in Patients Treated with Narcotics," *New England Journal of Medicine* 302 (1980):123.

Appendix 24-A Narcotic Use, Attitudes, and Knowledge

				Percentage of Respondents
(44)	1.	The appropriate end point of narcotic analgesia is:		
		a.	Complete relief of pain for the interval between doses	41
		b.	Relief of enough pain so that it is not distressing but still noticed	41
		c.	Decreased pain but prevention of addiction as proper goal	7
		d.	Decreased pain but toleration of it without creating a disturbance	2
		e.	Relief of pain during peak action of the narcotic	9
(45)	2.	For most clinical situations I feel my knowledge of narcotics is:		
		a.	More than adequate	9
		b.	Adequate	71
		c.	Less than adequate	18
		d.	Grossly inadequate	2
(44)	3.	Most patients at Mount Sinai Hospital on narcotics are:		
		a.	Undertreated	52
		b.	Overtreated	23
		c.	Correctedly treated	25
(45)	4.	The major source of your knowledge of pain management with narcotics is:		
		a.	Medical school	22
		b.	Fellow residents and interns	27
		c.	Attending physicians	4
		d.	*Physician's Desk Reference*	2
		e.	Bedside experience	44
		f.	Nursing staff	0

Note: Numbers in parentheses represent number of respondents.

			Percentage of Respondents
(44)	5.	Codeine, if given in large enough doses, can attain the same analgesic effects as meperidine and morphine for severe pain.	
		a. True	41
		b. False	59

Case 1

These questions refer to a fifty-five-year-old housewife who enters Mount Sinai Hospital in a painful sickle-cell crisis.

(43)	6.	You would treat this woman with ______ narcotics	
		a. Oral	12
		b. Intramuscular	86
		c. Subcutaneous	2
(46)	7.	Your drug of choice is:	
		a. Meperidine (Demerol)	76
		b. Methadone (Dolophine)	2
		c. Morphine	11
		d. Codeine	9
		e. Anileridine (Leritine)	0
		f. Hydromorphone (Dilaudid)	
(46)	8.	One day later you note that her mood is markedly improved and that she is sleeping frequently. You would:	
		a. Decrease the dose	80
		b. Maintain the dose	20
		c. Increase the dose	0
(46)	9.	Which of the following drugs are effective orally (circle as many as you wish)?	
		a. Meperidine	59
		b. Methadone	93
		c. Morphine	33
		d. Hydromorphone	76
		e. Anileridine	0

			Percentage of Respondents
(40)	10.	A parenteral dose of morphine constitutes ______ percent of an effective oral dose (in mg.).	
		a. 15	23
		b. 30	43
		c. 45	15
		d. 60	20
		e. 85	0
(45)	11.	A parenteral dose of meperidine constitutes ______ percent of an effective oral dose (in mg.).	
		a. 15	16
		b. 30	25
		c. 45	23
		d. 60	20
		e. 85	18
(46)	12.	If the patient experienced euphoria (an exaggerated and unfounded sense of well-being) it is wise to decrease the dose.	
		a. True	41
		b. False	59
(43)	13.	If the patient is kept entirely pain free without euphoria, she would be less likely to engage in drug-seeking behavior in the future.	
		a. True	40
		b. False	60

Case 2

The patient is a twenty-year-old East Harlem black man in severe pain due to a non-life-threatening gunshot wound. He denies any previous use of narcotics.

(45)	14.	You would treat him with ______ narcotics.	
		a. Oral	13
		b. Intramuscular	87
		c. Subcutaneous	0

			Percentage of Respondents
(44)	15.	Your drug of choice is:	
		a. Meperidine	71
		b. Methadone	0
		c. Morphine	16
		d. Codeine	11
		e. Anileridine	0
		f. Hydromorphone	2
(45)	16.	If the patient were receiving 75 mg. of meperidine intramuscularly every 4 hours and reported return of pain after three hours, you would change to:	
		a. 75 mg. every three hours	73
		b. 100 mg. every four hours	9
		c. Maintain same dose	18
(45)	17.	After treatment with 100 mg. meperidine intramuscularly every four hours for ten days, a hospitalized patient has what chance of becoming addicted to narcotics?	
		a. 0–1 percent	11
		b. 1–5 percent	36
		c. 6–15 percent	36
		d. 16–25 percent	11
		e. 25 percent or more	7
(45)	18.	After treatment with 100 mg. meperidine intramuscularly for ten days, what percentage of patients will develop withdrawal symptoms?	
		a. 0–1 percent	22
		b. 1–5 percent	29
		c. 6–15 percent	22
		d. 16–25 percent	11
		e. 25 percent or more	16
(44)	19.	What percentage of narcotic addicts become addicted in hospital settings?	
		a. 0–1 percent	27
		b. 1–5 percent	43
		c. 6–15 percent	18
		d. 16–25 percent	7
		e. 25 percent or more	5

			Percentage of Respondents
(42)	20.	70 mg. of meperidine intramuscularly relieves ______ percent of patients in severe pain.	
		a. Less than 70	19
		b. 70	36
		c. 80	12
		d. 90	26
		e. Almost 100	7
(45)	21.	The average duration of action of intramuscular meperidine is ______ hours.	
		a. 1	2
		b. 2	11
		c. 3	58
		d. 4	27
		e. 6	4
(45)	22.	Oral medications are preferable to intramuscular medications because they (circle as many as apply):	
		a. Cause less pain and are easy to administer	91
		b. Have prolonged duration of action	16
		c. Provoke less euphoria	20
		d. Are less likely to lead to addictive behavior	27
		e. Have less peak-and-valley effect	47
(42)	23.	Oral medications are inferior to intramuscular because (circle as many as apply):	
		a. Absorption is erratic	81
		b. They have less peak effect	52
		c. Onset of action is delayed significantly	88

Methadone

(42)	24.	The average duration of action of therapeutic (analgesic) doses of methadone is ______ hour(s).	
		a. 0–2	0
		b. 6–8	31
		c. 12–14	24
		d. 24	38
		e. 48	7

			Percentage of Respondents
(39)	25.	The peak activity of oral methadone occurs at ______ hour(s).	
		a. ½	3
		b. 1	15
		c. 2	21
		d. 4	30
		e. 8	26
(36)	26.	The onset of analgesia with intramuscular methadone is:	
		a. 0–10 minutes	10
		b. 10–20 minutes	42
		c. 30–45 minutes	42
		d. 1–2 hours	6
(44)	27.	Methadone for oral analgesic use is not available in the Mount Sinai Hospital pharmacy.	
		a. True	14
		b. False	86
(42)	28.	On a milligram-milligram basis; intramuscular methadone, compared to intramuscular morphine, is:	
		a. More potent	24
		b. Less potent	55
		c. The same	21
(40)	29.	The dose of narcotic you prescribe to a nonaddict depends upon:	
		i. Your perception of his potential to become an addict.	
		a. True	33
		b. False	66
		ii. In part, his socioeconomic status.	
		a. True	12
		b. False	88

Case 3

This patient is a forty-eight-year-old 70 kg. white man experiencing severe chest pain—perhaps due to coronary insufficiency.

			Percentage of Respondents
(35)	30.	If you choose intramuscular meperidine you would begin treatment with ______ mg.	
		a. 25	0
		b. 50	37
		c. 75	46
		d. 100	17
		e. 150	0
(40)	31.	Doses higher than 100 mg. intramuscular meperidine rarely if ever should be used because:	
		a. No additional analgesic effect is attained	17
		b. Serious side effects occur	15
		c. Both	53
		d. Neither	15
(43)	32.	The minimal effective adult intramuscular dose of meperidine is ______ mg.	
		a. 25	60
		b. 50	35
		c. 75	2
		d. 100	2
		e. 150	0
(43)	33.	If you had chosen intramuscular morphine to treat this man, you would start with ______ mg. every 4 hours	
		a. 1–2	33
		b. 4–6	40
		c. 8–10	23
		d. 14–16	4
		e. 20–22	0

The questionnaire reproduced here has been edited to produce clarity and consistency and to reduce brand names and medical jargon. We do not feel that the meaning or essence of any question was changed by such redaction. Some of the questions originally administered were dropped from this report when we belatedly sensed their ambiguity.

Despite changing our term of reference for these drugs to *opioids,* we have retained the use of the term *narcotic* in the questionnaire as it was in the original.

25 Antibiotic Prescribing in Office Practice: Modifying Inappropriate Use

William Schaffner, Wayne A. Ray, and *Charles F. Federspiel*

Numerous surveys have indicated that antibiotics are among the most frequently prescribed drugs in this country. Although antibiotics continue to be extraordinarily effective in treating many bacterial infections, physicians have become increasingly aware of problems associated with antibiotic use. These difficulties include allergic reactions, drug toxicities, complicating supra-infections, and the emergence of bacterial strains resistant to multiple antimicrobial agents. In addition, in this era of cost consciousness, some health-care planners are speculating that the widespread use of these medications may be more costly than cost-effective. While the original wonder drugs continue to give us cause to marvel, their use also has provided us with problems to ponder.

In response to the requirements of the Joint Commission on Accreditation of Hospitals, considerable recent effort has been directed to evaluating the use of antibiotics within hospitals. This activity is well intentioned, but it should be remembered that most prescriptions for antibiotics are written in physicians' offices and in ambulatory-care clinics. Likewise, although the emergence of antibiotic resistance often is considered primarily a hospital-related phenomenon, several bacterial pathogens have developed resistance to antimicrobial agents in the community, away from the hospital environment (table 25–1).

Clearly, then, a need exists for educational programs regarding appropriate use of antibiotics. Effective programs, however, cannot be designed from the armchair. It is important, first, to determine who is prescribing what antibiotics to whom and for which diagnoses. Only then, based on documented prescribing patterns, can educational programs be designed for the specific groups of physicians who have been identified as poor prescribers. Continuing surveillance of prescribing practices after the educational intervention can determine the effects (or lack thereof) of the program.

This work was supported by U.S. Public Health Service grant 1-R18-HS03899 and Tennessee Contract FA9284.

Table 25-1
Examples of Bacterial Pathogens that Have Developed Antibiotic Resistance outside of the Hospital Environment

Bacterial Pathogens	*Antibiotic*
Group A streptococci	Tetracycline, erythromycin
Meningococci	Sulfonamide
Pneumococci	Penicillin, tetracycline, others
Genococci	Penicillin, tetracycline, spectinomycin
Shigella	Multiple antiobiotics
Salmonella	Multiple antibiotics
Hemophilus influenzae	Ampicillin, chloramphenicol
Vibrio cholerae	Tetracycline

Delineation of Prescribing Patterns

Background and Methods

Because little was known concerning the prescribing habits of physicians in office (ambulatory) practice, the authors undertook a series of studies in this area. The populations studied were the Medicaid recipients in the state of Tennessee and the physicians who provided medical care under the auspices of that program. Approximately 400,000 persons are eligible for the Tennessee Medicaid Program (almost 10 percent of the state's population); over 5,000 physicians provide services to this population. Data collected for the normal adminstrative and fiscal purposes of Medicaid were used. These records contain demographic characteristics of Medicaid recipients, documentation of medical services rendered, and details of medications dispensed by pharmacists. Using a computer program, we also linked information available in the public record of the state's directory of licensed physicians. Details of these methods have been published.[1]

It is important to note that we made stringent efforts to protect the confidentiality of both patients and physicians. Individuals were identified only by number in the computer record; names were not used. Further, institutional committees for the protection of human subjects reviewed and approved all study protocols.

There are a number of advantages to using data from a well-administered Medicaid program, as shown in the following list:

One can study prescribing to a very large number of patients by a large number of physicians. This lends power to the study and tends to eliminate bias that may occur in smaller studies, particularly when doctors are requested to volunteer for a review of their prescribing habits. Large numbers also permit analysis of prescribing by physician specialty, board certification status, rural or urban location, year of graduation from medical school, and so forth.

Direct costs of the investigation are relatively low because the raw data already have been collected and validated by the Medicaid program.

There is a constant flow of timely data from the Medicaid program. This permits study of contemporary trends in prescribing (particularly important when new antibiotics are introduced) and the evaluation of intervention strategies.

Because neither patients nor physicians are disturbed by office record reviews or questionnaires, the method is unobtrusive. Patients and physicians also are unaware that investigations are being conducted. Thus, prescribing practices are not influenced by the conduct of the study.

In addition to the study of antibiotic use, the method lends itself to the investigation of prescribing patterns of other drugs.[2]

Under the Medicaid law, the state program is obliged to provide assurance that acceptable standards of medical care are met. Because of our association with the state Medicaid program, these investigations partially satisfy this obligation.

Of course, there also are certain disadvantages to using this data base for epidemiological research. For example:

We can measure prescribing to patients representing only the lowest socioeconomic stratum in our society. Fortunately, because the majority of Tennessee physicians participates in the state Medicaid program, the physician sample is not biased.

We have access to data from only a single state.

Telephone prescribing, prescription renewals, and imprecisely recorded diagnoses introduce limitations.

Although the prescriptions recorded are those actually dispensed by pharmacists, the method cannot detect prescriptions written but not filled, and it cannot measure patient compliance in taking the medications.

Finally, and importantly, the studies occasionally are jeopardized by political, economic, and administrative events that affect the Medicaid program.

All laboratory, clinical, and epidemiological studies have limitations. Rather than considering them deterrants to research, investigators should consider such limitations responsibly when analyzing data and discussing results.

We believe physicians are more receptive to issues pertinent to the quality of care than to financial considerations. Therefore, our investigations have emphasized the former. Indeed, if the magnitude of inappropriate antibiotic use could be reduced, we believe cost savings would result.

Summary of Previous Investigations

We have evaluated prescribing to ambulatory patients of two antibiotics that are contraindicated in these circumstances: the use of chloramphenicol in patients of all ages[3] and the prescribing of tetracycline to children less than 8 years of age.[4] Both antibiotics are associated with risks of serious toxic effects—namely, aplastic anemia due to chloramphenicol and the staining of teeth in young children due to tetracycline. The use of these drugs in treatment of the minor infections encountered in office practice is considered inappropriate because other less-hazardous, equally efficacious antibiotics are available. These constraints appear in standard texts, are emphasized in the drugs' package inserts, and should be widely known.

The result of these first studies indicated some important differences in the prescribing patterns of these two drugs. It was striking that whereas only 6 percent of physicians prescribed chloramphenicol, 27 percent of doctors treating young children gave them tetracycline. It would seem that the cautions regarding chloramphenicol were widely known and observed. In contrast, the contraindications regarding the use of tetracycline in young children either were not widely known or not believed. Recent medical-school graduates had significantly lower rates of prescribing tetracycline to children less than eight years of age than doctors whose formal education was more remote; no such difference could be shown in the study of chloramphenicol prescribing.

Similar patterns became evident, however, when prescribing practices were correlated with physician specialty and rural location of practice. Both the specialty of family practice and rural location of practice were associated independently with increased rates of prescribing both contraindicated drugs to ambulatory patients (figure 25–1). Of rural family practitioners, 21 percent prescribed chloramphenicol (in contrast to the low 6 percent overall rate), and 52 percent used tetracycline (double the 27 percent overall rate) in treating young children. Further, only twenty doctors wrote 55 percent of the chloramphenicol prescriptions to 47 percent of the recipients; likewise, only twenty-six doctors wrote 54 percent of the tetracycline prescriptions to

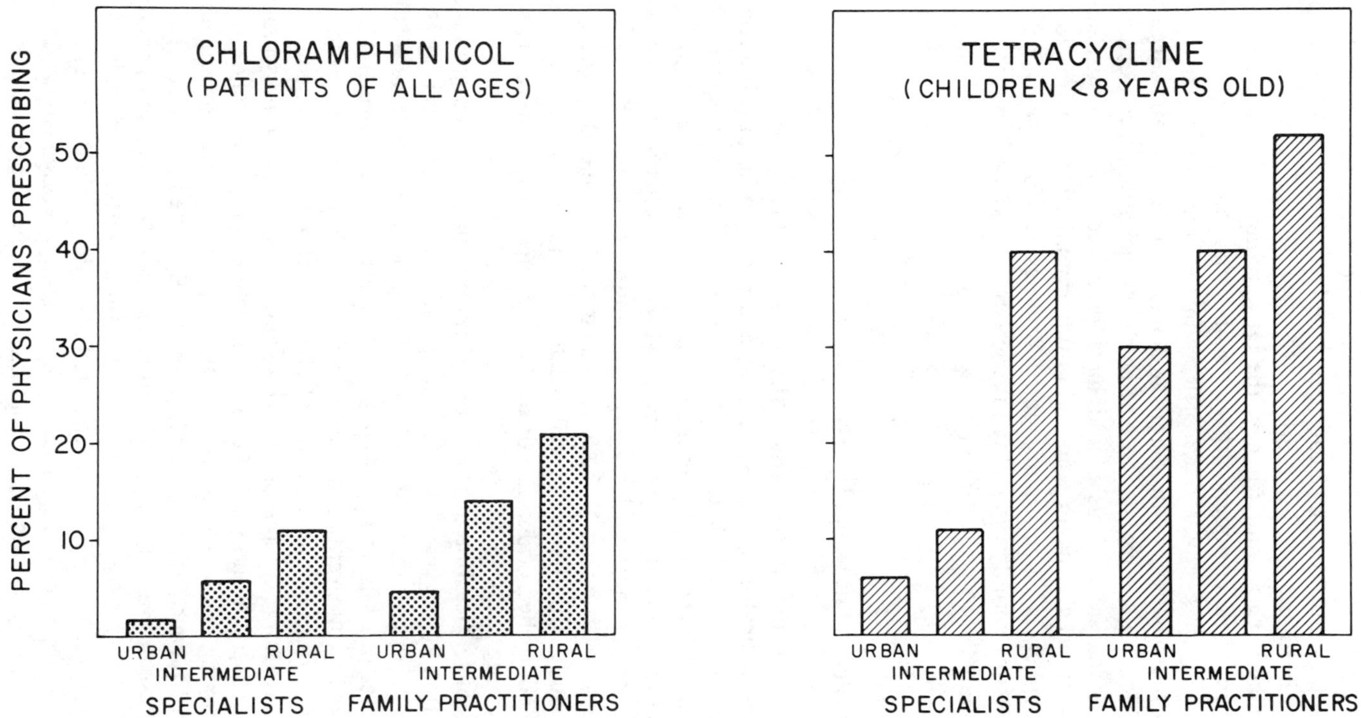

Figure 25-1. Percentage of Specialists and Family Practitioners in Urban, Intermediate, or Rural Counties Prescribing Chloramphenicol to Ambulatory Patients (All Ages) or Tetracycline to Ambulatory Children Less than Eight Years of Age

45 percent of the youngsters receiving this antibiotic. Thus, in both instances, specific groups of physicians could be identified who were in special need of remedial educational efforts.

To emphasize this point further, the tetracycline study also revealed that, after family practitioners, internists and surgeons prescribed more tetracycline to young children in office practice than other specialists (including pediatricians). It would appear that some internists and surgeons engage in office family practice more often than is acknowledged normally. It is unlikely that any of us would have predicted that internists and surgeons might need education in the antimicrobial treatment of young ambulatory children. Such unanticipated findings reinforce the need for documentation of actual prescribing practices before educational interventions are designed and undertaken.

An Uncontrolled Educational Intervention

Shortly after the results of the tetracycline study were known, the Tennessee commissioner of health and the state Medicaid program became interested in correcting this matter. The commissioner sent a letter regarding the appropriate use of tetracycline among young children to all physicians participating in the Medicaid program. Included with the letter was a reprint of a brief article on the same subject by the Committee on Drugs of the American Academy of Pediatrics.[5] The letter was mailed at the end of the third year of our study. Continuing surveillance during the subsequent year permitted an uncontrolled evaluation of the letter's impact on tetracycline prescribing to young children.

The use of tetracycline to treat young children had declined gradually during the first three years of the study; after the mailing this decline appeared more pronounced (figure 25–2). Note especially that there was no seasonal winter peak in tetracycline use (for respiratory infections) during the year after the intervention as had occurred regularly in prior years.

When analyzed by the specialty of the prescribing physicians (figure 25–3A), the greatest reduction in prescribing appeared among family practitioners, the group that most often used tetracycline inappropriately. Somewhat encouraging results also were evident when prescribing was analyzed by location of physicians' practices (figure 25–3B). The mailing seemed to have had its greatest effect among urban family practitioners and pediatricians. When the practices of the most frequent prescribers were analyzed, it was shown that their use of tetracycline fell after the mailing. Nonetheless, these doctors continued to use this antibiotic much too often (figure 25–4).

This necessarily uncontrolled natural experiment produced mixed

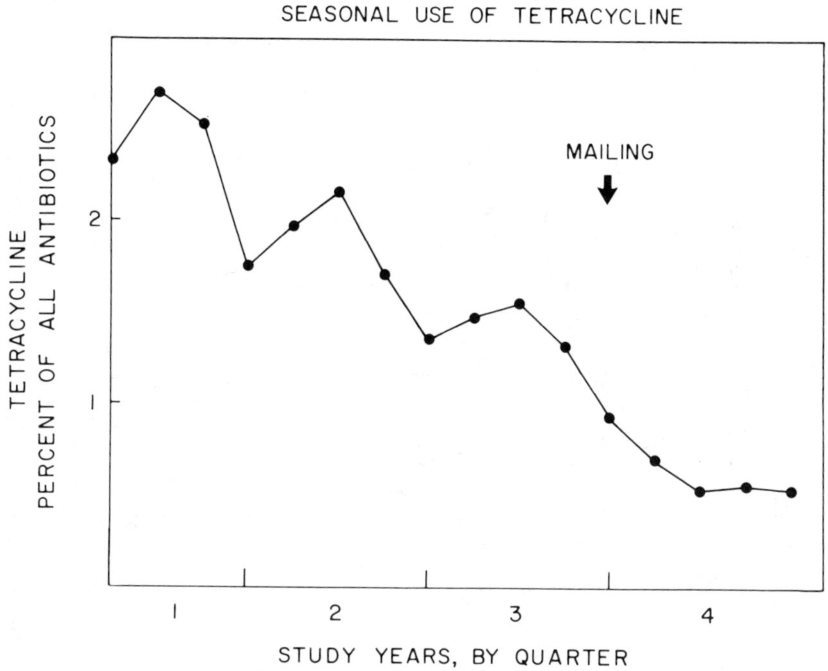

Figure 25-2. Use of Tetracycline to Treat Young Children before and after an Educational Mailing

results. Although it was encouraging that a simple, single educational mailing seemed to have a beneficial effect on the prescribing practices of some doctors, many others continued to use tetracycline in an inappropriate manner. Also, a strong recent trend in reduced tetracycline use was observed before the intervention—that is, it was shown that prescribing habits are not static but that they change over time. These changes may have been due to several influences including seasonal trends, the introductions of new oral antibiotics, and the consequent impact of pharmaceutical sales representatives. Clearly, then, if educational interventions were to be evaluated, two features seemed necessary. First, a control group that would not be influenced by the educational stimulus would enable us to measure contemporary changes in prescribing. The changes in prescribing produced by the educational stimulus then could be compared with these background changes among the controls. Second, although the mailing seemed to have an effect, it was small. Stronger stimuli apparently are necessary to produce significant results in medical practice. These features were incorporated into the next study undertaken by the authors.

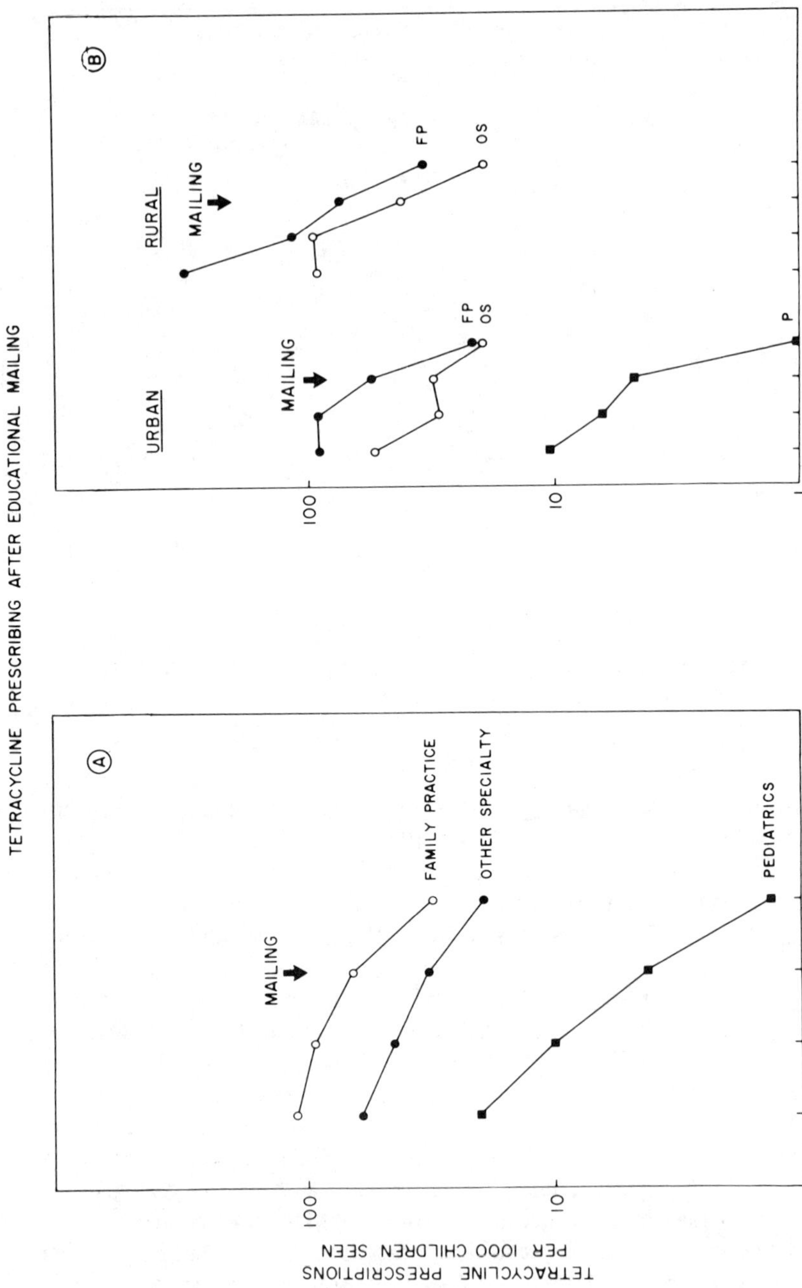

Figure 25–3. Influence of an Educational Mailing on the Prescribing of Tetracycline to Young Children

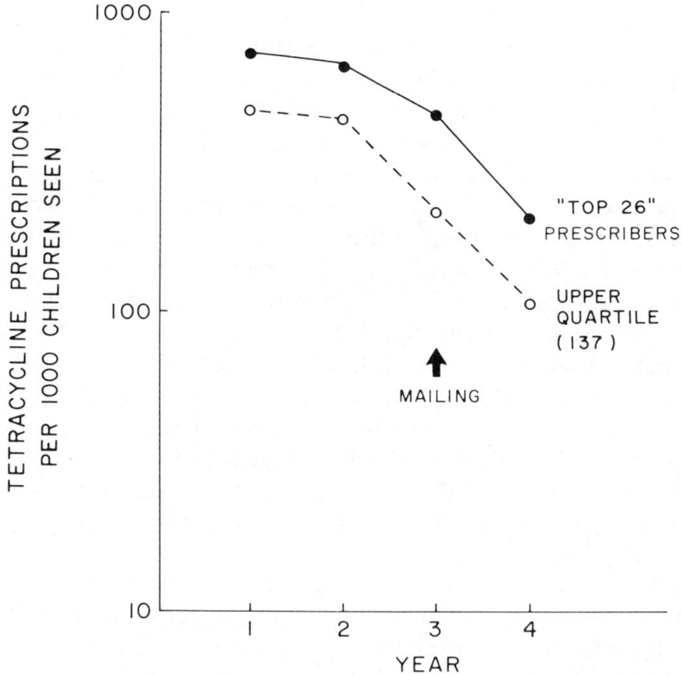

Figure 25-4. Influence of an Educational Mailing on Tetracycline Prescribing to Young Children by the Most Frequently Prescribing Doctors

The Current Educational Intervention—Design Features

A controlled statewide evaluation of three educational interventions on patterns of prescribing in ambulatory care is currently underway in Tennessee. A brief description of the goals and methods of the study follows.

The investigators are located at the Vanderbilt University School of Medicine. However, the university's name is not associated publicly with the project. It was thought inappropriate for academicians to appear to be imposing their views on the practicing-physician community. The Tennessee Medical Association kindly sponsored the project, and it became known as the Tennessee Medical Association Program in Prescribing Improvement. An active program advisory committee consists of representatives of the Tennessee Medical Association, the Tennessee Society of Internal Medicine, the Tennessee Department of Public Health, the Tennessee Academy of Family Physicians, and the Tennessee Chapter of the American Academy of Pediatrics. The committee reviews the content of the educational interventions and monitors the progress of the program. The program was announced in the state newsletters of the sponsoring professional societies. It was described as a professional service, not a research project.

Four antibiotics were selected as the subject for separate educational interventions: chloramphenicol, tetracycline (to children less than 8 years of age), clindamycin, and the group of orally administered cephalosporin drugs. The first three antibiotics are contraindicated for treatment of minor infections in ambulatory practice because of their risk of serious toxicity (clindamycin is associated with the development of pseudomembranous enterocolitis). The rationale for choosing these drugs was to improve the quality of care delivered; the goal was to eliminate the use of these antibiotics in office practice. In contrast, the oral cephalosporin antibiotics are both effective and safe drugs. The rationale against their widespread use is cost; they are many times more expensive than alternative, effective antibiotics such as oral penicillin and erythromycin. The goal of this intervention was to reduce use significantly. Thus, using these two different rationales we would be able to compare physician responses to the two issues of quality of care and costs.

In addition to a control group, three educational techniques were chosen (1) a specially designed mailed brochure, (2) visits to doctors by a trained drug-information specialist, and (3) visits to doctors by other recruited and trained physicians.

The brochures were written by the investigators, were amended and approved by the advisory committee, and were designed carefully for speedy and easy reading (figure 25–5). The brochures clearly indicate the sponsorship of the Tennessee Medical Association and also contain the names and affiliation of the advisory-committee members.

The content of the brochure was brief, and a scholarly tone was avoided. The hazards of the antibiotics were described, and very important reasonable alternatives were provided (including the advice to avoid antibiotic use in many instances such as viral upper-respiratory infections and nonspecific gastroenteritis). A set of practical frequently asked questions and answers was provided.

The drug-information specialist was a recent pharmacy graduate who was poised, was able to work independently and had an attractive and warm personality. This intervention was modeled after an existing educational device of known effectiveness—namely, the pharmaceutical sales representative. The drug-information specialist made appointments with doctors, was introduced as representing the Tennessee Medical Association, and had brief discussions (usually no longer than fifteen minutes) with doctors about the use of the antibiotic in question. Only a single antibiotic was the subject of each visit. Neither the doctor's personal prescribing record nor the Medicaid program was mentioned. If asked why he or she was being visited

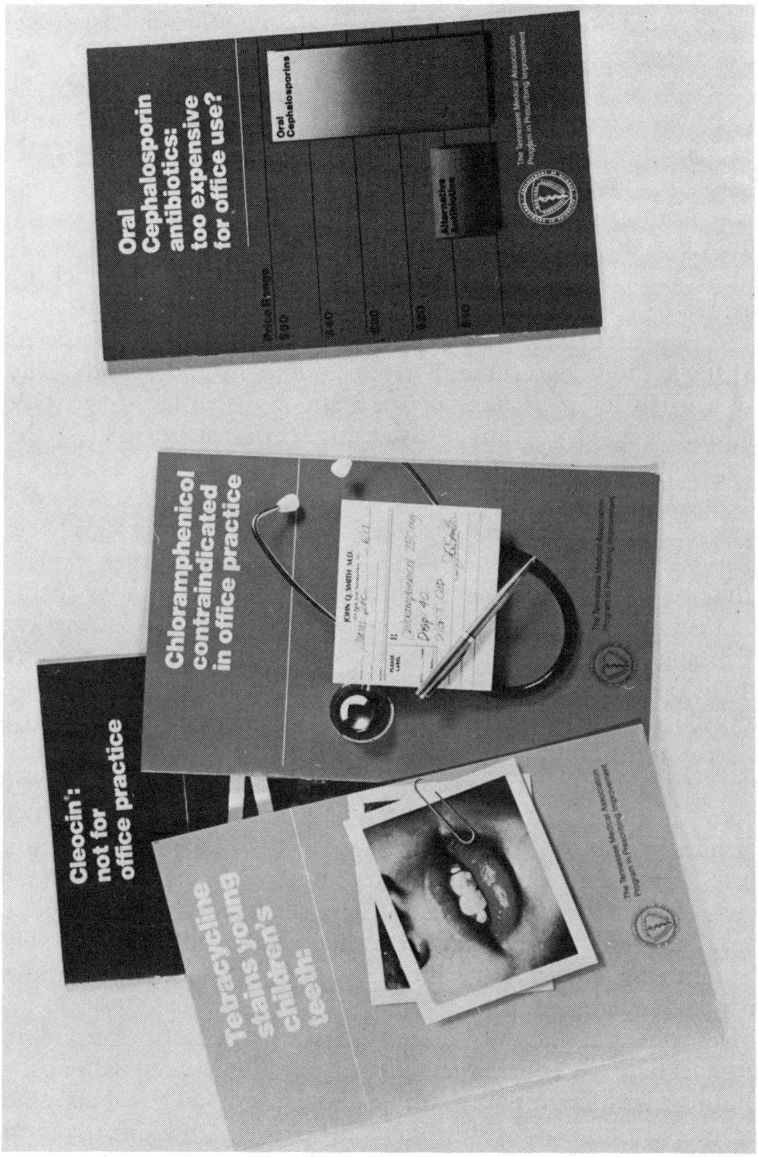

Note: Prominent Logo Identifies "Tennessee Medical Association Program in Prescribing Improvement."

Figure 25-5. Brochures Used in the Controlled Statewide Educational Project (a rare event), the doctor's record of Medicaid prescribing was acknowledged. At the conclusion of the interview, the doctor was given a copy of the relevant brochure.

The physician-visitors were recruited by members of the advisory committee and were senior members of the medical community in part-time practice. Both the physician-visitors and the drug-information specialist together underwent a one-day training course in relevant interviewing techniques to promote a positive and harmonious atmosphere in their visits with the doctors. They also received technical training in the various antibiotics in question. They both conducted their inverviews with prescribing doctors.

The state was divided into four geographic regions, each with a major metropolitan area surrounded by suburban and rural counties. Each of these regions was assigned a different educational technique (figure 25–6). With the exception of the control area, doctors in each region received educational information concerning the four antibiotics under study. The mailers were sent to all physicians in the region; the drug-information specialist and physician-visitors interviewed the heaviest prescribers of the study antibiotics.

The regional study design was chosen for two reasons. First, doctors over the whole state could have been selected for the four study groups. This design entailed the risk that the doctors might have compared their experiences with the prescribing-improvement program informally among themselves, found them to be different, and deduced that a study was underway. The second reason was a pragmatic one: Dividing the state into regions made it more convenient and less costly for the drug-information specialist and the physician-visitors to travel on their interviewing assignments.

Both the drug-information specialist and the physician-visitors completed a brief questionnaire after each interview that assessed the visited doctor's interest in the information and his or her receptivity of the program. Independently, two or three weeks after the visit, each visited doctor received a brief, structured telephone inquiry about the visit, asking about subsequent use of the antibiotic in question and the doctor's feelings about the program. Thus, we will be able to evaluate how doctors view this method of continuing medical education. We are assessing carefully the financial cost of this intervention.

Using Medicaid data, unobtrusive surveillance of antibiotic-prescribing practices subsequent to the educational interventions (compared with possible contemporary variation in the control group) will, of course, determine whether the intervention was worthwhile. This phase of the investigation currently is underway, and it is too early to predict results. However, anecdotal reports from the drug-information specialist and the physician-visitors as well as preliminary analysis of the follow-up questionnaires clearly

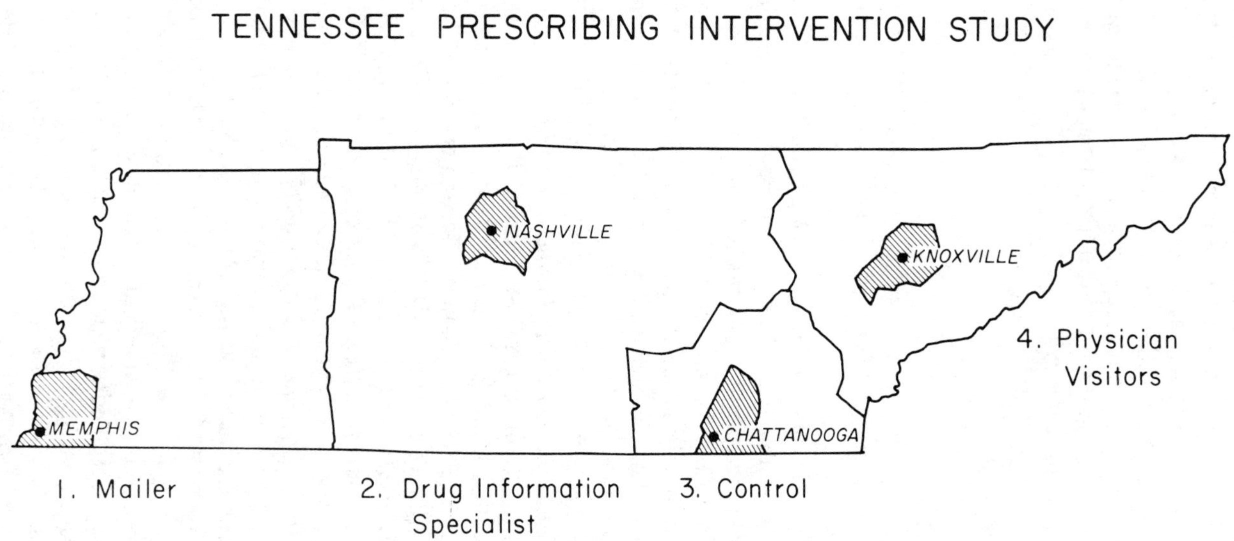

Figure 25-6. The Four Geographic Regions of Tennessee Used in the Program to Improve the Prescribing of Antibiotics in Office Practice

indicate that our visitors have not met with resentment or hostility. Indeed, practicing physicians have welcomed our visitors into their offices and professional lives. The doctors of Tennessee seem receptive to responsibly presented, helpful, and clear information about prescribing. They also are pleased that this is a program of their professional societies. Thus, it would appear that the program has been accepted; the challenge is for us to devise effective educational intervention. The results will determine whether or not we have succeeded in this attempt.

Notes

1. C.F. Federspiel, W.A. Ray, and W. Schaffner, "Medicaid Records as a Valid Data Source: The Tennessee Experience," *Medical Care* 14 (1976):166–172.

2. W.A. Ray, C.F. Federspiel, and W. Schaffner, "Prescribing of Chloramphenicol in Ambulatory Practice. An Epidemiologic Study among Tennessee Medicaid Recipients," *Annals of Internal Medicine* 84 (1976): 266–270; W.A. Ray, C.F. Federspiel, and W. Schaffner, "Prescribing of Tetracycline to Children less than 8 Years Old. A Two-Year Epidemiologic Study among Ambulatory Tennessee Medicaid Recipients," *Journal of the American Medical Association* 237 (1977):1069–2074; W.A. Ray, C.F. Federspiel, and W. Schaffner, "The Mal-prescribing of Liquid Tetracycline Preparations," *American Journal of Public Health* 67 (1977):762–763; J.C. Brocklebank et al., "Drug Prescribing during Pregnancy. A Controlled Study of Tennessee Medicaid Recipients," *American Journal of Obstetrics and Gynecology* 132 (1978):235–244; W. Schaffner, W.A. Ray, and C.F. Federspiel, "Surveillance of Antibiotic Prescribing in Office Practice," *Annals of Internal Medicine* 89 (1978):796–799; W.A. Ray, C.F. Federspiel, and W. Schaffner, "Surveillance of Prescribing Practices Utilizing Medicaid Claims-files: Analysis of Psychotropic Drug Use," *Annals of the World Association of Medical Informatics* (March 1979), pp. 454–459; W. Schaffner, W.A. Ray, and C.F. Federspiel, "Chloramphenicol and Tetracycline Usage in Outpatient Practice," *Quality Review Bulletin* 5 (1979):28–31; W. Schaffner, W.A. Ray, and C.F. Federspiel, "Changing Antibiotic Prescribing: Encouraging Early Results," in *Practical Aspects of Antibiotic Review,* ed. C.M. Kunin (Atlanta: American Health Consultants, 1979), pp. 341–345; W.A. Ray, C.F. Federspiel, and W. Schaffner, "A Study of Antipsychotic Drug Use in Nursing Homes: Epidemiologic Evidence Suggesting Misuse," *American Journal of Public Health* 70 (1980):485–491; and D.G. Blazer et al., "The Risk of Anticholinergic Toxicity in the Elderly: A Study of Prescribing Practices in Two Populations," *Journal of Gerontology* (in press).

3. Ray, Federspiel, and Schaffner, "Prescribing Chloramphenicol."

4. Ray, Federspiel, and Schaffner, "Prescribing Tetracycline."

5. Committee on Drugs of the American Academy of Pediatrics, "Requiem for Tetracyclines," *Pediatrics* 55 (1975):142–143.

26 Delivering Antihypertensive Therapy

R. Brian Haynes

Hypertension is one of the most important chronic medical conditions in our society. It affects about 10 percent of adults and leads to awesome morbidity and mortality if untreated, but its complications can be prevented by blood-pressure-lowering medications.[1] Unfortunately, under usual conditions of care only about 20–30 percent of individuals who know themselves to be hypertensive are under good control.[2]

The reasons for this tragic loss of therapeutic potential are thoroughly explored in a recent report.[3] The following list shows the six stages through which all hypertensive patients must pass if they are to achieve reduction of their blood pressure:

1. Detection (screening),
2. Linkage to a source of clinical care,
3. Clinical evaluation,
4. Prescription of therapy,
5. Compliance with therapy,
6. Lifelong follow-up.

Examination of each stage reveals imperfections in the ways in which we currently deliver antihypertensive care. For example, when detection of hypertension is performed through screening in the community up to 50 percent of patients fail to follow through on referral advice.[4] Since failure at any of the six steps prevents successful management, it is not difficult to understand why such a small proportion of hypertensive patients is treated adequately.

The subject of this chapter is the process of prescription of antihypertensive therapy and its role in blood-pressure lowering. It is clear from the list of stages that the prescription of treatment is but one step in the care of hypertensive individuals. Nevertheless, it is an essential step, not only in its own right but also in the influence it has on patient compliance and long-term follow-up. It is worth remarking here that although some of the ground we cover is unique to the treatment of hypertension, most of it is common to the management of any chronic condition that can be treated on an ambulatory basis.

Process versus Outcome in Antihypertensive Care

Two studies have shown that most of what physicians do in working up and treating hypertensive patients has no measurable impact on their blood pressure. Brook and Appel reviewed the clinical records of 173 hypertensive patients who had been discharged from the hospital.[5] Five methods of peer review were applied to assessment of the quality of care provided to these patients. In none of the assessments was the process of care found to be correlated with blood-pressure response. Similarly, Nobrega et al. found no positive correlations between blood-pressure lowering and the degree of performance of twenty-three items of clinical history, twenty-six items of physical examination, thirteen initial laboratory tests, nine special diagnostic tests, eight treatment procedures, and ten follow-up procedures.[6]

From a clinical perspective, these studies demonstrate the lack of therapeutic utility of many aspects of clinical care. However, these studies failed to investigate three factors of substantial importance. First, the studies limited themselves to patients who were already on drug therapy for hypertension, thus ignoring the initial decision to treat some but not other patients pharmacologically. Second, no assessment was made of the pharmacologic vigor of the regimens that were prescribed. Thus, patients who were treated with insufficient doses of medication were lumped with those on more-potent regimens. Third, no accurate measures of medication compliance were available in these studies.

A recent study that my colleagues and I completed in Hamilton, Ontario, provided an opportunity to assess the effect of these three factors.[7] In this investigation, workers at a large steel mill were screened for hypertension, and those with sustained, untreated elevation of blood pressure (diastolic blood pressure over 95 mm. Hg on three visits over three months) were referred to their personal physicians for care. Follow-through on the referral was guaranteed by making specific appointments for individuals being referred and contacting them periodically until they had attended an appointment. One year later, participants were assessed for blood-pressure control, and those on antihypertensive therapy were visited at home to assess compliance by pill count.

To assess the effect of the vigor of treatment prescribed, we constructed an empirical scale of relative potency of antihypertensive drugs based on controlled pharmacologic trials comparing various drugs with each other and setting 50 mg. of chlorthalidone per day as one unit of vigor.[8]

The results of this study are illustrated in three figures. Figure 26–1 shows that the decision of physicians to prescribe antihypertensive drugs had a clinically important and statistically significant effect on blood-pressure lowering. This is not particularly surprising until one considers the alternatives to prescribing antihypertensive drugs: Most of the patients not

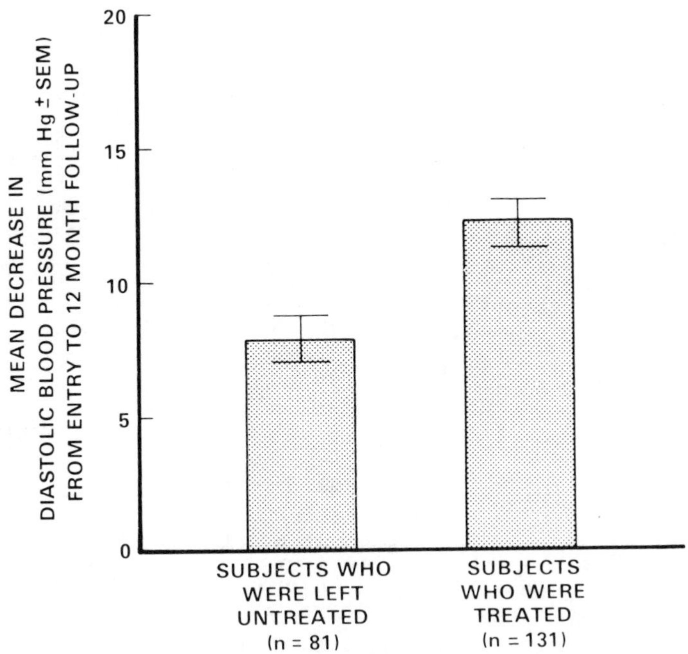

Figure 26–1. Response to Treatment with Antihypertensive Drugs

prescribed blood-pressure-lowering drugs were prescribed tranquilizers, sedatives, or a variety of nonpharmacologic treatments such as weight reduction, salt restriction, relaxation, or exercise. Many physicians prescribe these treatments first on the supposition that mild hypertensives can be managed by hygienic measures or mild sedation. To date, however, there has been no convincing demonstration that any of these measures is efficacious in isolation. Furthermore, the nonpharmacologic treatments are more difficult for patients to comply with than medication regimens.[9] Thus, the first message from our study is that the prescription of antihypertensive medications is more likely to result in blood-pressure lowering than prescription of alternative approaches.

The second conclusion of our study is derived readily from inspection of figure 26–2. Only when two or more units of vigor of therapy are prescribed does blood pressure begin to fall systematically ($p < .005$). Patients prescribed 1 to 1.9 units do not differ from those prescribed less than one unit, and comparison of figures 26–1 and 26–2 reveals that the blood-pressure responses in these two groups were not significantly different from those of patients who were not prescribed any pharmacologic treatments.

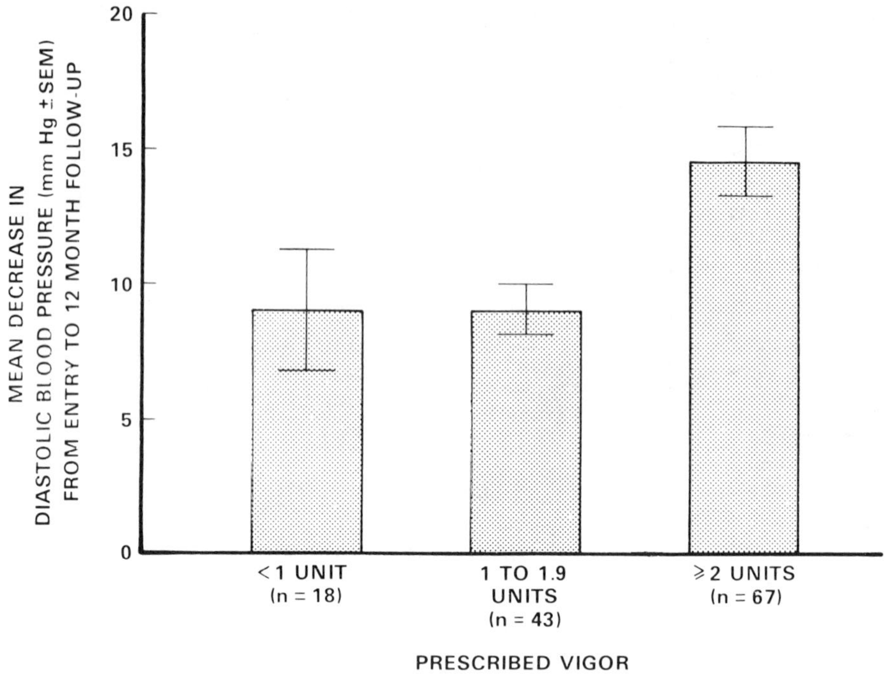

Figure 26–2. Response of Hypertensives to Vigorous Prescribing of Antihypertensive Drugs

Furthermore, although these latter three groups of patients did evidence a reduction in diastolic blood pressure of about 8 mm. Hg over the course of the study, this is not much more than the 6 mm. Hg that would be expected on placebo alone.[10] It is worth pointing out that fully two-thirds of the patients were on these insubstantial amounts of treatment.

Figure 26–3 completes the picture. In this, the patient's prescribed vigor of treatment was multiplied by his rate of compliance to derive the amount of medication consumed. The result is a much better correlation with treatment response. The implication is that there are at least two ways to overcome the effect of low compliance: (1) prescribe more medication (in the hope that the patient will maintain a constant rate of compliance) or (2) do something to improve patient compliance. In any event, the practitioner clearly must take compliance into account when prescribing.

In summary, studies of the process of antihypertensive care reveal that many of the procedures that physicians employ in caring for hypertensive patients have no observable influence on the success of that care but that the prescription of antihypertensive therapy, the pharmacologic vigor of that

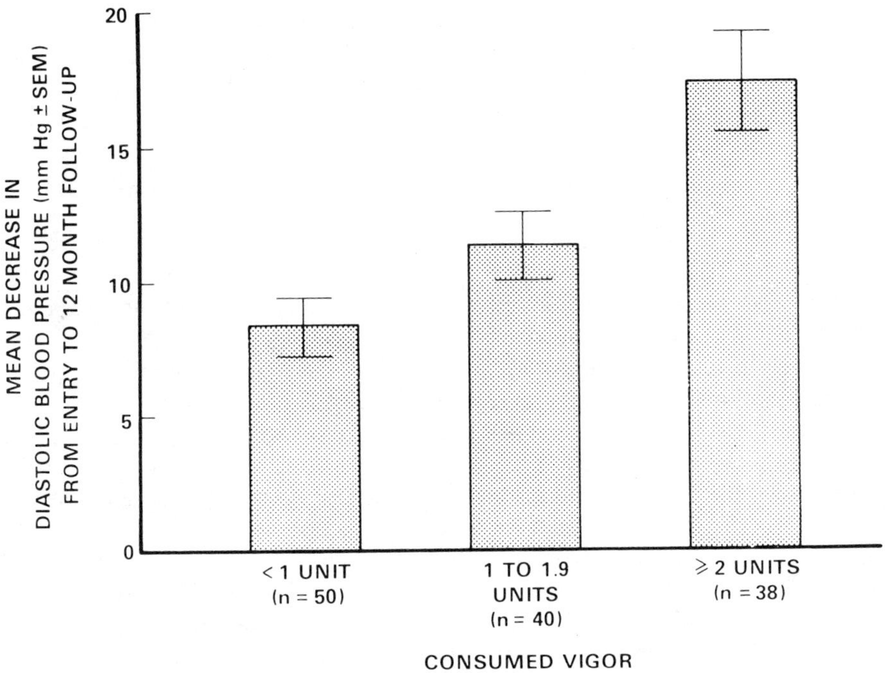

Figure 26–3. Response of Hypertensive Patients to Vigorous Consumption of Antihypertensive Drugs

prescription, and the practitioner's ability to obtain the cooperation of the patient with the regimen do affect outcome. The rest of this chapter focuses on the specific features of prescribing that are important to lowering blood pressure, including those features that influence patient compliance.

Elements of Success in Prescribing Antihypertensive Therapy

On the surface, treating hypertension is rather easy. Any fourth-year medical student can recite the management plan: weight reduction if the patient is obese, salt restriction in any event, and if pharmacologic treatment is required, a diuretic plus potassium supplementation. If the blood pressure still is not controlled, the student likely can name a number of other antihypertensive drugs than can be added.

In practice, this approach is demonstrably unsuccessful for the majority of patients despite the fact that the plan is rational and would work for virtually all patients if they and their physicians were able to follow it.[11] To achieve a high rate of success, some parts of the textbook plan must be dropped and some new maneuvers added. These maneuvers are described in the following sections, and they all must be addressed if the prescription is to achieve optimum results.

Selection of Appropriate Treatment

As a general approach, a stepped-care regimen has been outlined by the U.S. Joint National Commission on High Blood Pressure.[12] The regimen begins with a diuretic (step one), titrates the dose against blood-pressure response, and adds additional medications such as beta-blockers, reserpine, methyldopa, or clonidine (step two) and hydralazine, prazocin, or guanethidine (step three) as necessary. This incremental and flexible plan is designed to minimize side effects while achieving satisfactory blood-pressure control.

The stepped-care approach seems a reasonable one, but it has not been compared with alternative formal plans in a controlled trial. It has at least three potential limitations. First, it starts off with a common drug class (a diuretic) for virtually all patients. While the diuretics recommended for step one are inexpensive and ususally well tolerated by patients, they are not the best starting point for all patients. For example, patients with gout, maturity-onset diabetes mellitus, and certain forms of hyperlipidemia normally should not be prescribed diuretics for hypertension. Furthermore, patients with ischemic heart disease, especially if they have angina pectoris, are likely to be better served by a beta-blocker for their hypertension.

Second, the titration of a medication within a step to its maximum recommended dose before moving to the next step can be questioned. For example, there is evidence that most of the antihypertensive effect of diuretics can be achieved with doses that are about the middle of the recommended dose range and that increasing the dose beyond this level increases side effects but not the therapeutic effect.[13]

Third, patients may experience subjective side effects on certain antihypertensive medications. It may take more-creative prescribing than appears permissible with the stepped-care approach to find a regimen that is both effective and acceptable to the patient. These remarks are intended neither as an exhaustive list of exceptions to the stepped-care approach nor even a serious criticism of it; as a general approach it is both rational and efficacious. Instead, the point is that the treatment should be tailored to the patient's individual circumstances and that as much flexibility as possible should be employed in order to react optimally to the patient's responses to treatment, including changes in his or her blood-pressure level and any side effects that transpire.

Prescription of the Simplest Possible Regimen and Schedule

A key element of success in prescribing antihypertensive therapy is to keep the regimen as simple as is compatible with good blood-pressure control. As is shown by our study, most physicians did seem to have this principle in mind when prescribing medication, as most patients received no or little medication—so little, in fact, that the blood-pressure effect was minimal, suggesting that the drug regimens prescribed were too simple to do the job.[14] Conversely, many physicians in this study prescribed nonpharmacologic treatments. Indeed, a survey of physicians has shown that fully 98 percent recommend weight reduction in overweight patients and that over 90 percent state they prescribe salt restriction to control blood pressure.[15] These treatments are simple for the physician to prescribe but notoriously difficult for patients to follow.[16] In general, the success of nonpharmacologic means in controlling blood pressure is so poor that they should not be prescribed at all. If the patient is very keen to follow one or another such treatment, then two approaches can be recommended. The first is to bring the blood pressure under at least partial control by pharmacologic means and then to prescribe a nonpharmacologic treatment with the promise of reducing drug treatment if the nonpharmacologic therapy has observable physiological effects (for example, weight reduction or a decrease in urinary sodium excretion) and the blood pressure is lowered further. The second approach, which should be reserved for patients who insist on nonpharmacologic treatment first, is to prescribe nondrug therapy with specific goals for deciding on its continuation. For example, weight reduction might be prescribed with a goal of at least one-half-pound weight loss per week and with satisfactory lowering of blood pressure within six months. Failure to achieve either goal should result in negotiation for introduction of a drug regimen. In either of these two approaches, a specific program of intervention is required, and frequent follow-up is necessary if there is to be any hope for success. The command "Lose weight," even if backed up by a diet sheet, is not a credible prescription for the management of hypertension.[17]

Although drug regimens are much simpler than nondrug regimens for patients to follow, often these are prescribed in a more-complicated fashion than they need be. There is virtually no antihypertensive medication that need be prescribed more frequently than twice a day, and once-a-day treatment is possible with longer-acting drugs such as chlorthalidone, nadolol, atenotol, various sustained-release preparations, and even some drugs with short serum half-lives such as alpha-methyl-dopa.[18] It is often helpful in prescribing the dosage schedule to review the patient's daily routine in order to suggest specific times or events to which to attach medication taking so that it becomes part of the patient's usual routine rather than an add on to be fitted in if and when the patient remembers.[19]

Drug regimens also become more complicated than they need be when ancillary treatments are prescribed. The classic example here is the prescription of potassium supplements in tablet, liquid, or dietary form for patients on potassium-losing diuretics. Such supplements usually are unnecessary, particularly if therapeutic but nontoxic dosages of diuretics are prescribed as described earlier. For the few patients who do experience symptomatic hypokalemia, the most appropriate alternatives are to prescribe a potassium-sparing, potassium-losing combination diuretic pill or to discontinue the diuretic entirely and use another class of drug.

Competition by pharmaceutical companies for the lucrative antihypertensive market has resulted in the proliferation of medications for hypertension. While some of these drugs are undoubtedly me-toos with no practical advantages over previous medications, many of the new drugs have unique features that are of value in reducing side effects or simplifying the regimen. Because hypertension is a common disorder, the practitioner should make every effort to keep up with developments in therapy in this field in order to attain the best match of treatment and patient characteristics.

Informing the Patient

It is axiomatic that patients will be unable to follow their regimens unless they are told precisely what they must do. However, practitioners often tell patients things they do not need to know and omit telling them other things they do need to know. Furthermore, patients forget much of what they are told.[20] Few good studies have been done concerning what information is needed by patients who are prescribed antihypertensive regimens and how this information best can be conveyed. Nevertheless, there are some interesting findings from which guidelines can be derived.

First, Ley and co-workers have shown that patients forget almost half of what they are told by their physician.[21] They recall best the things they were told first in the interaction with their doctor, and their accuracy of recall can be increased by some simple measures such as arranging the information into categories, putting it in simple terminology, and providing specific, concrete, detailed advice rather than general recommendations.

Second, several studies have demonstrated that instruction alone is insufficient for gaining long-term cooperation with therapy even though knowledge is increased.[22]

Third, despite the poor showing of instructional approaches, 75 percent of physicians in a recent survey reported that they utilized one form or another of instruction to gain patient cooperation with antihypertensive therapy.[23]

Fourth, some preliminary evidence shows that instruction may have harmful effects in terms of causing increased dropout from care and increased sick-role behavior.[24]

Thus, while it is obvious that some information is essential if the patient is to follow the prescription, it would appear that intensive efforts to educate the patient are, at best, a waste of time and perhaps have some harmful effects; such efforts must not be relied upon to improve cooperation with care.

The following recommendations are offered as one possible course between the opposing evils of too little and too much information. They draw upon the wisdom of others and the clinical experience of the author. First, the prescriber should inform the patient that high blood pressure is normally a lifelong condition that can and should be treated. The condition is usually without symptoms until much damage has been done to the vessels. Because it causes no symptoms in its early stages, a person cannot use any sensations in his or her body to monitor blood-pressure level—specifically, the amount of stress or tension that a person feels has little to do with his or her blood pressure, and the only reliable way of assessing the blood pressure is to measure it. As the condition is lifelong, so its treatment must be taken on a daily basis for the rest of the person's life.

Next, the prescriber should broach the details of the treatment regimen—specifically, when it is to be taken, the need for regularity in taking the medication, what symptoms the patient is likely to feel (common side effects only), and what the future holds in terms of adjustments of medication and additional medication. A handy guideline here is that each medication will lower diastolic blood pressure by about 10 mm. Hg so that patients with a pretreatment diastolic blood pressure of more than 100 mm. Hg should be warned that it likely will require more than one medication to bring the blood pressure under full control. If patients are on more than one medication, they should be informed that the medications can be taken at the same time since many patients make their regimens unnecessary complex by spreading pills out over the course of the day. It is often desirable to identify specific events in the patient's daily schedule and to prescribe the pills for these times (for example, to be taken with breakfast rather than once a day). The patient also should be told what to do if a dose is missed or if he or she runs out of pills between visits and exactly how to reach the prescriber or his substitute in case of an emergency or an unusual symptom. It is helpful if this key information is printed on a small card that the patient can keep in his or her wallet, to be updated as the occasion arises. Beyond these instructions, the patient should be encouraged to ask whatever questions he or she may have and to write down any questions that arise in the interval between visits so that they can be dealt with at the next visit.

These instructions can be handled in a few minutes. They are as important to the success of prescribing as choosing an appropriate medication and completing the prescription chit in a legible hand.

Physicians can expect that the patient will forget most of what has been said.[25] The need for regular medication consumption should be underscored and the key points reiterated on subsequent visits.

Monitoring the Patient's Response

With a stepped-care approach to prescribing for hypertension, it is essential that the prescriber utilizes a well-defined system of monitoring if success is to be assured. There are, no doubt, many ways to monitor hypertensive patients; the following system is based on my own experience.

The first parameter to monitor is attendance at appointments. Over 50 percent of hypertensive patients simply drop out of care within the first year of treatment,[26] unless special measures are taken.[27] To permit attendance-monitoring, patients must be given definite follow-up appointments at each visit rather than an instruction to call back later, and any patients who miss scheduled appointments must be identified—say, by reviewing the charts of nonattenders at the end of each clinic day.

Next, the blood pressure must be monitored in such a fashion that trends are obvious in relation to the pretreatment blood pressure and the treatment goal. Writing the blood pressure in arabic numerals in the patient's notes hardly accomplishes this in an optimal fashion. A graph on which the blood pressure can be charted and medications indicated provides a visual display that illustrates the effect of changes in therapy to both the practitioner and patient. If more than one health-care practitioner is involved (for example, specialist and family practitioner or private physician and company nurse), a copy of the graph can be given to the patient to facilitate communication.[28] The main uses of the graph, however, are to assist in titrating therapy if progress has been made toward the treatment goal but the goal has not been reached; to illustrate to patients what is being done and to reward them for what has been accomplished, recognizing that they have done most of the work; and to warn when noncompliance may be interfering with success, as shown by failure of the blood pressure to fall despite successive increases in the vigor of therapy prescribed. In the latter instance, it should be noted that lack of blood-pressure lowering is not an infallible indicator of noncompliance but that it signals when noncompliance should be considered as a possible problem.

The third matter to be monitored is the occurrence of side effects. The relationship of side effects to patient satisfaction is not clear, but with the variety of antihypertensive drugs available today, there is little need for patients to persist with drugs that are having adverse effects on them.[29]

The fourth issue that merits regular monitoring is patient satisfaction with the therapy. Although this overlaps with side effects it is not coincident, there is a much more-consistent relationship between noncompliance and dissatisfaction with treatment than with the occurrence of side effects.[30] Elements of dissatisfaction include the price of medication, the complexity of the schedule, having to attend appointments (especially if the waiting time is long), and simply having to take any treatment at all. Patients must be given the opportunity to voice and discuss these dissatisfactions if the prescriber is to be able to expect their ongoing cooperation.

Finally, patient cooperation with therapy must be monitored. Ideally, this should be done by periodic serum drug-level assessments.[31] Unfortunately, these are not available at the present time so less-satisfactory methods must be employed. The best of these assessments in terms of convenience and accuracy is asking the patient, keeping in mind that the admission of missing any pills at all is associated with an average compliance rate of less than 50 percent.[32] In practice, questions about compliance are most timely when it is apparent that progress toward the therapeutic goal has been halted despite increments in therapy and/or when patients express dissatisfaction with therapy.

Maintaining High Compliance

The monitoring procedures of watching for nonattenders, watching for nonresponders, and asking patients about their compliance will detect the majority of patients who are not following the treatment as prescribed. The successful prescriber then will have a variety of strategies at his or her disposal in order to promote and maintain high compliance. These have been described in detail elsewhere.[33] Three generic strategies are worth outlining here. First, barriers to compliance should be reduced as much as possible, through making appointments as convenient as feasible and treatment programs as simple as can be achieved. Second, there must be adequate supervision of the patient, with attention focused directly on the problems that most patients have in following prescribed treatments. In most instances, this means seeing patients more frequently than the traditional three or four times per year that most hypertensives currently are seen by primary-care practitioners. In addition, more time at each visit should be set aside for discussing matters of compliance.[34] This need not mean longer visits so much as a shifting of the emphasis during visits. Finally, any efforts that the patient makes to follow the treatment program should be rewarded or reinforced through recognition of his or her attempts and praise and encouragement for following the regimen.[35] Reinforcement is essential to long-term maintenance. Simple praise from the prescriber is a strong reinforcer, and lengthening the time between follow-up visits can be used as a reward for good blood-pressure control.

Conclusion

The provider of antihypertensive therapy has a challenging task that goes far beyond the prescription of a blood-pressure-lowering treatment. Included in this task are optimum selection of the treatment and schedule to suit the patient's unique characteristics, avoiding the twin evils of two little and too much information, monitoring the patient's therapeutic and personal response, adjusting the treatment according to this response, and maintaining high compliance with therapy. Utilizing this more-comprehensive approach to therapy, the practitioner can expect to achieve a much higher success rate in control of the blood pressure of his patients than is currently the usual case in our communities.

Notes

1. Hypertension Detection and Follow-up Program Cooperative Group, "Five Year Findings of the Hypertension Detection and Follow-up Program. I. Reduction in mortality of persons with high blood pressure, including mild hypertension," *Journal of the American Medical Association* 242 (1979):2562–2571; and Australian Therapeutic Trial in Mild Hypertension, "Report by the Management Committee," *Lancet* 1 (1980): 1261–1267.

2. T. Baitz and A. Shimizu, "Blood Pressure Surveys: Are They Worth It?" *Canadian Family Physician* 23 (1977):70–72; and N. Borhani, "Implementation and Evaluation of Community Hypertension Programs," in *Epidemiology and Control of Hypertension,* ed. O. Paul (Miami: Symposia Specialists, 1975), pp. 627–661.

3. "Hypertension. A Report of the Ontario Council of Health" (Toronto, 1977).

4. F.A. Finnerty, L.W. Shaw, and C.K. Himmelsbach, "Hypertension in the Inner City. II. Detection and Follow-Up," *Circulation* 47 (1973): 76–78; and J.A. Wilber and J.G. Barrow, "Hypertension—A Community Problem," *American Journal of Medicine* 52 (1972):653–663.

5. R.H. Brook and F.A. Appel, "Quality of Care Assessment: Choosing a Method for Peer Review," *New England Journal of Medicine* 288 (1973):1323–1329.

6. F.T. Nobrega et al., "Quality Assessment in Hypertension: Anal-

ysis of Process and Outcome Methods,'' *New England Journal of Medicine* 296 (1977):145–148.

7. R.B. Haynes et al., ''Process versus Outcome in Hypertension: A Positive Result,'' *Circulation* 65 (1982):28–33.

8. Ibid.

9. R.B. Haynes, ''Determinants of Compliance: The Disease and the Mechanics of Treatment,'' in *Compliance in Health Care,* eds. R.B. Haynes, D.W. Taylor, and D.L. Sackett (Baltimore: Johns Hopkins University Press, 1979), pp. 49–62.

10. ''Randomized Controlled Trial of Treatment for Mild Hypertension: Design and Pilot Trial.'' Report of the Medical Research Council Working Party on Mild and Moderate Hypertension, *British Medical Journal* 1 (1977):1437–1440.

11. Borhani, ''Implementation and Evaluation.''

12. U.S. Joint National Commission on High Blood Pressure Control, ''Recommendations on the Treatment of High Blood Pressure,'' *Journal of the American Medical Association* 237 (1977):255–261.

13. M.G. Tweeddale, R. Ogilvie, and J. Ruedy, ''Antihypertensive and Biochemical Effects of Chlorthalidone,'' *Clinical Pharmacology and Therapeutics* 22 (1977):519–527.

14. Haynes et al., ''Process versus Outcome.''

15. I. Soltero et al., ''A Survey of Patterns of Nonpharmacologic Care for Hypertensive Patients, Including Recommendations for Their Children,'' *Hypertension* 2 (1980):215–220.

16. R.B. Haynes, ''A Critical Review of the Determinants of Patient Compliance with Therapeutic Regimens,'' in *Compliance with Therapeutic Regimens,* eds. D.L. Sackett and Haynes (Baltimore: Johns Hopkins University Press, 1976), pp. 26–39.

17. L.E. Ramsay et al., ''Weight Reduction in a Blood Pressure Clinic,'' *British Medical Journal* 2 (1978):244–245.

18. J.M. Wright, P.J. McLeod, and W. McCullough, ''Antihypertensive Efficacy of a Single Bedtime Dose of Methyldopa,'' *Clinical Pharmacology and Therapeutics* 20 (1976):733–737.

19. R.B. Haynes et al., ''Improvement of Medication Compliance in Uncontrolled Hypertension,'' *Lancet* 1 (1976):1265–1268.

20. P. Ley et al., ''Improving Doctor-Patient Communication in General Practice,'' *College of General Practice Journal* 26 (1976):720–724.

21. Ibid.

22. Haynes et al., ''Improvement of Medication Compliance''; M.A. Swain and S.B. Steckel, ''Influencing Adherence among Hypertensives,'' *Research in Nursing and Health* (March 1981):213–222; R.D. Caplan et al., *Adhering to Medical Regimens—Pilot Experiments in Patient Education and Social Support* (Ann Arbor: Institute for Social Research, University of

Michigan, 1976); and D.M. Tagliacozzo et al., "Nurse Intervention and Patient Behaviour," *American Journal of Public Health* 64 (1974):596–603.

23. A.S. Logan, *Investigation of Toronto General Practitioners' Treatment of Patients with Hypertension,* Report #D-8471 (Toronto: Canadian Facts, 1978).

24. R.B. Haynes et al., "Increased Absenteeism from Work after Detection and Labeling of Hypertensive Patients," *New England Journal of Medicine* 299 (1978):741–744.

25. Ley et al., "Improving Doctor-Patient Communication."

26. Wilber and Barrow, "Hypertension."

27. J. Takala et al., "Improving Compliance with Therapeutic Regimens in Hypertensive Patients in a Community Health Center," *Circulation* 59 (1979):540–543.

28. R.B. Haynes, D.L. Sackett, and D.W. Taylor, "Practical Management of Low Compliance with Antihypertensive Therapy: A Guide for the Busy Practitioner," *Clin. Invest. Med.* 1 (1979):175–180.

29. Haynes, "Determinants of Compliance."

30. Ibid.

31. R.B. Haynes, "Strategies to Improve Compliance with Referrals, Appointments, and Prescribed Medical Regimens," in *Compliance in Health Care,* eds. Haynes, D.W. Taylor, and D.L. Sackett (Baltimore: Johns Hopkins University Press, 1979), pp. 121–143.

32. R.B. Haynes et al., "Can Simple Clinical Measures Detect Patient Noncompliance?" *Hypertension* 2 (1980):757–764.

33. Haynes, Sackett, and Taylor, "Practical Management"; Haynes, "Strategies to Improve Compliance"; and Haynes, "A Review of Tested Interventions for Improving Compliance with Antihypertensive Treatment," in *Patient Compliance with Antihypertensive Treatment,* eds. Haynes and M.E. Mattson, NIH Publication 80-2102 (Washington, D.C.: U.S. DHHS, 1980), pp. 85–111.

34. T. Inui, E. Yourtee, and J. Williamson, "Improved Outcomes in Hypertension after Physician Tutorials," *Annals of Internal Medicine* 84 (1976):646–651.

35. Haynes, "Strategies to Improve Compliance."

27 Undertreatment: Who Is to Blame?

Michael Weintraub

Undertreatment, as I define it, is the lack of appropriate therapy to prevent, cure, or palliate the symptoms of a medical condition. The prescriber, the patient who receives the prescription, the nature of the treatment (for example, medication, changes in life-style, or preventive measures), and the nature of the disease being treated all can play a part in undertreatment.

The Role of the Prescriber

Prescribers—who are usually physicians, but who also may be other health professionals—can undertreat patients by not prescribing needed medication. This may occur if the diagnosis is downgraded from one necessitating treatment to one not requiring a prescription. For example, if a physician fails to diagnose acute otitis media by ascribing the pain to transient temporomandibular joint dysfunction, serious undertreatment would result. An equally serious problem would occur if the otitis media were diagnosed but judged to be due to a viral infection and therefore not amenable to antibiotics. In the elderly, tuberculosis and legionella (Legionnaire's disease) are not uncommonly overlooked or, at least initially, are diagnosed as conditions that do not require specific drug treatment. Therefore, physicians may undertreat because they downgrade the diagnosis, often with the complicity of the patient. Unfortunately, we do not have data on the frequency of downgrading. Complex studies involving several examiners and assessing the patient's role will be necessary to document the amount and impact of downgrading—hypertension (fixed to labile), sore throats (bacterial to viral), or angina pectoris (cardiac to gastrointestinal disorders or other problems).

A major reason why undertreatment occurs is fear, not only of the seriousness of the condition but also of the treatment itself. In the case of early cancer signs or symptoms of acute myocardial infarction, patients may fear the diagnosis and avoid professional counsel by downgrading the diagnosis to one not requiring either diagnostic or therapeutic intervention. Patients may thus ascribe their symptoms to a self-treatable or self-limited disease such as constipation or heartburn instead of colonic cancer or myocardial ischemic pain.

Medical schools teach students about the horrible specter of hospitals filled with patients who cannot be treated because their illnesses are due to antibiotic-resistant bacteria. We overemphasize the harm these medications can do and devalue their efficacy. Thus, medical students learn to make erroneous risk-benefit analyses and to withhold active indicated therapy. Some years ago, an article in the *British Medical Journal*[1] discussed five patients who died when the physician withheld an admittedly toxic medication, amphotericin B, despite life-threatening disseminated fungal infections, in order to avoid the hepatic and renal toxicity that this agent is known to produce. In this article. Symmers coined the term "pharmacophobia" to describe this behavior.* An example of fear-related undertreatment from my own experience occurred when an infectious disease specialist repeatedly delayed treatment for a patient who had a life-threatening *Pneumocystis carinii* infection. The physician pointed out the potential for serious adverse effects (sterile abcesses, hypoglycemia, and hypotension) from the intramuscular injection of the only appropriate medication available at the time (pentamidine isothionate), and approved treatment only after much urging. This physician did not lack intelligence, but he feared the consequences of *intervening.* In fact, he was more afraid of the possible undesirable effects arising from his actions than of the undesirable effects of the untreated disease.

Prescribers may also undertreat a patient by choosing a second-line or less efficacious drug in order to avoid adverse effects associated with a more potent medication (in analgesic selection, for example, inappropriately substituting codeine when morphine is indicated, or in antibiotic selection, avoiding chloramphenicol even if it might be the most effective treatment of typhoid fever). At other times, physicians will prescribe low dosages of a medication, or spread the dosages out during the day, with the mistaken idea that decreasing the total dose will preserve the benefits and decrease drug toxicity. We observed a variant of this form of undertreatment in a study of emergency room patients treated for status epilepticus. Some of the patients had received a smidgen of one drug (diazepam [Valium]) and a partial dose of another (phenytoin), without receiving the benefit of either. Only when more experienced and vigorous therapists were asked to help did the patients receive fully effective doses of anticonvulsant medication. I have spoken to neurologists specializing in epilepsy who confirm my own observation that this phenomenon still occurs in major centers today.

Medical school faculty members (including myself) are partly to blame for prescribers' attitudes leading to undertreatment. Among other faults of omission, we have failed to emphasize the necessity for exploring the

---

* Pharmacophobia, at least involving amphotericin B, still exists, as attested to by two recent publications. An editorial in the *British Medical Journal* called the fear of amphotericin use difficult to explain,[2] and Baum attributed amphotericin underuse to fear of toxicity, noting that the greatest danger arises from not using the drug when it is indicated.[3]

dose-effect relationship. If we do discuss dose response, we too often counsel, "Dose low—go slow," that is, begin with low doses and increase them slowly. Titrating medications in this way often makes perfectly good sense, but at times it does not. This approach may result in continual undertreatment, as we chase after the disease, attempting to catch up but always remaining a step or two behind. Giving low doses of analgesics or prescribing with large dosing intervals when treating acute postsurgical pain is a good example.

Medical educators also do not sufficiently stress the importance of evaluating the effects of treatment. We do not teach students to use the tools for such evaluation—the flowcharts, simple office tests, activity diaries and cusums.[4] Thus, prescribers whose training has not emphasized the necessity of evaluating drug therapy may never be aware that they are undertreating.

Prescribers may undertreat because they do not know of or believe in the value of a treatment for a particular disease. This commonly occurs in situations where the data are controversial, for example, the treatment of mild hypertension, venereal disease contacts, obesity, and influenza. The prescribers believe the issues are not settled, and, therefore, they do not treat.

The Role of the Patient

If the patient is not convinced of the necessity of treatment, he or she may not come in for evaluation, may not take the trouble to learn the results of diagnostic tests, or may not follow the prescribed treatment plan. In addition, both the patient and the prescriber often have a "fear of addiction," which fosters undertreatment. This fear leads physicians to prescribe too-small doses of narcotics and leads patients to neglect to take analgesics or follow other treatment regimens. (In one study,[5] my colleagues and I found that 10 percent of patients being treated with digoxin, a cardiac glycoside, were not taking their medication for fear of becoming "addicted.") Health professionals may focus on the major manifestations of a disease such as renal disease, cancer, diabetes, or hypertension (chronic conditions where a major variable can be followed and the others, often patient symptoms, neglected), and undertreat concomitant symptoms, such as nausea or itching. Some patients—perhaps out of a puritanical belief, shared with the prescriber, that suffering improves character—neither request nor use prescribed symptomatic therapy. In hospitals, the nurses' views on the value of "biting the bullet" and "keeping a stiff upper lip" may also compound the problem. In the outpatient setting, the pharmacist's words or facial expression can convey the similar impression that the patient is "weak" for using symptomatic treatment.

While we must not denigrate the patient's decision whether or not to accept treatment for what is, after all, his or her own body, public health considerations and scientific data can help differentiate between intelligent noncompliance and unintelligent or irrational noncompliance. Patients can choose not to fill prescriptions or follow diets, or they may only partially adhere to the prescribed treatment. I have found numerous instances in which elderly patients made excellent decisions in not blindly following the treatment plan.[6-9] Nevertheless, when I am on a bus, I certainly hope that the person sitting next to me has taken *all* of his isoniazid that day so that I won't get tuberculosis or be exposed to resistant strains of the bacillus, the appearance of which has been promoted by undertreatment. (Several drug-resistant strains of microorganisms have developed because of undertreatment, for example, underuse of antimalarials.) I also hope that people around me have not become overly suspicious of drugs, "chemicals," and other "nonnatural" treatments from press or television reports. If only selfishly, I want my driver to take his antihypertensive medication, in its appropriately prescribed dosage, so that he won't have a stroke and either harm me or make my Blue Cross premiums and Social Security taxes go up to pay for his possibly preventable hospitalization and disabilities. The data on undertreatment of hypertension are especially upsetting because the risk-benefit assessments of such treatment are quite convincing.[10]

The patient thus plays an important role in undertreatment by being unwilling to discuss the severity of symptoms, deciding not to get a vaccination, rejecting prescribed treatment for fear of adverse effects or "addiction," or worrying about using unnatural chemicals or products of "evil" technology.

The Nature of the Treatment

The nature of the treatment also affects patient acceptance. Treatments with a high nuisance value—bad taste, inconvenience, minor but annoying side effects—will not be followed as often. If the effect of a treatment is not convincing, or if the major benefits are either poorly defined or realized only in the distant future (for example, antihypertensive therapy, prophylactic treatment or chronic therapy with psychotropics), patients are less likely to comply with therapy. Occasionally, the necessary therapeutic agents are not available. At other times, the serious toxicity caused by the available agents outweighs their therapeutic advantages.

The influence of treatment expense, whether for diet counseling, programs to stop smoking, vaccines, or drugs, varies with different people. For example, if "expensive" is perceived as *better* by both prescriber and patient, high cost will not deter the patient's acceptance and use of a treatment. On the other hand, the expense may cause the patient to refuse treatment.

The Disease

Diseases themselves may produce physiological or psychological changes that lead to undertreatment. If a patient is depressed, he or she may not wish to discuss a medical problem, or both patient and prescriber may decide that the problem is related to the depression and undertake neither appropriate diagnostic procedures nor treatment for the symptoms. A disease may decrease the effect of a medication to the extent that the standard dosages are ineffective; without monitoring and dose adjustment, the patient may remain undertreated. For example, we recently saw a patient whose signs and symptoms had not resolved despite unusually high doses of an oral anticoagulant. We found that concomitant renal disease had diminished her response to the medication so that she needed even higher doses and could safely tolerate them.

In Conclusion

Undertreatment, then, is not a simple phenomenon. It can be affected by such disparate factors as newspaper articles, psychology, physiology, disease, medical or general education, and diagnostic errors. Scientific knowledge and clinical trial data about a treatment and its value are important, but prescribers and patients must accept the therapeutic intervention before it can be implemented. The physician's decision to prescribe and the patient's decision to follow the prescription are often based on emotional grounds rather than on scientific evidence. We need to consider the socioeconomic and psychological factors of prescribing and drug use, as well as the scientific ones if we are to avoid undertreatment.

References

1. Symmers, W.C.S. "Amphotericin Pharmacophobia." *British Medical Journal* 4 (1973):460.

2. Editorial. "Treatment of Systemic Fungal Infections." *British Medical Journal* 280 (1980):688.

3. Baum, G.L. "Treatment of Systemic Fungal Infections." *Postgraduate Medical Journal* 55 (1979):587.

4. Weintraub, M.; R.A. Jacox; E.A. Atwater; et al. "Piroxicam in Rheumatoid Arthritis. A Controlled Clinical Trial with Novel Assessment Techniques." *Journal of Rheumatology* 4 (1977):393–404.

5. Weintraub, M.; W.Y.W. Au; L. Lasagna. "The Determinants of Compliance with Digoxin." *Journal of the American Medical Association* 224 (1973):481–485.

6. Moore, S.R. "Medication Taking in the Elderly." *Drug Intelligence and Clinical Pharmacy* 12 (1978):739–741.

7. Spriet, A.; B. Beiler; J. Dechorgant; et al. "Adherence of Elderly Patients to Treatment with Pentoxyfylline." *Clinical Pharmacology and Therapeutics* 27 (1980):1–7.

8. Turakha, H. and H. Enlund, "Drug Use and Prescribing Compliance by Elderly Patients." *Journal of Clinical Pharmacology* 3 (1978): 103–112.

9. Lundin, D.V.; P.A. Eros; J. Melloh; et al. "Education of Independent Elderly in the Responsible Use of Prescription Medication." *Drug Intelligence and Clinical Pharmacy* 14 (1980):355.

10. Morgan, J.P. "The Politics of Medication." In *Controversies in Therapeutics,* edited by L. Lasagna (Philadelphia: W.B. Saunders, 1980), pp. 16–22.

Index

About the Contributors

James C. Anthony, Ph.D., is assistant professor of mental hygiene and epidemiology at the School of Hygiene and Public Health, Johns Hopkins University. He is an epidemiologist interested in applications of this field to drug- and alcohol-induced problems. His recent work has focused on models of control of hazardous psychoactive medication.

Mitchell B. Balter, Ph.D., is chief of the Applied Therapeutics and Health Practices Program, National Institute of Mental Health. He has worked in the general area of social psychology and epidemiology of psychopharmacology and, in recent years, he coordinated a national program of research on the extent and nature of psychotherapeutic-drug prescribing and use.

Patricia J. Bush, Ph.D., is assistant professor, Department of Community and Family Medicine, Georgetown University School of Medicine. In addition to the Ph.D. in social and administrative pharmacy, Professor Bush holds degrees in medical sociology and pharmacy. Her work often combines these disciplines as it is directed to determinants and social perspectives in the use of and prescribing of medication.

Ruth Cooperstock is a medical sociologist, Epidemiology Section, Policy Research Department, Addiction Research Foundation, Toronto. She studies, writes, and speaks on the epidemiology of the use and misuse of psychotherapeutic drugs. She has principally focused on the social aspects of the medical utilization of psychoactive drugs.

J. Richard Crout, M.D., is currently associate director for Medical Applications of Research, National Institutes of Health, Bethesda, Maryland. He was previously the director of the Bureau of Drugs of the Food and Drug Administration. He brought to that job an extensive background in investigative clinical pharmacology, particularly in the area of cardiovascular drugs.

Thomas G. Davis, M.D., is vice-president and medical director of Smith, Kline and French Laboratories, Philadelphia. Dr. Davis trained in internal medicine at the University of Pennsylvania and was affiliated with that school of medicine and engaged in private practice, before beginning his industrial career.

Marlin Demlinger, M.S., M.L.S., is the acting chief librarian of Public Services and the chief librarian of the Science Engineering Division, City College Library, City University of New York. He has worked in corporate, industrial, and academic libraries.

Carolee DeVito, Ph.D, R.Ph., is assistant professor in the Department of Family Medicine, University of Miami School of Medicine. She is trained in pharmacy, health-service administration, and medical-care organization. Her principal research interest is in the structure and evaluation of drug-product-selection legislation.

Charles F. Federspiel, Ph.D., is professor of biostatistics in the Department of Preventive Medicine, Vanderbilt University School of Medicine. Professor Federspiel's academic interests involve mathematics and biostatistics. He applies these skills to health-services research, particularly in those areas related to public health-care programs.

Theodore Goldberg, Ph.D., is professor and chairman of the Department of Community Medicine, Wayne State University School of Medicine. His early academic interests encompassed political science and economy. Moving to the economy of health care, he has been the principal investigator of a national program to evaluate the impact of drug-substitution legislation.

R. Brian Haynes, M.D., Ph.D., is currently assistant professor, Department of Clinical Epidemiology and Biostatistics, and Department of Medicine, McMaster University Faculty of Health Sciences, Hamilton, Ontario. His background and training in epidemiology and clinical medicine have well-suited him to take a broad approach to hypertensive disease and the scholarship of the variables affecting its therapy.

Stephen Janofsky, M.L.S., is medical librarian, Sophie Davis School of Biomedical Education, City College of the City University of New York, and is committed to teaching drug-information skills to medical students and medical scientists.

Robert L. Lantos, M.S., is director, Continuing Pharmaceutical Education; and assistant to the executive dean, Arnold and Marie Schwartz College of Pharmacy and Health Sciences, Long Island University. Mr. Lantos has worked as a retail and hospital pharmacist and, in his current position, in education and expansion of the role and responsibilities of pharmacists.

William F. McGhan, Pharm.D., Ph.D., is associate professor of pharmacy practice, University of Arizona College of Pharmacy, Tucson. Professor

McGhan has a background in clinical pharmacy and in social and administrative pharmacy. He has been active in health-services research, particularly that involving drug use and misuse, and the evaluation of pharmacist drug prescribers.

Glen D. Mellinger, Ph.D., is executive director and president of the Board of Directors, Institute for Research in Social Behavior, Oakland, California. He is a social psychologist with principal interests in patterns of national use of psychotherapeutic agents.

Louis A. Morris, Ph.D., is head of the Patient Labeling Branch, Food and Drug Administration (FDA), Rockville, Maryland. Dr. Morris was involved extensively in the FDA's patient-information programs. He has continuing research interests in the psychology of medication use and consumer information in health care.

Stuart L. Nightingale, M.D., is associate commissioner for Health Affairs of the Food and Drug Administration. Dr. Nightingale trained in internal medicine with a concentration on drug-abuse care and methadone maintenance, and served in a variety of clinical and academic settings. He entered government service and has been affiliated with the Special Action Office for Drug Abuse Prevention, National Institute on Drug Abuse, and the FDA.

David L. Pleet, M.D., will begin his fellowship in gastroenterology at Temple University Hospital in June 1983. He graduated from Mount Sinai School of Medicine in 1980, where he carried out the analgesic study described in this book while completing his rotation in community and public health.

David L. Rabin, M.D., M.P.H., is professor and associate chairman of the Department of Community and Family Medicine, Georgetown University School of Medicine. Dr. Rabin is trained in clinical medicine and is interested in public health and the broader aspects of medical care, particularly as they apply to the use of prescription medications.

Wayne A. Ray. Ph.D., is research assistant professor of biostatistics, Department of Preventive Medicine, Vanderbilt University School of Medicine. His interests in biostatistics and computer science have recently been applied to health-services research and epidemiology, particularly in the area of prescribing.

T. Donald Rucker, Ph.D., is professor in the Division of Administrative and Social Sciences, College of Pharmacy, and professor in preventive medicine, College of Medicine, The Ohio State University. Professor Rucker is interested in and has published widely on the structure of drug evaluation, particularly the functions of hospital formularies and pharmacy and therapy committees, and the broader issues of drug-utilization review.

William Schaffner, M.D., is professor, Departments of Medicine and Preventive Medicine, Vanderbilt University School of Medicine. Dr. Schaffner was trained in clinical medicine and infectious disease, and worked in epidemiology. He has recently attempted to apply epidemiological analysis to drug-prescribing patterns and attempts to modify them.

Leroy L. Schwartz, M.D., practices pediatrics in Staten Island, New York. His interest in the determinants of health-care policy and the impact of regulation on medical practice led him to found The Princeton Institute for Health Policy, Inc., where a number of studies regarding these issues are in progress.

Richard B. Seymour, M.A., is currently director of training for Haight-Ashbury Training and Education Projects, a division of Youth Projects, Inc., and the Haight-Ashbury Free Medical Clinic, San Francisco. He has had extensive consulting, editorial, and educational roles in the area of alcohol and substance abuse. With his coauthor, David Smith, he writes a monthly column on drug-abuse facts for *High Times.*

David E. Smith, M.D., is associate clinical professor of toxicology, University of California School of Medicine; founder and medical director, Haight-Ashbury Free Medical Clinic. Dr. Smith has extensive clinical, consulting, and academic experience in the field of the use and misuse of psychoactive drugs and alcohol.

Mickey C. Smith, Ph.D., R.Ph., is professor, Department of Health Care Administration, and assistant director, Bureau of Pharmaceutical Services, School of Pharmacy, University of Mississippi. Professor Smith's research interests encompass pharmaceutical marketing, media attitudes toward prescription medication, retail-pharmacist behavior, and the character of prescription-drug advertising.

Andrew A. Sorensen, Ph.D., is associate professor of preventive, family, and rehabilitation medicine, University of Rochester School of Medicine and Dentistry. Professor Sorensen's academic background is in public health and sociology. His research interests include health-service evaluation, particularly the social and administrative structure of Health Maintenance Organizations, the care of alcohol- and drug-misusing patients, and the evaluation of prescribing.

Glen L. Stimmel, Pharm.D., is associate professor of clinical pharmacy, associate clinical professor of psychiatry and behavioral sciences, University of Southern California (USC), Los Angeles. Professor Stimmel's research activities include clinical psychopharmacology and pharmacy education. He is the project director of the USC pharmacist-prescribing project.

Peter Temin, Ph.D., is professor of economics, Massachusetts Institute of Technology. His research interests have ranged widely in the field of economics, including applications to the historical economy of the postbellum South, the Great Depression, industrial growth, and labor scarcity. He has recently turned his attention to the economics of drug prescribing, the pharmaceutical industry, and drug regulation.

William M. Wardell, M.D., Ph.D., is associate professor, Pharmacology and Toxicology; assistant professor, Department of Medicine; and director, Center for Study of Drug Development, University of Rochester School of Medicine and Dentistry. Dr. Wardell's interest in drug therapy led to the doctorate in pharmacology, in addition to training in medicine and clinical pharmacology. His interest in documenting the character of medication development and the influences of regulation led to the establishment of the influential Center for the Study of Drug Development.

Michael Weintraub, M.D., is associate professor of pharmacology and toxicology and associate professor of medicine at the University of Rochester School of Medicine and Dentistry. He trained in internal medicine and clinical pharmacology and has since worked on clinical drug evaluation, clinical trial methodology, and the characteristics and teaching of drug therapy.

Albert I. Werthheimer, Ph.D., is professor and director of the Department of Social and Administrative Pharmacy, School of Pharmacy, University of Minnesota in Minneapolis. He has published over 100 papers on various aspects of pharmacy and medical care in the United States, while maintaining active teaching, consulting, and editorial roles involving the character of drug use.

Charles Winick, Ph.D., is professor, Department of Sociology, City College of the City University of New York. Professor Winick has published extensively on the social context of drug abuse in this culture, including evaluation of patterns of use, media reflections of drug abuse, and the social philosophy of intervention and care for drug-abusing patients.

About the Editors

John P. Morgan, M.D., is medical professor and director of the Pharmacology Program at the Sophie Davis School of Biomedical Education, City College of New York. He is also an associate professor of pharmacology and internal medicine at Mount Sinai School of Medicine, New York. Dr. Morgan's training in internal medicine and clinical pharmacology led to his current interests in the cultural and social context of drugs and medications.

Doreen V. Kagan, received the M.S. from the Columbia University School of Social Work and has worked in program development and administration in drug misuse, emergency care, and other hospital-service programs. She is currently a research associate in the Pharmacology Program at the Sophie Davis School of Biomedical Education, City College of New York.